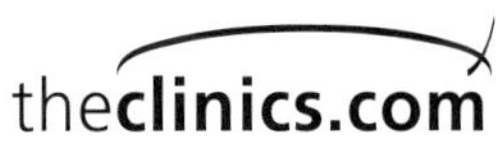

Robert A. Smith, DVM, MS
CONSULTING EDITOR

VETERINARY CLINICS OF NORTH AMERICA

Food Animal Practice

Update in Soft Tissue Surgery

GUEST EDITOR
André Desrochers, DMV, MS

March 2005 • Volume 21 • Number 1

SAUNDERS

An Imprint of Elsevier, Inc.
PHILADELPHIA LONDON TORONTO MONTREAL SYDNEY TOKYO

W.B. SAUNDERS COMPANY
A Division of Elsevier Inc.

The Curtis Center • Independence Square West • Philadelphia, Pennsylvania 19106

http://www.vetfood.theclinics.com

THE VETERINARY CLINICS OF NORTH AMERICA: FOOD ANIMAL PRACTICE
March 2005
Editor: John Vassallo

Volume 21, Number 1
ISSN 0749-0720
ISBN 1-4160-2849-8

The Veterinary Clinics of North America: Food Animal Practice (ISSN 0749-0720) is published in March, July, and November by W.B. Saunders Company. Corporate and editorial offices: The Curtis Center, Independence Square West, Philadelphia, PA 19106-3399. Accounting and circulation offices: 6277 Sea Harbor Drive, Orlando, FL 32887-4800. Subscription prices are $115.00 per year for US individuals, $182.00 per year for US institutions, $58.00 per year for US students and residents, $137.00 per year for Canadian individuals, $238.00 per year for Canadian institutions, $160.00 per year for international individuals, $238.00 per year for international institutions and $80.00 per year for Canadian and foreign students/residents. To receive student/resident rate, orders must be accompained by name of affiliated institution, date of term, and the *signature* of program/residency coordinator on institution letterhead. Orders will be billed at individual rate until proof of status is received. Foreign air speed delivery is included in all *Clinics* subscription prices. All prices are subject to change without notice. POSTMASTER: Send address changes to *The Veterinary Clinics of North America: Food Animal Practice*, Elsevier, Customer Service Department, 6277 Sea Harbor Drive, Orlando, FL 32887-4800, USA; phone: (+1)(877) 8397126 [toll free number for US customers], or (+1)(407)3454020 [customers outside US]; fax: (+1) (407) 3631354; e-mail: usjcs@elsevier.com

Reprints. For copies of 100 or more, of articles in this publication, please contact the Commercial Reprints Department, Elsevier Inc., 360 Park Avenue South, New York, New York 10010-1710. Tel.: (212) 633-3813; Fax: (212) 462-1935; e-mail: Reprints@elsevier.com

The Veterinary Clinics of North America: Food Animal Practice is covered in *Current Contents/Agriculture, Biology and Environmental Sciences, Index Medicus, and Excerpta Medica.*

Printed in the United States of America.

CONSULTING EDITOR

ROBERT A. SMITH, DVM, MS, Diplomate, American Board of Veterinary Practitioners; Veterinary Research and Consulting Services, LLC, Greely, Colorado

GUEST EDITOR

ANDRÉ DESROCHERS, DMV, MS, Diplomate, American College of Veterinary Surgeons; Associate Professor, Department of Clinical Sciences, Université de Montréal, Faculté de Médecine Vétérinaire, St Hyacinthe, Québec, Canada

CONTRIBUTORS

DAVID E. ANDERSON, DVM, MS, Diplomate, American College of Veterinary Surgeons; Associate Professor and Section Head, Food Animal Medicine and Surgery, Department of Veterinary Clinical Studies, College of Veterinary Medicine, The Ohio State University, Columbus, Ohio

PASCALE AUBRY, DMV, Assistant Professor, Department of Clinical Sciences, Faculté de Médecine Vétérinaire, Université de Montréal, Saint-Hyacinthe, Québec, Canada

MARIE BABKINE, DMV, DES, Clinical Instructor, Centre Hospitalier Universitaire Vétérinaire, Faculté de Médecine Vétérinaire, Université de Montréal, St Hyacinthe, Québec, Canada

LUDOVIC BOURÉ, Méd Vét, MSc, DES, Diplomate, European College of Veterinary Surgeons; Diplomate, American College of Veterinary Surgeons; Assistant Professor of Large Animal Surgery, Department of Clinical Studies, Ontario Veterinary College, University of Guelph, Guelph, Ontario, Canada

UELI BRAUN, Dr med vet, Dr med vet h c, Diplomate, European College of Bovine Health Management; Professor of Internal Diseases of Cattle, Department of Farm Animals, University of Zürich, Zürich, Switzerland

YVON COUTURE, DVM, Professor, Department of Clinical Sciences, Université de Montréal, Faculté de Médecine Vétérinaire, St Hyacinthe, Québec, Canada

ANDRÉ DESROCHERS, DMV, MS, Diplomate, American College of Veterinary Surgeons; Associate Professor, Department of Clinical Sciences, Université de Montréal, Faculté de Médecine Vétérinaire, St Hyacinthe, Québec, Canada

JENNIFER M. IVANY EWOLDT, DVM, MS, Scott County Animal Hospital, Eldridge, Iowa

GILLES FECTEAU, DMV, Diplomate, American College of Veterinary Internal Medicine; Professor, Department of Clinical Sciences, Université de Montréal, Saint-Hyacinthe, Québec, Canada

THOMAS GEISHAUSER, Dr med vet, Dr med vet habil, FTA, MSc, Adjunct Professor, Department of Population Medicine, Ontario Veterinary College, University of Guelph, Guelph, Ontario

WILLIAM W. MUIR, DVM, PhD, Diplomate, American College of Veterinary Anesthesiologists; Department of Veterinary Clinical Sciences, College of Veterinary Medicine, The Ohio State University, Columbus, Ohio

PIERRE-YVES MULON, DMV, Resident, Large Animal Surgery, Department of Clinical Sciences, Université de Montréal, Faculté de Médecine Vétérinaire, St Hyacinthe, Québec, Canada

KENNETH D. NEWMAN, DVM, Clinical Instructor, Food Animal Medicine and Surgery, Department of Veterinary Clinical Studies, College of Veterinary Medicine, The Ohio State University, Columbus, Ohio

JULIA QUERENGÄSSER, Dr med vet, Tierärztliche Klinik Babenhausen, Babenhausen, Germany

KLAUS QUERENGÄSSER, Dr med vet, Tierärztliche Klinik Babenhausen, Babenhausen, Germany

CONTENTS

GOAL STATEMENT

The goal of the *Veterinary Clinics of North America: Food Animal Practice* is to keep practicing veterinarians up to date with current clinical practice in food animal medicine by providing timely articles reviewing the state of the art in food animal care.

ACCREDITATION

The *Veterinary Clinics of North America: Food Animal Practice* will be offering continuing education credits, to be awarded by a school of veterinary medicine, contract pending.

The aforementioned school of veterinary medicine is a designated provider of continuing veterinary education. Veterinarians participating in this learning activity may earn up to 6 credits per issue up to a maximum of 18 credits per year. Credits awarded may not apply toward license renewal in all states. It is the responsibility of each participant to verify the requirements of their state licensing board.

Credit can be earned by reading the text material, taking the examination online at ***http://www.theclinics.com/home/cme***, and completing the program evaluation. Each test question must be answered correctly; you will have the opportunity to retake any questions answered incorrectly. Following successful completion of the test and the program evaluation, you may print your certificate.

TO ENROLL

To enroll in the *Veterinary Clinics of North America: Food Animal Practice* Continuing Education program, call customer service at 1-800-654-2452 or sign up online at ***http://www.theclinics.com/home/cme***. The CME program is available to subscribers for an additional annual fee of $49.95.

FORTHCOMING ISSUES

July 2005

Bovine Theriogenology
Grant Frazer, BVSc, MS, *Guest Editor*

November 2005

Emergency Medicine and Critical Care
Sheila M. McGuirk, DVM, PhD and
Simon Peek, BVSc, PhD, *Guest Editors*

RECENT ISSUES

November 2005

Managing the Transition Cow to Optimize Health and Productivity
Nigel B. Cook, BVSc, MRCVS, and
Kenneth V. Nordlund, DVM, *Guest Editors*

July 2004

Ruminant Neurologic Diseases
Peter D. Constable, BVSc, MS, PhD,
Guest Editor

March 2004

Bovine Viral Diarrhea Virus: Persistence is the Key
Kenny V. Brock, MS, DVM, PhD, *Guest Editor*

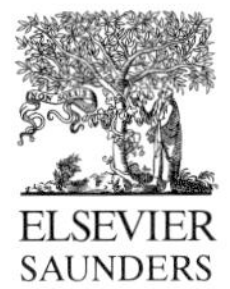

VETERINARY
CLINICS
Food Animal Practice

Vet Clin Food Anim 21 (2005) xi–xii

Preface

Update in Soft Tissue Surgery

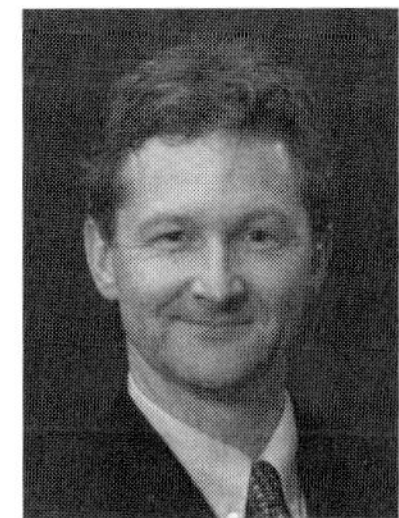

André Desrochers, DMV, MS
Guest Editor

As a guest editor, my personal goal was to demonstrate the paradox in food animal surgery. One day, a surgeon can perform a laparoscopic abomasopexy and the day after castrates so many calves in a feedlot and finishes the day by performing a cesarean section. Two major differences exist in food animal surgery compared with equine and small animal surgery: profit-driven industry and surgical theater. Economics is important in every species, even human surgery, but nothing compared with food animal. The surgical theater is the biggest difference compared with other species. Trying to suture a cesarean section on a moving and kicking target is more a matter of stunt ability than surgical training. Also, surgical procedures are performed in unclean and hostile environments containing dust, wind, flies, and herd mates.

Food animal surgery has progressed over the years, adapting state-of-the-art technology (eg, laparoscopy, theloscopy, and ultrasound) to field conditions. Welfare issues raised by the general public, veterinarians, and farmers have led to changes in pain management, which previous took into consideration economic concerns only. Not long ago, it was common practice to dehorn calves without analgesia and sedation. Today, based on research, veterinarians know this practice is not acceptable. Food animal surgeons should be proactive and participate actively in promoting good surgical practice for routine surgery and develop new techniques with collaborative work between universities and private practice.

0749-0720/05/$ - see front matter
doi:10.1016/j.cvfa.2004.12.009

I would like to acknowledge all the authors for their outstanding contributions. It was a pleasure to read these articles and, most of all, to have the privilege of corresponding with these authors. Food animal surgery has made much progress and has a bright future. I also wish to thank Dr. Bob Smith for giving me this opportunity to serve as a guest editor. This issue could not be possible without the outstanding work of John Vassallo and the editorial staff of the *Veterinary Clinics*. Thanks to all pioneers in food animal surgery and especially to Dr. Bruce Hull and Dr. Guy St-Jean, who are great ambassadors of food animal surgery and great teachers to me. This issue is for you.

André Desrochers, DMV, MS
Department of Clinical Sciences
Université de Montréal
Faculté de Médecine Vétérinaire
3200, Sicotte, St Hyacinthe
Québec, J2S 6K9, Canada

E-mail address: andre.desrochers@umontreal.ca

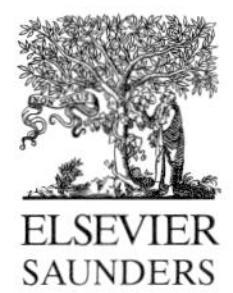

ELSEVIER
SAUNDERS

Vet Clin Food Anim 21 (2005) 1–17

VETERINARY
CLINICS
Food Animal Practice

General Principles of Surgery Applied to Cattle

André Desrochers, DMV, MS

Food Animal Medicine and Surgery, Department of Clinical Sciences, Faculty of Veterinary Medicine, Université de Montréal, 3200 Sicotte, Saint-Hyacinthe, Québec, Canada J2S 7C6

Doing surgery almost everyday, we have a tendency to forget simple principles that can make a big difference in the final outcome. Those principles are the same whatever the species and always should be remembered and applied when doing surgery; practice makes perfect. A French study reported that 7 out of 10 veterinary legal proceedings in France are related to an obstetric procedure [1]. Of the 400 records that were studied between 1992 and 1996, the results of autopsy following a prosecution showed that 40% of legal cases were from a defect of the uterine suture, 20% were from hemorrhage, and 10% were from peritonitis. According to this study, the surgeon is required to achieve a perfect uterine suture; therefore, there is an obligation of result. Otherwise he has to prove that something was wrong with the uterus. Batra et al [2] compared knot security between board certified surgeons and medical students after appropriate training sessions. Students' tying technique was judged to be superior to that of experienced surgeons. According to a study, only 25% of the surgeons correctly used the appropriate knot construction [3]. The food animal surgeon is no exception to this rule. Applying basic surgical principles can make a big difference in surgical wound complication, and therefore, prevent wound abscess, dehiscence, herniation, or retroperitoneal abscess. Economics and contaminated surgical theaters in food animal surgery are a reality that makes this basic principal even more important. This articles reviews the basic principles of preoperative preparation, suture material, and knot-tying techniques.

E-mail address: andre.desrochers@umontreal.ca

doi:10.1016/j.cvfa.2004.12.006 *vetfood.theclinics.com*

Preoperative considerations

Surgical site preparation

By the middle of the nineteenth century, postoperative sepsis infection accounted for the death of almost half of the human patients who underwent major surgery. A common report by surgeons was that the operation successful but the patient died. In 1865, Louis Pasteur suggested that decay was caused by living organisms in the air, which, on entering matter, caused it to ferment. A meticulous researcher and surgeon, Lister recognized the relationship between Pasteur's research and his own. He considered that microbes in the air likely were causing the putrefaction and had to be destroyed before they entered the wound [4].

Preoperative site preparation is important to reduce the incidence of surgical wound infection. An ideal preoperative solution should decrease the number of microorganisms rapidly immediately after the scrub at the surgical site and maintain a residual effect for an extended period of time. Therefore, self-infection of patients by the transfer of potential pathogens from the skin to the underlying tissues with a scalpel, needle, or implants is prevented [5,6].

Preoperative skin preparation is essential in preventing surgical wound infection (SWI) [5,7,8]. Although it is impossible to sterilize the skin, a small number of microorganisms at incision time will decrease the chances of infection. The population of microorganism can be divided into two distinctive categories—resident and transient. Transient microflora are eliminated efficiently by preliminary cleaning with soap and water [9,10]. The resident microflora are the normal inhabitants of the skin. Bacteria are found superficially on the epidermis which compromise the efficacy of certain disinfectants [9,11,12]. The ultimate goal of disinfectants is to decrease cutaneous microorganisms significantly—more specifically, the resident microflora—just before skin incision [9,13].

Extensive research has been performed to find the best preoperative preparation protocol in humans, as well as in dogs [8,14–19]. All of those protocols were effective in decreasing the number of microorganisms. Large animal preoperative preparation protocols are extrapolated from other species; however, their environment as well as skin microflora are different. Whatever the species, preparation of the surgical site is divided in three basic parts: hair removal, site cleaning, and sterile preparation.

Hair removal

By clipping or shaving the surgical site, contact of the disinfectant solution with the skin is improved, and ultimately, decreases the population of resident microorganisms. In humans, shaving the surgical site was proven to damage the natural epidermal skin barrier that favors bacterial growth [20,21]. As a consequence, the use of razor has been associated with a higher frequency of SWI when compared with depilatory cream or clippers as a hair-removal technique. Animal hair density is different than humans; therefore, we need to be careful with interspecies extrapolation. Cattle hair being dense, shaving seems to be the best hair-removal technique for increasing disinfectant contact efficacy. Lloyd et al [22] compared the effect of shaving and clipping on bovine epidermal structure. Their conclusion was that shaving and clipping removed several cell layers of the stratum corneum and a protective lipid layer. They also reported that a 1-minute scrub on finely-clipped skin removed more cell layers than a 2-minute scrub on coarsely-clipped skin. In humans, shaving the skull before head surgery is not significantly superior to not shaving at all in the prevention of SWI [23,24]. Bedard et al [25] compared four protocols of preoperative preparation in cattle. Surgical wound infection frequency was the same for cattle who underwent clipping or shaving although more skin reactions were observed when povidone-iodine and chlorhexidine were used on shaved skin (47.8%) compared with clipping only (8.7%).

Whatever the hair removal technique is used, it should be done just before the surgery and not the previous day, which increases SWI [21]. The instrument should be sharp and lubricated to avoid any skin trauma. A clipper blade number 40 (Oster, Sunbeam Products, Inc., Boca Raton, FL) is used routinely used in our clinic. For cattle with a thick winter coat, a larger blade can be used first, followed by a number 40 blade (Oster). The surface to be clipped should be wide enough to account for surgical drape sliding, manipulation around the incision, and lengthening of the incision if needed. We recommend clipping 20 cm to 30 cm on each side of the planned incision.

Disinfectants

Many disinfectant have been used for the surgical site preparation. Table 1 compares the different disinfectants that are used commonly for surgical site preparation. The most popular disinfectants are the povidone-iodine (0.75% to 1% of free iodine) and chlorhexidine gluconate 4%. Povidone-iodine is composed of polyvinylpyrolidone and iodine which allows a slow release of iodine, which consequently decreases its irritating and staining effect; however, its contact time with the skin should be longer than iodine solution to be efficient [26]. Adding alcohol to povidone-iodine improves its efficacy and efficiency [18]. Povidone-iodine is the most popular disinfectant in bovine surgery. Its major advantages are a broad spectrum of action against bacteria, viruses, fungi, and some spores. It is inexpensive. Its slow onset of action (2 minutes) compared with alcohol and chlorhexidine, the skin irritation that occurs on certain patients, and a decreased efficacy with the presence of organic material are disadvantages [27,28].

Chlorhexidine gluconate has not been used in surgery as long as iodine compounds and alcohol. The major advantages of this disinfectant are its rapid onset of action; its residual effect for up to 6 hours because of proteins

Table 1
Skin disinfectants

	Mechanism of action	Advantages	Disadvantages
Hexachlorophene	Bacteriostatic Inactivation of essential enzyme systems in microorganisms	Good against gram + and *S aureus* 3% solution Good residual effect for several hours Cumulative effect after multiple scrubbings	Inefficient against gram − , spores, and fungus 3% solution are absorbed through the skin Teratogenic Long contact time to be effective
Benzalkonium chloride	Permeability	Good against gram + and some gram −, and fungi Safe for topical use Excellent for urogenital disinfection	Strong concentration may damage mucosa Poor activity in presence of soap and organic materials Long contact time to be effective More bacteriostatic than bactericidal
Chloroxylenol (PCMX)	Inactivation of bacterial enzymes and alteration of cell walls	Good against gram + and most gram − Safe No skin reaction Active in presence of organic material	Variable efficacy depending on if it combines with other disinfectant combination, EDTA, and concentration Not as rapid as chlorhexidine and iodine compounds
Triclosan	Enters bacterial cells and affects the cytoplasmic membrane and synthesis of RNA, fatty acids, and proteins	Good against gram + and some gram − Poor activity against fungi Effective concentration between 0.2% and 2% Incorporated into soaps	Safe Good residual activity like chlorhexidine Not affected by organic matter
Povidone-iodine	Bactericidal	Organic compounds cause less skin reaction and stain	Skin reaction

	Penetrates cell wall of microorganisms and inactivates cells by forming complexes with amino acids and unsaturated fatty acids, resulting in impaired protein synthesis and alteration of cell membranes	Broad spectrum Povidone solution of 10% Concentrations between 0.75% and 3% are combined in a detergent Residual activity	Activity decreased in presence of organic material Residual effect shorter than chlorhexidine (1–2 hours)
Chlorhexidine gluconate	Its bactericidal effect is based on damaging the bacterial cytoplasmic membrane precipitating intracellular proteins	Good against gram +, gram −, some fungi Frequently combined with alcohol No skin reaction Residual effect up to 6 hours Active in presence of organic material Best concentrations are 2% to 4%	Possible contamination of low concentration solution (0.02 – 0.1%) Effect not as rapid as alcohol Could be inactivated by normal soap, inorganic anions, hand cream Dilution with tap water may cause contamination with resistant germ (eg, *Pseudomonas*)
Alcohol	Damage to lipid portion of the cell wall and precipitation of its contents	Bactericidal Variable concentration from 70% to 90% Broad spectrum	High concentrations are less effective Skin irritation with repeated usage No residual effect

Abbreviations: EDTA, ethylenediaminetetraacetic acid; gram +, gram-positive; gram −, gram-negative.

Data from Boyce JM, Pittet D. Guideline for hand hygiene in health care settings. MMWR Morb Mortal Wkly Rep: Recommendations and Reports 2002;51:1–45; and Block SS, editor. Sterilization and preservation. 4th edition. Philadelphia: Lea & Febiger; 1991.

that bind to the stratum corneum; and its constant activity, even with organic material [5,6,28]. Its major disadvantages are its price, decreased foaming effect, and possible contamination if concentrations are altered by diluting the product. Contamination has been reported with solutions less than 1% [28]. Bacterial counts after surgical preparation on animals that were treated with chlorhexidine were less than from dogs and cattle that were treated with povidone-iodine [17,29]. Even with significantly smaller numbers of bacteria, however, SWI frequency was the same. In dogs, skin reaction was significantly more frequent with povidone-iodine than chlorhexidine [30]; this was not observed in cattle [29].

Surgical preparation involved the alternate use of chlorhexidine or povidone-iodine and isopropylic alcohol to combine rapid onset of action with residual effect. A disinfectant that combines those two characteristics will save time. Dura Prep (3M Canada Inc., London, Ontario, Canada) is an iodine compound with 0.5% of free iodine in a solution of isopropylic alcohol. Once applied on the skin, a waterproof bactericidal film is formed that acts as a physical and chemical barrier. Its spectrum of action is similar to povidone-iodine, although it has a rapid onset of action combined with a residual effect. According to veterinary and human literature, there is not a significant advantage to this preparation compared with more traditional preoperative protocols regarding the number of colony formation units (CFUs), frequency of SWI, and skin reaction. The only significant difference was the preparation duration time in favor of Dura Prep [15,18,31]. Galuppo et al [32] evaluated two preoperative protocols in horses; the first used a combination of povidone-iodine and alcohol and the second used Dura Prep. Dura Prep preparation time was shorter but no significant differences were found in the number of CFUs perioperatively. It is distributed as 6 mL to 26 mL surgical skin prepping solution with a sterile applicator; however, the amount that is needed to prepare a cattle flank is cost prohibitive.

Alcohol has been used for a long time as a disinfectant. Its bactericidal action is rapid and efficient. Alcohol dissolves fat which compromises skin lipid protective layers after repeated application. Alcohol solutions that contain 60% to 95% alcohol are the most effective; stronger concentrations are less potent because proteins are not denatured easily in the absence of water [33]. The major disadvantage of alcohol is its lack of residual effect compared with other disinfectants; however, regrowth of bacteria on the skin occurs slowly after the use of alcohol-based hand antiseptics, presumably because of the sublethal effect that alcohols have on some of the skin bacteria. For this reason, it is essential to combine chlorhexidine or povidone-iodine with a preoperative skin preparation protocol [27].

Patient scrubbing time

Duration of the preparation is as important as the disinfectant itself. In 1986, the Centers for Disease Control suggested that the preoperative preparation should last between 3 and 6 minutes for SWI prevention [34]. Scrubbing time longer than 10 minutes damaged the skin and buried bacteria popped up to the surface [27]. In cattle, povidone-iodine and chlorhexidine gluconate were compared as skin preoperative protocols and were significantly efficient in decreasing the number of CFUs. The preparation time for this study was five minutes of sterile scrub and 5 minutes of alternate passages of isopropylic alcohol and povidone-iodine or chlorhexidine gluconate. Chlorhexidine gluconate was more effective in reducing the number of CFUs compared with povidone-iodine, although the infection rate was similar (10.7% and 9.8%) [29]. Bedard et al [25] compared four preoperative protocols in cleaning the paralumbar fossa laparotomy in cattle: shaving and chlorhexidine gluconate, clipping and chlorhexidine gluconate, shaving and povidone-iodine, and clipping and povidone-iodine. The duration of the preparation was 6 minutes—3 minutes of cleaning with a disinfectant detergent, 3 minutes of sterile scrub, and 3 alternate strokes of a selected disinfectant and isopropylic alcohol. The four protocols were effective in decreasing the number of CFUs before the surgery with a bacterial reduction of 99.7% to 99.9%. The infection rate between the treatment groups was not statistically different and varied from 0% to 8.7%. The residual effect of disinfectants was not demonstrated in this study [25] compared with others in different species [28,30]. Recently, Zubrod et al [35] evaluated four protocols of skin preparation with povidone-iodine before arthrocentesis of the coffin joint in horses. The four povidone-iodine preparations included a 10-minute scrub, 5-minute scrub, three 30-second scrubs, or commercial one-step iodophor surgical solution. They were equally effective in reducing the number of bacteria at the site of arthrocentesis.

Scrubbing technique

Scrubbing action is important to mechanically remove skin debris and decrease microorganisms. This fact was well-accepted for a long time but was questioned recently with new research on hand washing and scrubbing in humans [36,37]. Again, we have to be cautious in extrapolating results from another species. In cattle, scrubbing is essential to remove dirt and organic materials.

The first step is to scrub the animal with a soft bristle brush to avoid damaging the epidermis. It is essential to use the same disinfectant category throughout the surgical preparation. Disinfectants with detergent are used first. Their foaming action keeps debris in suspension which will be eliminated later with rinsing. There is no particular pattern when cleaning the animal other than working on a large surface and rinsing with clean water. In cattle, before extrapolating from another species, the surgeon needs to consider the planned surgical site dimension and cleanliness of the animal. Some protocols take less than 2 minutes without any scrubbing action. It is the author's opinion that the scrubbing should last at least 3 minutes in cattle for the cleaning portion of the preparation. Bedard et al [25] demonstrated that after 3 minutes of cleaning, the percentage bacteria was reduced between 95.7% and 98%, depending on the preoperative protocol that was used.

The second step is the sterile scrub. With a soft bristle brush or sponge, scrubbing should start from the center and proceed in a circular manner toward the periphery of the planned surgical site without coming back to the center. The surgical site may be divided into three distinctive portions; the first portion is directly on the surgical site, the second portion surrounds the planned incision, and the third portion is at the junction of the clipped and nonclipped hair. Based on previous principles, we start with the first zone, followed by the second, and finally, the third. Sixty to 90 seconds of scrubbing are performed on each zone. After scrubbing, the surgical site is cleaned with alcohol on gauze or sterile saline, if available.

The last step consists of three alternate passages with isopropylic alcohol and a disinfectant without detergent because it is reported to be toxic [26]. The alternate passages are performed the same way as described for the sterile scrub.

The alternate usage of alcohol and chlorhexidine gluconate in dogs was questioned by Osuna et al [17]. It was reported that the number of skin bacteria at the surgical site after the surgery was significantly greater if alcohol was used to rinse chlorhexidine, instead of sterile saline. Therefore, the residual effect of chlorhexidine may have been altered by the alcohol. To the author's knowledge, this finding was not reported in any other study. In cattle, the use of alcohol is more practical because the same container can be reused without contamination, instead of using a different bottle of sterile saline every time.

Surgeon preparation

Surgeon preparation, if performed in a hospital environment, should follow the same principles of aseptic surgery; however, in field practice, it is illogical to wear head covering and a face mask in a highly contaminated area. We should talk of a clean environment instead of a sterile environment. The use of a surgical mask was questioned recently in human medicine because of major improvements in air filtering system with 20 changes per hour in a surgery suite. As Belkin [38] stated, mask usage "managed to escape criticism and simply survived the ages by being perpetuated by the 'that's the way we've always done it' syndrome." Still, it does not mean that all principles should be forgotten. It is the author's opinion that gloves should be worn when performing surgery in a food animal. An impervious gown should be worn if the abdominal cavity of an adult cow is invaded.

Gloves

The use have of sterile gloves have been accepted in veterinary medicine since the late 1950s [39]. It is part of our food animal culture to operate without gloves. Cattlemen are more and more concerned about cross contamination between farms. Wearing gloves or avoiding contamination, by any means, when we leave a farm and go to another should be a priority for food animal veterinarians. Again, we have to be logical. Wearing sterile gloves for dehorning may be questionable, although wearing sterile gloves when performing an umbilical hernia repair on a calf is not questionable. Latex gloves are more resistant than nonlatex gloves in a hospital environment, although both of them avoid disease transmission [40,41].

The latex glove can be worn over a plastic sleeve (rectal palpation type) when performing invasive abdominal surgery in cattle. The tips of the plastic sleeve fingers can be cut off to provide better sensation and prehension when latex gloves are worn over them (Fig. 1).

Hand scrubbing

Surgical hand scrubs should decrease the number of resident microorganisms on the skin and maintained a small number for as long as possible. There is some distinctive concept to remember when describing surgical hand scrubbing [42]. Hand washing removes the soil and transient microorganisms. It can be accomplished in 10 to 15 seconds. Hand antisepsis involves some antimicrobial agent. There is a minimum contact time, at least 10 to 15 seconds. Each antimicrobial agent has its own characteristic. Alcohol works quickly, but other agents might take a minute. This means that people who use antimicrobial agents must make sure that they follow the minimal antimicrobial agent contact time. Surgical hand scrub destroys transient and resident microorganisms. This is used to prevent the resident bacteria of the skin from getting into the patient's body during surgery or invasive care.

Different disinfectants have been used by surgeons to scrub and wash their hands. Alcohol is probably the oldest disinfectant. It is fast and effective but lacks any residual effect. Therefore, it is used frequently with chlorhexidine and iodine to combine their residual effect. Alcohol has poor efficacy if hands are dirty [43]. Applying small volumes (eg, 0.2–0.5 mL) of alcohol to the hands is not more effective than washing hands with plain soap and water [44]. One study documented that 1 mL of alcohol was substantially less effective than 3 mL [45]. The ideal volume of product to apply to the hands is not known and may vary for different formulations; however, if hands feel dry after rubbing them together for 10 to 15 seconds, an insufficient volume of product likely was applied.

Wan et al [46] compared different protocols of hand scrubbing for large animal veterinarians considering that their hands can be contaminated heavily (mouth, feet, rectum) and they go to the surgery room right away.

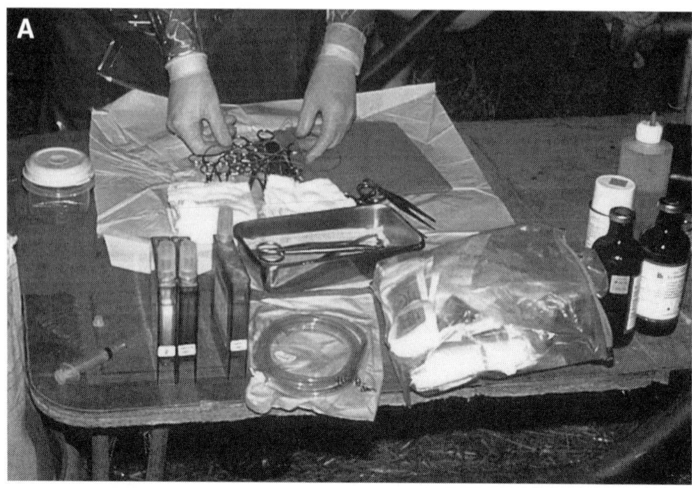

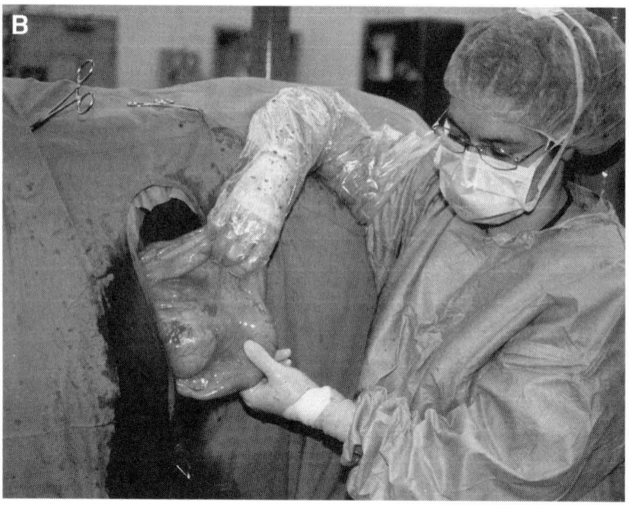

Fig. 1. (*A*) The surgeon in the field is wearing latex gloves over plastic sleeves. A clean table with proper instruments are prepared and ready to use. It is important to plan in advance the instruments that will be needed during the surgery and possible complication. (Courtesy of Dr Denis Harvey, Saint-Hyacinthe, Quebec, Canada.) (*B*) Abdominal surgery on a cow in a hospital setting.

Their objective was to determine the effectiveness of a 5-minute surgical scrub using a one-brush or a two-brush technique in clean and dirty surgical procedures, and to compare the efficacy of povidone-iodine with chlorhexidine as surgical scrub solutions. All protocols were equally effective in reducing the number of CFUs after scrubbing and up to 120 minutes after.

Several studies demonstrated that scrubbing for 5 minutes reduced bacterial counts as effectively as a 10-minute scrub [47,48]. In other studies, scrubbing for 2 or 3 minutes reduced bacterial counts to acceptable levels [49,50]. Pereira et al [51] showed that an initial 2-minute scrub with chlorhexidine gluconate and a consecutive scrub of a 30-second application of ethanol 70% and chlorhexidine gluconate 0.5% was as effective as a traditional protocol that consists of an initial scrub of 5 minutes and a consecutive scrub of 3.5 minutes with chlorhexidine gluconate 4% [51]. The shorter protocols with alcohol solution had a drying effect on the hands. Recent studies corroborate these findings and propose new protocols of hand scrubbing that consists of scrubbing around the nails with brushes and rubbing the hands and arms with antiseptic from the elbow to the antebrachium [36,37]. These protocols are appealing for bovine practitioners because of the time savings.

Use of a surgical drape

The use of a surgical drape in field practice is debatable. The goal of a surgical drape is to limit the surgical site to a minimum, thereby avoiding contamination with a nonsterile portion of the skin; however, it may give a false sense of security if it is not used adequately. The surgical drape should be stable—either fixed with towel clamps or any other mean. If the surgical drape keeps moving during the surgery, dust underneath the drape, and consequently, microorganisms, eventually will migrate toward the incision (Fig. 2). A sticky drape would be an appealing solution. Adhesive incise drapes that may or may not be impregnated with disinfectant have been used in other species to avoid this migration of microorganisms by patient manipulation and movement of the surgical drapes [32,52–54]. Poor intraoperative drape adherence is a common finding that allows bacterial migration, harboring, and proliferation during surgery [55]. In dogs, drape peeling was present in 66% of them without a significant increase in bacterial count underneath it; however, inadequate adherence was reported as a risk factor of incisional drainage in horses [32]. There also is a recolonization underneath the drape with or without impregnated disinfectant [56]. The appropriate use of adhesive spray as well as adequate placement of the drape is essential. Iodine-impregnated drapes do not seem to decrease SWI rate, although bacterial growth is reduced [53,54]. To the author's knowledge, no study has been done in cattle. It is not used routinely because of its price and the poor adherence to cattle skin. We do use it for orthopedic surgery and some umbilical surgery when scars or fistulas are present.

Surgical wound infection in cattle

Increased susceptibility to wound infection is related to five basic factors. (1) The presence of necrotic tissue is an excellent growth medium for

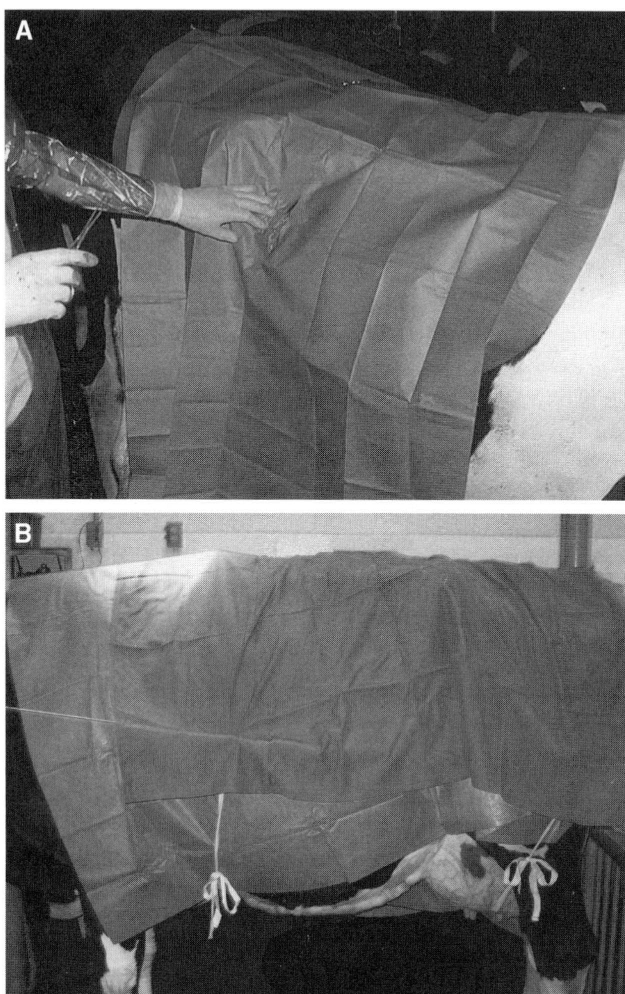

Fig. 2. (*A*) Abdominal surgery on a cow in a farm environment. The surgeon wears a disposable gown with plastic sleeves and latex gloves. A clean, disposable paper drape covers the animal and is fixed with towel clamp. (Courtesy of Dr Denis Harvey, Saint-Hyacinthe, Quebec, Canada.) (*B*) A fenestrated surgical drape envelopes the animal and is attached with two strings.

bacteria, and specifically, anaerobes. Poor to nonexistent vascularization decreases antibiotic efficacy and the natural defense mechanism. (2) Phagocytosis and humoral immunity are significantly decreased in damaged tissue. (3) It is difficult to eliminate microorganisms from an infected foreign body (sutures, implants) by medical means. Therefore, surgical removal is necessary. (4) Hematoma or blood in any disrupted anatomic space significantly decreases the number of microorganisms that is necessary to establish an infection. Blood serves as an excellent growth medium and, because it clots, interferes with the perfusion of the body's defense mechanisms. (5) The creation of dead space lends itself to infection because it has no defense mechanism.

Because the surgical environment in cattle is unique, it is not useful to compare it with what was reported in other species. Seger et al [57] reported a 37.7% wound complication rate in 252 cattle that underwent Cesarean section; however, only 9% were considered to be infected and needed drainage. The condition of the fetus (alive or dead) did not have any effect on the wound complication rate. In another study in cattle, the wound infection frequency for clean surgery was 10%; however, the infection rate for the ventral abdominal approach was much higher compared with a flank approach (35.7% versus 2.4%) [29]. Bedard et al [25] reported an infection rate of approximately 5% for cattle that underwent clean flank surgery. Nevertheless, those studies were conducted in a veterinary teaching hospital set-up. The results would be different, but not necessarily worse, in a field environment. Experimented practitioners are faster and the animal is open for a shorter period of time ("time is trauma"). The animal staying on the farm decreases the stress effect of a new environment with a different microflora. More studies are needed.

Basic principles of suture materials

Using suture is a second nature for every surgeon. Our choice of material and pattern frequently is based on our graduate training, tradition, and intuition. For many years, catgut, cotton (umbilical tape), and polyamid (Supramid, Serag Wiessner GmbH, Naila, Germany) have been used in bovine surgery for two good reasons—those were the only sutures that were available on the market and they were inexpensive. With the discovery of new synthetic molecules over the last 10 years, we have the choice between different monofilament, braided, absorbable and nonabsorbable sutures, with their advantages and disadvantages. Despite the sophistication of today's suture materials and surgical techniques, closing a wound involves the same basic procedure that was used by surgeons to the Roman emperors.

Several factors may influence the surgeon's choice, including training and experience in veterinary school, professional experience, knowledge of the healing characteristics of tissues and organs to suture, knowledge of the physical and biologic characteristics of various suture materials, and animal factors (age, weight, overall health status, presence of infection). For the characteristics of commonly-used suture material in cattle surgery, see Table 1 in the article by Newman and Anderson elsewhere in this issue.

Size denotes the diameter of the suture material. The accepted surgical practice is to use the smallest diameter suture that adequately holds the mending wounded tissue. This practice minimizes trauma as the suture is passed through the tissue to affect closure. The accepted rule is that the tensile strength of the suture need never exceed the tensile strength of the tissue; however, sutures should be at least as strong as normal tissue through which they are being placed. This is not always possible to achieve in large animal surgery. Our preliminary research demonstrated that the abdominal wall of a 300-kg Holstein bull is 30% stronger than a USP 2 suture (Lequient and Desrochers, Université de Montréal, unpublished data, 1997). Keeping this important fact in mind, we are walking a fine line when we suture the ventral abdominal wall of a 600-kg animal. Appropriate suture material and pattern, proper suture handling, and knot security are essential to avoid a catastrophic outcome.

Tying suture knots to obtain reliable tissue apposition is a basic, but important, skill in veterinary surgery. When closing a wound, the knot usually is the weakest point of the suture loop [58]. Because knot failure may have disastrous consequences, surgeons must assure total security of their knots. Tying secure knots while leaving the smallest amount of material in the wound should not be a matter of guesswork or tradition. Knot security and strength depends on the size and the type of suture material used, number of throws, and knot configuration [59,60]. Two studies tested in vitro breaking strength of large USP suture materials frequently used in large animal surgery [61,62]. Trostle et al [61] found that size 5 polyester was the strongest suture tested followed by size 3 polyglactin 910 and size 2 polyglycolic acid. Ninety-three percent of suture loops failed by breakage at the knot. Although the suture materials tested were different, Campbell and Bailey [62] showed a superior breaking strength of size 5 polyester with an overall loop breakage rate at the knot of 93.6%. Both studies used a reinforced surgeon knot and neither of them evaluated the number of throws that is necessary to obtain a secure knot with these different and larger suture sizes. A secure knot commonly is defined as a knot that does not slip more than 3 mm when the loop is submitted to an increasing load. If the knot holds, eventually breakage of the suture material will occur at the knot as a result of shear stress. The symmetric square knot is the most recommended knot; however, it seems that this knot is not always executed. Because of the difficulty of discerning the cause of a ligature failure or a dehiscence, in vivo performances of asymmetric knots were not evaluated. With a large diameter suture, each surgical knot should be constituted of five throws for a interrupted pattern. If a continuous pattern is used, one additional throw at the beginning and two additional throws at the end of the suture will improve the security of the knot. Knots are difficult to tighten under excessive tension. Different knot configurations can be used to avoid this problem. A needle holder or hemostats commonly are placed on the first throw to hold it tight. Needle holder jaws with teeth produce distinct structural changes in synthetic sutures that cause a marked reduction in the suture-breaking strength [63]. Huber et al [64] evaluated the effect of knotting method on the structural properties of large-diameter nonabsorbable monofilament sutures. According to their results, square knot, sliding half-hitch, and surgeon's knot influenced the structural properties of suture materials, whereas the clamped square knot did not.

Summary

Basic principles of surgery are important to review, even for experienced surgeons. Although aseptic surgical principles are not always applicable in the field, we have to respect some guidelines. Recent research will influence the way that we do things, based on what we have been taught and our experience. Respecting those simple principles can make a big difference in the final outcome.

References

[1] Mangermartin G. L'opération césarienne chez la vache et la responsabilité civile professionnelle du vétérinaire. [Caesarian section in cattle and the professional liability of the veterinarian.] Bulletin des Groupements Techniques Vétérinaires 1998;321–5.

[2] Batra EK, Franz DA, Towler MA, et al. Influence of surgeon's tying technique on knot security. J Appl Biomater 1993;4(3):241–7.

[3] Thacker JG, Rodeheaver GT, Kurtz L, et al. Mechanical performance of sutures in surgery. Am J Surg 1977;133:713–5.

[4] Bendiner E. Liberator of surgery from shackles of sepsis. Hosp Pract 1986;21:126C.

[5] Larson E. Guideline for use of topical antimicrobial agents. Am J Infect Control 1988;16(6): 253–66.

[6] Ayliffe GA. Surgical scrub and skin disinfection. Infect Control 1984;5(1):23–7.

[7] Cruse PJ, Foord R. The epidemiology of wound infection. A 10-year prospective study of 62,939 wounds. Surg Clin North Am 1980;60(1):27–40.

[8] Kaul AF, Jewett JF. Agents and techniques for disinfection of the skin. Surg Gynecol Obstet 1981;152(5):677–85.

[9] Lowbury EJ. Skin disinfection. J Clin Pathol 1961;14:85–90.

[10] Lilly HA, Lowbury EJ. Transient skin flora: their removal by cleansing or disinfection in relation to their mode of deposition. J Clin Pathol 1978;31(10):919–22.

[11] White JJ, Wallace CK, Burnet LS. Skin disinfection. Johns Hopkins Med J 1970;126(3): 169–76.

[12] Selwyn S, Ellis H. Skin bacteria and skin disinfection reconsidered. BMJ 1972;1(793):136–40.

[13] Smeak DD, Olmstead ML. Infections in clean wounds: the roles of the surgeon, environment, and host. Comp Cont Educ 1984;6(7):629–33.

[14] Brown TR, Ehrlich CE, Stehman FB, et al. A clinical evaluation of chlorhexidine gluconate spray as compared with iodophor scrub for preoperative skin preparation. Surg Gynecol Obstet 1984;158(4):363–6.

[15] Gibson KL, Donald AW, Hariharan H, et al. Comparison of two pre-surgical skin preparation techniques. Can J Vet Res 1997;61(2):154–6.

[16] Newsom SW, Rowland C. Studies on perioperative skin flora. J Hosp Infect 1988; 11(Suppl B):B21–6.

[17] Osuna DJ, DeYoung DJ, Walker RL. Comparison of three skin preparation techniques. Part 2: Clinical trial in 100 dogs. Vet Surg 1990;19(1):20–3.

[18] Rochat MC, Mann FA, Berg JN. Evaluation of a one-step surgical preparation technique in dogs. J Am Vet Med Assoc 1993;203(3):392–5.

[19] Ritter MA, French ML, Eitzen HE, et al. The antimicrobial effectiveness of operative-site preparative agents: a microbiological and clinical study. J Bone Joint Surg Am 1980;62(5): 826–8.
[20] Alexander JW, Fischer JE, Boyajian M, et al. The influence of hair-removal methods on wound infections. Arch Surg 1983;118(3):347–52.
[21] Seropian R, Reynolds BM. Wound infections after preoperative depilatory versus razor preparation. Am J Surg 1971;121(3):251–4.
[22] Lloyd DH, Dick WD, Jenkinson DM. The effects of some surface sampling procedures on the stratum corneum of bovine skin. Res Vet Sci 1979;26(2):250–2.
[23] Tang K, Yeh JS, Sgouros S. The influence of hair shave on the infection rate in neurosurgery. A prospective study. Pediatr Neurosurg 2001;35(1):13–7.
[24] Gil Z, Cohen JT, Spektor S, et al. The role of hair shaving in skull base surgery. Otolaryngol Head Neck Surg 2003;128(1):43–7.
[25] Bedard S, Desrochers A, Fecteau G, et al. Comparaison de quatre protocoles de préparation préopératoire chez le bovin. [Comparison of four protocols for preoperative preparation in cattle]. Can Vet J 2001;42(3):199–203.
[26] Rodeheaver G, Bellamy W, Kody M, et al. Bactericidal activity and toxicity of iodine-containing solutions in wounds. Arch Surg 1982;117(2):181–6.
[27] Altemeier WA. Surgical antiseptics. In: Block SS, editor. Disinfection, sterilization, and preservation. 3rd edition. Philadephia: Lea & Febiger; 1983. p. 493–504.
[28] Denton GW. Chorhexidine. In: Block SS, editor. Disinfection, sterilization, and preservation. 4th edition. Philadelphia: Lea & Febiger; 1991. p. 274–89.
[29] Desrochers A, St-Jean G, Anderson DE, et al. Comparative evaluation of two surgical scrub preparations in cattle. Vet Surg 1996;25(4):336–41.
[30] Osuna DJ, DeYoung DJ, Walker RL. Comparison of three skin preparation techniques in the dog. Part 1: Experimental trial. Vet Surg 1990;19(1):14–9.
[31] Gilliam DL, Nelson CL. Comparison of a one-step iodophor skin preparation versus traditional preparation in total joint surgery. Clin Orthop 1990;(250):258–60.
[32] Galuppo LD, Pascoe JR, Jang SS, et al. Evaluation of iodophor skin preparation techniques and factors influencing drainage from ventral midline incisions in horses. J Am Vet Med Assoc 1999;215(7):963–9.
[33] Larson EL, Morton HE. Alcohols. In: Block SS, editor. Disinfection, sterilization and preservation. 4th edition. Philadelphia: Lea and Febiger; 1991. p. 642–54.
[34] Garner JS, Favero MS. CDC guidelines for the prevention and control of nosocomial infections. Guideline for handwashing and hospital environmental control, 1985. Supersedes guideline for hospital environmental control published in 1981. Am J Infect Control 1986; 14(3):110–29.
[35] Zubrod CJ, Farnsworth KD, Oaks JL. Evaluation of arthrocentesis site bacterial flora before and after 4 methods of preparation in horses with and without evidence of skin contamination. Vet Surg 2004;33(5):525–30.
[36] Grabsch EA, Mitchell DJ, Hooper J, et al. In-use efficacy of a chlorhexidine in alcohol surgical rub: a comparative study. ANZ J Surg 2004;74(9):769–72.
[37] Furukawa K, Ogawa R, Norose Y, et al. A new surgical handwashing and hand antisepsis from scrubbing to rubbing. J Nippon Med Sch 2004;71(3):190–7.
[38] Belkin NL. The surgical mask: is it still necessary? Surgery 1997;122(3):641–2.
[39] Clem MF. Preparation for surgery. In: Auer JA, editor. Equine surgery. Philadelphia: W.B. Saunders Company; 1992. p. 111–9.
[40] Korniewicz DM, Garzon L, Seltzer J, et al. Failure rates in nonlatex surgical gloves. Am J Infect Control 2004;32(5):268–73.
[41] Korniewicz DM, Garzon L, Plitcha S. Health care workers: risk factors for nonlatex and latex gloves during surgery. AIHA J (Fairfax, Va) 2003;64(6):851–5.
[42] Boyce JM, Pittet D. Guideline for hand hygiene in health-care settings. MMWR Morb Mortal Wkly Rep: Recommendations and Reports 2002;51:1–45.

[43] Larson E, Bobo L. Effective hand degerming in the presence of blood. J Emerg Med 1992;10(1):7–11.
[44] Mackintosh CA, Hoffman PN. An extended model for transfer of micro-organisms via the hands: differences between organisms and the effect of alcohol disinfection. J Hyg (Lond) 1984;92(3):345–55.
[45] Larson EL, Eke PI, Wilder MP, et al. Quantity of soap as a variable in handwashing. Infect Control 1987;8(9):371–5.
[46] Wan PY, Blackford JT, Bemis DA, et al. Evaluation of surgical scrub methods for large animal surgeons. Vet Surg 1997;26(5):382–5.
[47] O'Farrell DA, Kenny G, O'Sullivan M, et al. Evaluation of the optimal hand-scrub duration prior to total hip arthroplasty. J Hosp Infect 1994;26:93–8.
[48] Galle PC, Homesley HD, Rhyne AL. Reassessment of the surgical scrub. Surg Gynecol Obstet 1978;147(2):215–8.
[49] Hingst V, Juditzki I, Heeg P, et al. Evaluation of the efficacy of surgical hand disinfection following a reduced application time of 3 instead of 5 min. J Hosp Infect 1992;20(2):79–86.
[50] Wheelock SM, Lookinland S. Effect of surgical hand scrub time on subsequent bacterial growth. AORN J 1997;65(6):1087–92 [discussion 1094–8].
[51] Pereira LJ, Lee GM, Wade KJ. An evaluation of five protocols for surgical handwashing in relation to skin condition and microbial counts. J Hosp Infect 1997;36(1):49–65.
[52] Chiu KY, Lau SK, Fung B, et al. Plastic adhesive drapes and wound infection after hip fracture surgery. ANZ J Surg 1993;63(10):798–801.
[53] Dewan PA, Van Rij AM, Robinson RG, et al. The use of an iodophor-impregnated plastic incise drape in abdominal surgery—a controlled clinical trial. ANZ J Surg 1987;57(11):859–63.
[54] Osuna DJ, DeYoung DJ, Walker RL. Comparison of an antimicrobial adhesive drape and povidone-iodine preoperative skin preparation in dogs. Vet Surg 1992;21(6):458–62.
[55] Beck WC, Geffert JP, Hansen M. The incise drape—boon or hazard: an experimental study. Am Surg 1981;47(8):343–6.
[56] Fleischmann W, Meyer H, von Baer A. Bacterial recolonization of the skin under a polyurethane drape in hip surgery. J Hosp Infect 1996;34(2):107–16.
[57] Seger VT, Grunert E, Ahlers D. Wound complications following cesarean section in cattle. Dtsch Tierärztl Wochenschr 1994;101:309–11.
[58] Trimbos JB. Security of various knots commonly used in surgical practice. Obstet Gynecol 1984;64(2):274–80.
[59] Thacker JG, Rodeheaver G, Moore JW, et al. Mechanical performance of surgical sutures. Am J Surg 1975;130(3):374–80.
[60] Fayolle P. Le materiel de suture. Point Vétérinaire 1993;150:709–13.
[61] Trostle SS, Wilson DG, Stone WC, et al. A study of the biomechanical properties of the adult equine linea alba: relationship of tissue bite size and suture material to breaking strength. Vet Surg 1994;23(6):435–41.
[62] Campbell EJ, Bailey JV. Mechanical properties of suture materials in vitro and after in vivo implantation in horses. Vet Surg 1992;21(5):355–61.
[63] Stamp CV, McGregor W, Rodeheaver GT, et al. Surgical needle holder damage to sutures. Am Surg 1988;54(5):300–6.
[64] Huber DJ, Egger EL, James SP. The effect of knotting method on the structural properties of large diameter nonabsorbable monofilament sutures. Vet Surg 1999;28(4):260–7.

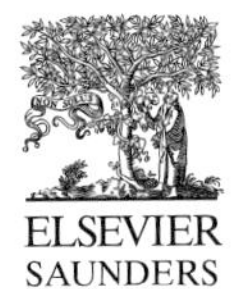
ELSEVIER
SAUNDERS

Vet Clin Food Anim 21 (2005) 19–31

VETERINARY CLINICS
Food Animal Practice

Pain Management in Ruminants

David E. Anderson, DVM, MS*,
William W. Muir, DVM, PhD

Department of Veterinary Clinical Sciences, College of Veterinary Medicine, The Ohio State University, 601 Tharp Street, Columbus, OH 43210, USA

Pain and the biologic responses to it are part of a highly integrated multidimensional system that causes all animals to react, respond (fight, flight, freeze), and protect themselves from their environment. Whether or not animals "feel" pain the same as humans is immaterial, and regardless of how pain is processed, many if not most of the neural elements and biologic consequences of pain are the same among all mammalian species. One clinically useful definition of animal pain states is that "pain is an aversive feeling or sensation associated with actual or potential tissue damage and resulting in physiologic, neuroendocrine, and behavioral changes that are indicative of a "stress" response." [1] The sensation of pain is part of everyday life and is essential for survival, as evidenced by the high morbidity and mortality of humans with congenital insensitivity to pain [2]. Affected humans sustain all forms of undetected tissue damage, including destruction of the joints, pressure sores, internal organ trauma, and self-mutilation. The importance of the sensation of pain in maintaining and protecting the normal physiologic condition of the body has led to its consideration as a homeostatic emotion that initiates feeling and motivation [3]. The latter consideration is the basis for why pain perception (*nociception*) is not considered to represent the pain experience fully and helps to explain the relationship between painful experiences and pain behaviors in animals. In this context, pain can be categorized broadly as either adaptive or maladaptive [4]. Adaptive pain increases the potential for survival by protecting the animal from injury and promoting healing. In contrast, maladaptive pain is a disease created by pathologic processes that result in the persistence of pain for long after the initiating cause has been removed.

* Corresponding author.
E-mail address: Anderson.670@osu.edu (D.E. Anderson).

doi:10.1016/j.cvfa.2004.12.008 *vetfood.theclinics.com*

The pain system includes sensors, neural pathways, and processing centers [5]. This conglomeration of neural elements is responsible for detecting, transmitting, and actualizing biologic and behavioral responses to noxious events. Understanding the physiologic and pathophysiologic processes responsible for pain and its consequences (stress, distress) is key to restoring normal physiologic (homeostatic) pain responses and developing rational pain therapies [6,7].

Physiologic pain versus pathologic pain

Pain signals the potential for or development of tissue damage, protecting the recipient from further injury. Nociception refers to the neurophysiologic processes whereby noxious stimuli are transduced, transmitted, modulated, projected, and perceived (Fig. 1). Noxious mechanical, chemical, or thermal stimuli are *transduced* into electrical signals (action potentials) by high-threshold pain receptors (nociceptors) located on the peripheral terminals of thin, uninsulated or minimally insulated (myelinated) C and A delta nerve fibers. The nerve action potentials are *transmitted* centrally to the superficial layers of the dorsal horn of the spinal cord, where they are modified (*modulated*) by local and descending facilitatory and inhibitory neurons and *projected* to the brain (*perception*) (see Fig. 1). Increases in temperature, respiration, heart rate, and arterial blood pressure are physical signs indicating disease. Similarly, increased responses to noxious and non-

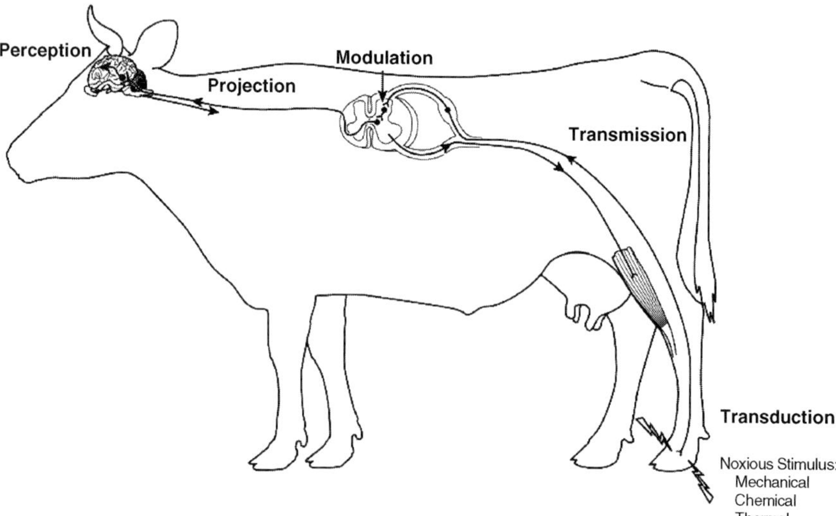

Fig. 1. Physiologic (nociceptive) pain. Noxious stimulus is tranduced, transmitted, modulated, projected, and perceived. The brain also generates responses that travel via descending nerve pathways that facilitate or inhibit (modulate) sensory input to the spinal cord.

noxious stimuli as exemplified by hyperalgesia (increased response to a stimulus that is normally painful) and allodynia (pain caused by a stimulus that is normally nonpainful) indicate disease and should be considered the "fifth clinical sign."

Physiologic, or "ouch," pain is nociceptive pain that uses normal sensory pathways and serves to protect the recipient from tissue damage [7]. The free nerve endings of afferent sensory pain processing fibers encode noxious stimuli depending on the modality, intensity, duration, and location of the stimulus. In the absence of tissue damage, pain is considered to be "physiologic," warning the animal of potentially harmful stimuli. The intensity of the stimulus is considerably greater than that required to elicit innocuous sensations, is the most important factor determining the severity of pain, and can be defined quantitatively by a stimulus intensity-response relationship similar to other sensations.

Pathologic pain generally is produced by tissue or nerve damage and frequently involves the development of peripheral sensitization, central sensitization, structural reorganization of neural elements within the central nervous system (CNS), and disinhibition (Fig. 2) [5]. It can be nociceptive

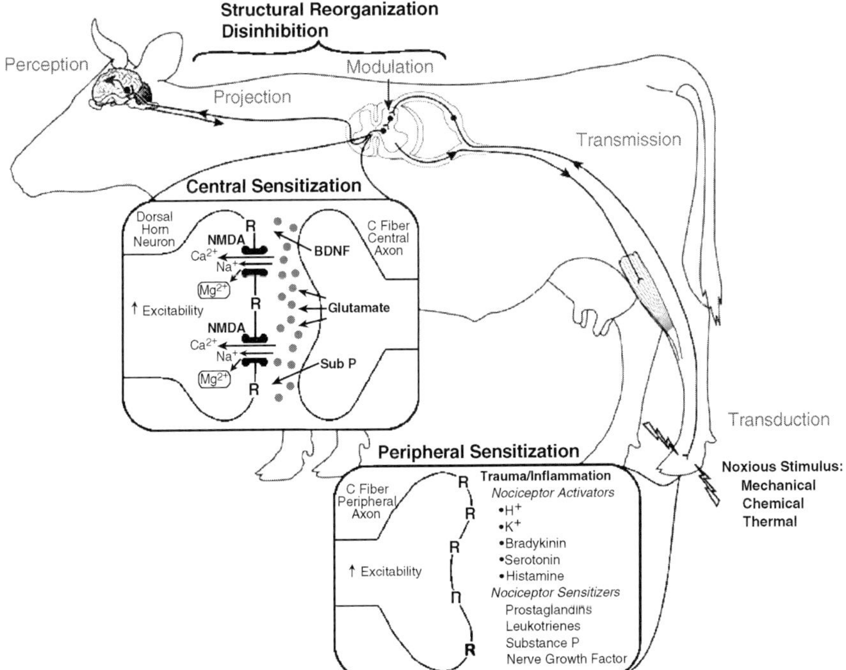

Fig. 2. Pathologic pain. Peripheral sensitization, central sensitization, structural reorganization, and disinhibition are several of the more prominent mechanisms responsible for the development of moderate, severe, and chronic pain conditions. BDNF, brain-derived neurotrophic factor; NMDA, *N*-methyl-D-aspartate.

(activation of high-threshold nociceptors) or nonnociceptive (structural reorganization and phenotypic switches of neurons) [5,8–10]. Tissue damage and the associated inflammatory response are responsible for producing a wide variety of chemicals that function as nociceptor activators or sensitizers and include hydrogen and potassium ions, prostaglandins, histamine, bradykinin, nerve growth factor, cytokines, and chemokines. Together, these factors act as a "sensitizing soup" changing high-threshold nociceptors to low-threshold nociceptors and activating quiescent or "silent" nocireceptors, resulting in *peripheral sensitization* and a zone of primary hyperalgesia [10]. Severe tissue or nerve damage and chronic activation of peripheral pain fibers produce action potentials that continue to bombard dorsal horn neurons causing biochemical (transcriptional) changes within dorsal horn neurons, resulting in *central sensitization,* the potential for a change in the neurons' phenotype (neuroplasticity) [5,10]. Central sensitization is highly dependent on the activation of glutamate-activated *N*-methyl-D-aspartate (NMDA) receptors and is responsible for the development of a zone of secondary hyperalgesia and allodynia in noninjured tissues [5]. Other potential causes for pathologic pain include abnormalities within the nervous system (function pain), structural reorganization of the CNS, and disinhibition [4,11]. An understanding of the pathologic neurophysiologic processes that sensitize, activate, modify, and produce permanent alterations in how sensory inputs are processed is paramount to the development and implementation of effective pain therapy [7].

Peripheral sensitization

Tissue damage and inflammation result in activation and release of intracellular components from damaged cells, inflammatory cells (lymphocytes, neutrophils, macrophages), and the primary nerve fiber itself. The local release and spread of ions (H^+, K^+), prostaglandins (prostaglandin E_2), bradykinin, cyclooxygenase (COX), neurotrophic growth factors, and cytokines (interleukin [IL]-1, IL-6, tumor necrosis factor α) sensitize pain fibers to subsequent painful and nonpainful stimuli (Fig. 2) [5,10]. Mast cell degranulation increases the local concentration of 5-hydroxytryptamine (serotonin) and histamine. Together, these substances produce a sensitizing soup, which lowers the threshold of nociceptors and activates "silent" nociceptors (10–40% of total nociceptor population), amplifying the pain response. Local vasodilation and plasma extravasation result in a further amplification of the inflammatory response and the spread of hypersensitivity to surrounding tissues (secondary hyperalgesia).

Central sensitization

Central sensitization occurs when the cumulative effects of frequent (chronic) or severe peripheral nociceptor input releases excessive quantities of CNS nuerotransmitters (substance P, neurokinin A, brain-derived neurotrophic fator), including glutamate, which remove the normally present magnesium (Mg^{2+}) block of NMDA, activating these and other receptors in the superficial layers of the dorsal horn of the spinal cord, resulting in an increase in their sensitivity (see Fig. 2) [10]. Activation of NMDA receptors leads to an increase in calcium (Ca^{2+}) in dorsal horn neurons, resulting in increased excitability and spontaneous ectopic discharge. During various disease states, the increase in dorsal horn sensory neuron excitability also is contributed to by the production of sensitizing substances (eg, prostaglandins) by glial cells in response to increases in cerebrospinal fluid cytokines (tumor necrosis factor α, IL-1) [11]. Sensitization of dorsal horn neurons can last for hours and is believed to be responsible for pain outside the area of tissue injury (secondary hyperalgesia) and allodynia. Central sensitization is fundamentally different from peripheral sensitization in that it enables low-intensity stimuli to produce pain sensations; when pain is chronic, it enables sensory fibers that normally transmit nonpainful stimuli (low-threshold A beta fibers) to produce pain as a result of changes in sensory processing in the spinal cord. Central sensitization increases the responsiveness of dorsal horn neurons to sensory inputs (allodynia), expands the receptive field, and is believed to be responsible for the intense pain produced by severe injury. Chronic pain is responsible for activity-dependent plasticity and long-term structural changes (neuroplastic) within the CNS. The extension of central sensitization from the spinal cord to the brain leads to the development or modification of memory patterns and are responsible for changes in animal behavior. Together the development of peripheral sensitization, wind-up, and central sensitization represents a continuum of the pain process, which exists as a consequence of continuous, unrelenting, and untreated pain.

Structural reorganization

Normally the central terminals of nociceptive (high-threshold) neurons (pain neurons) terminate in the superficial layers of the dorsal horn of the spinal cord before projecting painful information to the brain. The low-threshold sensory fibers activated by touch, pressure, vibration, and movement (shear) terminate in deeper layers (laminae) of the dorsal horn. Peripheral nerve injury occasionally can lead to the death of neurons in the superficial layers and the sprouting of the central terminals of low-threshold sensory neruons located in the deeper laminae into zones normally occupied only by nociceptor terminals [12]. This rewiring of the spinal cord results in the perception of pain by normally nonpainful stimuli, such as touch.

Disinhibiton

The brain continuously receives sensory information from ascending projections, but modulates this input by descending facilitatory and inhibitory influences. Inhibitory influences from the brain and brainstem mediated by the release of serotonin and norepinephrine activate inhibitory neurons within the spinal cord that release the inhibitory neurotransmitters glycine and γ-aminobutyric acid. These inhibitory neurotransmitters hyperpolarize dorsal horn neurons, making them less sensitive to afferent nociceptive input. The loss of these inhibitory influences (*disinhibition*) secondary to central (cancer, CNS trauma) or peripheral (neurodegenerative disease, toxemia) nerve injury can result in hypersensitivity, hyperalgesia, and allodynia [13].

Stress and distress

Pain is responsible for stress and can lead to distress [14,15]. Stress is an adaptive pattern of behavioral, neural, endocrine, immune, hematologic, and metabolic changes directed toward the restoration of homeostasis. The stress response prepares the animal for an emergency reaction and fosters survival in circumstances of immediate threats (fight or flight). Acute pain is capable of producing a significant stress response by initiating activation of the sympathetic nervous system, secretion of glucocorticoids (primarily cortisol), hypermetabolism, sodium and water retention, and altered carbohydrate and protein metabolism [16–18]. The maintenance of normal homeostatic balance to an acute stress-producing event (pain) is by negative feedback controls that act at multiple levels within the brain (amygdala) and sympathoadrenal and hypothalamic-pituitary-adrenal (HPA) axes, thereby elevating catecholamines and glucocorticoids and leading to enhanced arousal, appraisal, cardiorespiratory, and cognitive performance to deal with the immediate threat. Increases in corticotropin-releasing hormone, plasma cortisol, and vasopressin often directly correlate with the stressful or painful event and help to restore homeostasis. Severe or prolonged pain resulting in severe stress eventually becomes maladaptive, however, producing depression and immunosuppression (sickness syndrome), which, if not controlled, can lead to distress and the activation of self-sustaining cascades of neural and endocrine responses that derail physiologic homeostasis [19]. Prolonged stress impairs the animal's ability to interact and learn and changes the animal's behavioral phenotype [1]. Severe pain produces behavioral, autonomic, neuroendocrine, and immunologic responses that can result in self-mutilation, immune incompetence, and a poor quality of life potentially leading to gradual deterioration and death.

Clinical management of pain in ruminants

The easiest type of pain to treat is that which is induced. The magnitude of surgical pain is influenced by the procedure, the methods used, and the experience and skill of the practitioner. Some strategies to minimize pain before it occurs (eg, preemptive) are obvious—local anesthesia, general anesthesia, sedation, and tranquilization. Some thought should be given to the physiologic processes that are induced by tissue injury and may lead to "pathologic" pain after surgery. Sedatives, tranquilizers, narcotics, and anesthetics inhibit detection of or intensity of pain by interfering with pain pathways, but these drugs do not treat the processes (eg, inflammation) to stop continued noxious stimuli. Nonsteroidal anti-inflammatory drugs (NSAIDs) are a crucial link to multimodal treatment of pain. Often a surgical stimulus (eg, castration in young calves) is so brief that little difference can be observed or measured between animals having or not having local anesthesia applied. NSAIDs can provide prolonged post-operative analgesia, however, and a quantifiable benefit can be found.

General anesthesia may be thought of as a "gold standard" for pain-free surgery. In research comparing various methods of castration, however, general anesthesia consistently stimulated the most severe rise in serum cortisol (Anderson and Grubb, unpublished data, 2000). These studies have suggested that general anesthesia may be intensely distressful to a patient despite the absence of pain stimulus from surgery. In ruminant surgery, economic pressures and limitations of field surgery have caused selection against general anesthesia. The behavior and demeanor of cattle favor use of sedatives, local or regional anesthesia, or epidural anesthesia.

Local anesthetics are the most commonly used preemptive analgesic drugs used in food animal practice [21]. These drugs, especially lidocaine 2% HCl, are used to prevent incisional pain during surgery. These drugs act locally or regionally when perineural anesthesia is performed, but have no systemic or behavioral effect. Local anesthetics block nerve fibers (B fibers > C fibers > A fibers) [22]. These nerve fiber types represent motor/touch (B fibers), nonmyelinated pain and temperature sensation (C fibers), and motor and proprioceptive (A fibers). The acuteness or severity of the perception of pain is influenced by the stimulus, and perception diminishes pain → cold → warmth → touch → deep pressure. Local anesthetic drugs act by inhibiting sodium channels to impede nerve conduction by preventing depolarization of the nerve fiber. These drugs must disassociate in an alkaline environment for this to occur. In infected tissues, quality of local anesthesia is often poor because the relatively more acidic environment prevents disassociation of drug. An example of this effect is septic cellulitis associated with complicated sole ulcer complex in dairy cattle. The acidic environment associated with the cellulitis may cause local administration of lidocaine to be ineffectual with continued pain sensation. One solution to this problem is to administer the "block" remote to infected tissues. Lidocaine 2% HCl is painful in and of itself, but this noxious characteristic can be eliminated by adding sodium bicarbonate to neutralize the solution.

Local anesthetics can be used in a variety of techniques, including surface active, local block, ring block, selected peripheral nerve block, and regional blocks (eg, paravertebral, epidural). The authors have tried various topical products for inducing local anesthesia, including topical lidocaine spray and lidocaine sustained-release pads. The topical sprays, designed for application on human skin, failed to provide sufficient anesthesia to obtund the response to needle insertion for paravertebral blocks. Bovine skin, especially dorsal skin, may be too thick or resistant to absorption of the anesthetic to induce anesthesia. Lidocaine sustained-release patches were designed for topical use in humans for relief of isolated pain confined to superficial areas. These patches release lidocaine over 12 to 24 hours. The authors prospectively evaluated these patches in cows after surgery for cruciate ligament surgery, septic arthritis, and incisional pain. Results were highly variable, with most cows showing minimal detectable response.

Epidural anesthesia has been the focus of attention of many research projects in cattle in an attempt to minimize pain of surgery [23–29]. Caudal epidural anesthesia is applied easily in cattle, and a variety of drugs have been shown to be beneficial (Table 1). Of particular interest are drugs (eg, α_2-agonists) that optimize analgesia, but minimize motor nerve interference such that the patient may remain standing and stable throughout surgery.

NSAIDs inhibit COX. COX acts on arachidonic acids to liberate prostaglandins and other mediators of inflammation. COX inhibitors prevent production of these factors. Nonspecific COX inhibitors include flunixin, ketoprofen, and phenylbutazone. Selective COX-2 inhibitors are rapidly evolving and include etodolac and carprofen. NSAIDs have differential activity because of the presence of variable receptors and variable drug effects. Clinical observations suggest that flunixin provides excellent visceral analgesia but has less potent effects for many musculoskeletal injuries. Alternatively, phenylbutazone seems to provide excellent

Table 1
Use of epidural anesthesia for paralumbar analgesia or laparotomy in cattle

Drug	Dosage	Onset of analgesia	Duration of analgesia
Lidocaine 2%	0.2 mg/kg (5 mL)	5 min	10–115 min
Xylazine	0.05 mg/kg (5 mL in saline) 0.07 mg/kg 1.0 mg/kg	20–40 min	2–3 h
Clonidine	2–3 μg/kg diluted to 8 mL in saline	2-μg dose: 19 min 3-μg dose: 9 min	2-μg dose: 192 min 3 μg dose: 311 min Peak effect during 60–180 min
Ketamine 5%	5 mL (250 mg) 10 mL (500 mg) 20 mL (1000 mg)	5 mL: 6.5 min 10 mL: 5 min 20 mL: 5 min	5 mL: 17 min 10 mL: 34 min 20 mL: 62 min
Procaine HCl 5%	300 mg (6 mL)	8–20 min	45–127 min; mean 83 min
Medetomidine	15 μg/kg (5 mL)	5 min	412 min
Detomidine	40 μg/kg		
Romifidine plus morphine	R: 50 μg/kg M: 0.1 mg/kg		12 h maximum

musculoskeletal pain relief, but offers little benefit for treatment of visceral pain. The authors have used etodolac for several years for management of chronic musculoskeletal pain in ruminants. The authors' clinical experience suggests that although these drugs may be safer for long-term use (eg, COX-2 inhibition is less likely to interfere with homeostasis of abomasal muscosa or renal perfusion), COX-2 inhibitors provide less potent analgesia.

Much of the pain research performed has shown tremendous benefits of preemptive analgesia. There is a consistently less impressive effect of administration of analgesic medication after the noxious stimulus has become established. Zulauf et al [30] showed that if NSAIDs were administered before castration with Burdizzo, during first the 72 hours, lower serum cortisol, greater feed intake, and less scrotal swelling occurred. Stafford et al [31] compared various surgical castration techniques (ring versus band versus surgery versus clamp) with or without local anesthesia or NSAIDs. Local anesthesia alone did not prevent cortisol increase, but local anesthesia plus NSAID did obtund cortisol response. Mellor et al [32] showed that there was a marked increase of cortisol and noradrenaline after castration, dehorning, and tailing amputation and that local anesthesia obtunded this response, but only so long as the local anesthesia was present. When the local anesthesia had resolved, these calves could not be distinguished from calves that did not receive local anesthesia. Faulkner and Weary [33] showed that dehorning calves 4 to 8 weeks old under sedation and local anesthesia was beneficial only when combined with an NSAID. Calves that had NSAIDs administered for castration had less head shaking, head rubbing, and ear flicking and gained more weight compared with calves that received sedation and local anesthesia alone. Grondahl-Nielsen et al [34] compared cornual nerve block versus sedation (xylazine plus butorphanol) and found that the cornual nerve block significantly decreased pain responses as evidenced by lower serum cortisol and lower heart rate. McMeekan et al [35] used long-acting local anesthesia (bupivicaine, 3–4 hours' duration) for scoop dehorning. The cortisol response was obtunded only when period local anesthesia was active.

Age does not seem to have as profound an effect on stress of minor surgical procedures in cattle compared with swine. Taschke and Folsch [36] examined dehorning stress in calves newborn to 4 months. Age had no effect, but anesthesia significantly reduced cortisol and adverse responses. Eicher and Dalley [37] studied tail docking in 3- to 5-week-old calves. Calves showed increased activity after banding for about 2 hours, the tail was heat sensitive distal to band for 2 hours, and more fly avoidance behaviors were observed (caused by increased fly attacks) on calves that had tail docks. Ruminants, especially cattle, differ in behaviors associated with pain. Ruminants often become subdued, spend more time lying down and less time eating and ruminating, and fail to clean the nostrils as frequently when in pain or stressed. Galindo and Broom [38] observed that lame cows had more lying time, less eating time, and more lying time outside of cubicles and performed fewer aggressive behavior actions despite having the same frequency of receiving aggressive behavior interactions. These lame cows licked other cows less and were licked more themselves. Many social and environmental factors influence pain perception and responses in cattle. Whay et al [39] reported that heifers developed hyperalgesia in the periparturient period. Rushen et al [40] showed that cows subjected to social isolation, with or without naloxone therapy, had increased vocalization, heart rate, and cortisol. These cows also showed increased hypoalesgia, however (stress-induced analgesia?).

Future directions

Many advances in drug therapy are being made. Food animal veterinarians are partly responsible for the preservation of a safe food product. To that end, veterinarians must be cautious with cross-species applications of drugs and therapies. What is the cost-benefit relationship? Pertinent data include the roles of various hormones and cellular mechanisms of pain signal interference. Estradiol modulates L-type voltage-gated calcium channels. Can this hormone be used to decrease sensitivity of peripheral nerves to pain? *N*-arachidonyl γ-aminobutyric acid is present in the brain of cows and is known to inhibit pain. Can drugs be used to increase the presence of this molecule? Pinheiro Machado et al [41] studied the analgesic effects of amniotic fluids in cows. This study compared amniotic fluids versus water and morphine versus saline. Amniotic fluids increased periparturient opioid-mediated analgesia, and cows ingesting amniotic fluid had higher thermal threshold 1 hour postpartum.

The authors have been measuring skin impedance in ruminants in an attempt to quantify "clinical pain." This relatively new technology has been able to show differences with the intensity of "pain" or "distress." The most severely distressing diseases seemed to involve neurologic or respiratory disease or septicemia (Fig. 3). Surgical conditions of the gastrointestinal

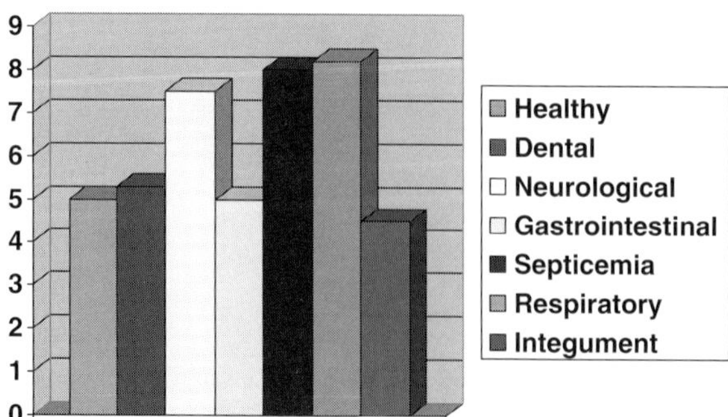

Fig. 3. Comparison of skin impedance values among ruminants with diseases of various body systems (1–10 scale; 1 = no pain, 10 = severe pain).

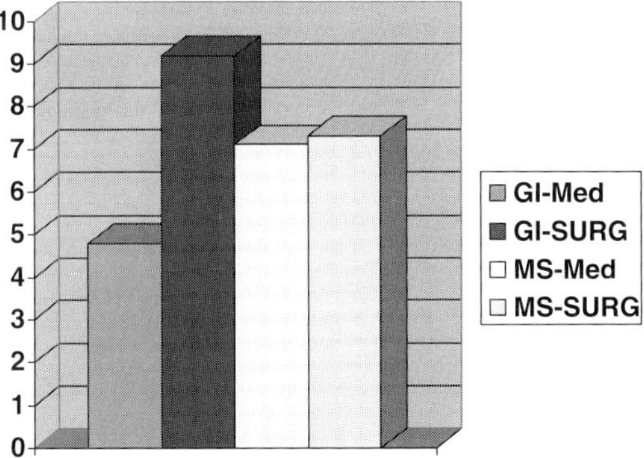

Fig. 4. Comparison of medical (Med) and surgical (SURG) conditions of the gastrointestinal (GI) and musculoskeletal (MS) systems.

tract seemed to be more intensely painful than medical diseases of the gastrointestinal tract (Fig. 4). Understanding the clinical intensity of noxious stimuli associated with various body systems may help guide decisions for the need or type of preemptive analgesia used.

Summary

Based on the available literature, the most important tool available in modern veterinary medicine is preemptive analgesia. Veterinarians must capture "opportunities" to prevent the onset of pain, prevent noxious stimuli or their perception, and limit the pain-stress-distress cascade that results in altered behavior and deviation from physiologic norms. Rational treatment of pain requires an appreciation of its consequences, a fundamental understanding of the mechanisms that are responsible for its production, and a practical appreciation of the analgesic drugs that are available. The goal of pain treatment should be to restore normal (physiologic) pain responses and to eliminate pathologic pain processes. In this context, pain therapy should be directed at the multiple mechanisms (multimodal therapy) responsible for its production, and analgesic therapies should be instituted before (preemptive therapy) pain is initiated (eg, surgery) whenever possible [7,20].

References

[1] Broom DM. The evolution of pain. Vlaams Diergeneeskundig Tijdschrift 2000;69:385–411.

[2] Miranda C, Di Virgilio M, Selleri S, et al. Novel pathogenic mechanisms of congenital insensitivity to pain with anhidrosis genetic disorder unveiled by functional analysis of neurotrophic tyrosine receptor kinase type 1/nerve growth factor receptor mutations. J Biol Chem 2002;277:6455–62.

[3] Craig AD. Pain mechanisms: labeled lines versus convergence in central processing. Annu Rev Neurosci 2003;26:1–30.

[4] Woolf CJ. Pain: moving from symptom control toward mechanism-specific pharmacologic management. Ann Intern Med 2004;140:441–51.

[5] Muir WW, Woolf CJ. Mechanisms of pain and their therapeutic implications. J Am Vet Med Assoc 2001;219:1346–56.

[6] Carstens E, Mober GP. Recognizing pain and distress in laboratory animals. ILAR J 2000; 41:62–71.

[7] Scholz J, Woolf CJ. Can we conquer pain? Nature 2002;5:1062–7.

[8] Hunt SP, Mantyh PW. The molecular dynamics of pain control. Nat Rev Neurosci 2001;2: 83–91.

[9] Julius D, Basbaum AI. Molecular mechanisms of nociception. Nature 2001;413:203–10.

[10] Woolf CJ, Slater MW. Neuronal plasticity: increasing the gain in pain. Science 2000;288: 1765–9.

[11] Watkins LR, Milligan ED, Maier SF. Glial activation: a driving force for pathological pain. Trends Neurosci 2001;24:450–5.

[12] Woolf CJ, Shortland P, Coggeshall RE. Peripheral nerve injury triggers central sprouting of myelinated afferents. Nature 1992;355:75–8.

[13] Moore KA, Koho T, Karchewski LA, et al. Partial peripheral nerve injury promotes a selective loss of GABAergic inhibition in the superficial dorsal horn of the spinal cord. J Neurosci 2002;22:6724–31.

[14] Clark JD, Rager DR, Calpin JP. Animal well-being: I. general considerations. Lab Anim Sci 1997;47:564–70.

[15] Clark JD, Rager DR, Calpin JP. Animal well-being: II. stress and distress. Lab Anim Sci 1997;47:571–85.

[16] Carr DB, Goudes LC. Acute pain. Lancet 1999;353:2051–8.

[17] Desborough JP. The stress response to trauma and surgery. Br J Aneasth 2000;85:109–17.

[18] Weissman C. The metabolic response to stress: an overview and update. Anaesthesia 1999; 73:308–27.

[19] Chapman CR, Gavin J. Suffering: the contributions of persistent pain. Lancet 1999;353: 2233–7.

[20] Woolf CJ, Max MB. Mechanism-based pain diagnosis: issues for analgesic drug development. Anesthesiology 2001;95:241–9.

[21] Muir WW, Hubbell JAE, Skarda R, Bednarski RM. Local anesthesia in cattle, sheep, goats, and pigs. In: Muir WM, Hubbell JAE, Skarda R, Bednarski RM, editors. Handbook of veterinary anesthesia. 2nd edition. St Louis: Mosby; 1995. p. 53–77.

[22] Muir WW, Hubbell JAE, Skarda R, Bednarski RM. Local anesthetic drugs and techniques. In: Muir WM, Hubbell JAE, Skarda R, Bednarski RM, editors. Handbook of veterinary anesthesia. 2nd edition. St Louis: Mosby; 1995. p. 39–52.

[23] St-Jean G, Skarda RT, Muir WW, Hoffsis GF. Caudal epidural analgesia induced by xylazine administration in cows. Am J Vet Res 1990;51:1232–6.

[24] Caron JP, LeBlanc PH. Caudal epidural analgesia in cattle using xylazine. Can J Vet Res 1989;53:486–9.

[25] DeRossi R, Bucker GV, Varela JV. Perineal analgesic actions of epidural clonidine in cattle. Vet Anesth Analg 2003;30:64–71.

[26] Lee I, Yoshiuchi T, Yamagishi N, et al. Analgesic effect of caudal epidural ketamine in cattle. J Vet Sci 2003;4:261–4.

[27] Fierheller EE, Caulkett NA, Bailey JV. A romifidine and morphine combination for epidural analgesia in the flank in cattle. Can Vet J 2004;45:917–23.

[28] Prado ME, Streeter RN, Mandsager RE, Shawley RV, Claypool PL. Pharmacologic effects of epidural versus intramuscular administration of detomidine in cattle. Am J Vet Res 1999; 60:1242–7.

[29] Lin HC, Trachte EA, DeGraves FJ, Rodgerson DH, Steiss JE, Carson R. Evaluation of analgesia induced by epidural administration of medetomidine to cows. Am J Vet Res 1998; 59:162–7.

[30] Zulauf M, Gutzwiller A, Steiner A, Hirsbrunner G. The effect of a pain medication in bloodless castration of male calves on the concentrated feed intake, weight gain and serum cortisol level. Schweiz Arch Tierheilkd 2003;145:283–90.

[31] Stafford KJ, Mellor DJ, Todd SE, Bruce RA, Ward RN. Effects of local anaesthesia or local anaesthesia plus a non-steroidal anti-inflammatory drug on the acute cortisol response of calves to five different methods of castration. Res Vet Sci 2002;73:61–70.

[32] Mellor DJ, Stafford KJ, Todd SE, et al. A comparison of catecholamine and cortisol responses of young lambs and calves to painful husbandry procedures. Aust Vet J 2002;80: 228–33.

[33] Faulkner PM, Weary DM. Reducing pain after dehorning in dairy calves. J Dairy Sci 2000; 83:2037–41.

[34] Grondahl-Nielsen C, Simonsen HB, Lund JD, Hesselholt M. Behavioural, endocrine and cardiac responses in young calves undergoing dehorning without and with use of sedation and analgesia. Vet J 1999;158:14–20.

[35] McMeekan CM, Mellor DJ, Stafford KJ, Bruce RA, Ward RN, Gregory NG. Effects of local anaesthesia of 4 to 8 hours' duration on the acute cortisol response to scoop dehorning in calves. Aust Vet J 1998;76:281–5.

[36] Taschke AC, Folsch DW. Ethological, physiological and histological aspects of pain and stress in cattle when being dehorned. Tierarztl Prax 1997;25:19–27.

[37] Eicher SD, Dalley JW. Indicators of acute pain and fly avoidance behaviors in Holstein calves following tail-docking. J Dairy Sci 2002;85:2850–8.

[38] Galindo F, Broom DM. Effects of lameness of dairy cows. J Appl Anim Welf Sci 2002;5: 193–201.

[39] Whay HR, Waterman AE, Webster AJ, O'Brien JK. The influence of lesion type on the duration of hyperalgesia associated with hindlimb lameness in dairy cattle. Vet J 1998;156: 23–9.

[40] Rushen J, Boissy A, Terlouw EM, de Passille AM. Opioid peptides and behavioral and physiological responses of dairy cows to social isolation in unfamiliar surroundings. J Anim Sci 1999;77:2918–24.

[41] Pinheiro Machado FLC, Hurnik JF, Burton JH. The effect of amniotic fluid ingestion on the nociception of cows. Physiol Behav 1997;62:1339–44.

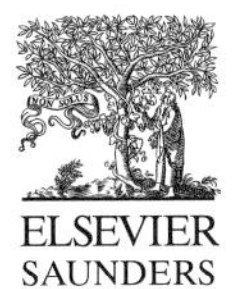
ELSEVIER
SAUNDERS

Vet Clin Food Anim 21 (2005) 33–53

VETERINARY
CLINICS
Food Animal Practice

Ultrasound as a Decision-Making Tool in Abdominal Surgery in Cows

Ueli Braun, Dr med vet, Dr med vet h c

Department of Farm Animals, University of Zurich, Winterthurerstrasse 260, CH-8057 Zürich, Switzerland

Until relatively recently, exploratory laparotomy was performed in many cattle with unexplained illness. Today, most owners consent to this invasive procedure only when the prognosis is good, and there is a reasonable chance that the animal can be cured. Exploratory laparotomy should be avoided in cattle with a poor prognosis because it inflicts additional pain, it is expensive, and the animal usually cannot be slaughtered for human consumption for some time after the operation. Abdominal surgery should be reserved for therapeutic rather than diagnostic purposes. Whether abdominal surgery would benefit an ill animal must be decided before the operation; in some cattle, surgery is advised, whereas in others, euthanasia or slaughter is a better alternative.

The results of a clinical examination often do not provide enough information to make such a decision. Analysis of blood, urine, and ruminal fluid usually yields information about the severity but not the nature of the disease. Elevated concentrations of gamma globulins and fibrinogen indicate marked inflammatory processes [1], and an elevated concentration of ruminal chloride is associated with severe abomasal reflux [2]. Such results do not always reflect a poor prognosis, however; elevated concentrations of gamma globulins and fibrinogen may be due to a reticular or liver abscess, which can be lanced and drained, and abomasal reflux may be caused by a duodenal bezoar, which can be removed surgically.

Ultrasonography, sometimes in combination with radiography, is well suited for evaluating abdominal disease in cattle. The most important diseases are foreign body–associated lesions in the reticulum and peritoneum, left and right displacement of the abomasum, ileus of the small intestine, dilation and displacement of the cecum, abdominal

E-mail address: ubraun@vetclinics.unizh.ch

doi:10.1016/j.cvfa.2004.11.001 *vetfood.theclinics.com*

abscesses, and various disorders of the liver and urinary tract. Ultrasound examinations are done using a 3.5-MHz linear transducer on standing, nonsedated animals. The author prefers to use a linear transducer because it gives a realistic image, which is easier to interprete than that of a sector transducer. When a tentative diagnosis has been made based on the clinical findings, often only the region in question is examined. In cases with suspected traumatic reticuloperitonitis, the examination is performed in the sternal and parasternal regions, and in cattle suspected of having cholestasis, only the costal part of the abdominal wall on the right side is examined.

Even experienced clinicians may not be able to pinpoint the organ affected and make a diagnosis in patients in which abdominal disease is suspected. In such cases, both sides of the abdomen are examined. The hair from the shoulder to the wing of the ilium and on the ventral abdomen on both sides is clipped. For optimal transduction, alcohol is applied to the skin followed by transducer gel. Alternatively, remaining hair may be removed using a razor or depilatory cream. The following areas normally are examined ultrasonographically: The reticulum [3,4], spleen [3–5], rumen [4], and parts of the abomasum [6,7] are seen on the left side, and the liver [8–10], omasum [11], parts of the abomasum [6,7], small intestine [12,13], large intestine [14,15] and right kidney [16] are seen on the right. The uterus may be seen on either side depending on the stage of pregnancy. Transrectal ultrasonography often is required for examining the left kidney, left ureter, urinary bladder, and pelvic cavity [17]. This article discusses diseases in which ultrasonography can be used to determine whether or not surgical treatment is indicated.

Traumatic reticuloperitonitis

Traumatic reticuloperitonitis occurs when ingested foreign bodies, such as nails or wire, enter the reticulum and penetrate its wall; subsequent reticular contractions cause the foreign body to travel deeper into the wall or perforate it [18,19]. The position of the foreign body in the reticular wall, perforation of the reticular wall, peritonitis, and abscesses cannot be diagnosed accurately by a physical examination alone. In cattle with traumatic reticuloperitonitis that do not respond within 2 to 4 days to the standard treatment with a magnet and antibiotic administration, exploratory laparoruminotomy or slaughter is recommended [18]. Whenever possible, the reticulum should be examined ultrasonographically and radiographically before a decision is made [20]. Radiography is a reliable method of visualizing metal foreign bodies and magnets inside and outside the reticulum [21–26]. Radiography can be used to determine whether the foreign body is attached to a magnet or has penetrated the reticular wall and whether the magnet is in the wrong location (eg, in the craniodorsal blind sac of the rumen or in the rumen) [26,27]. If indicated, a second magnet can be administered, or the animal can be operated on or slaughtered.

The contour of the reticulum, reticular contractions, fibrinous adhesions, abscesses, and involvement of the organs adjacent to the reticulum can be assessed via ultrasonography [28]. The normal reticulum, which is examined from the parasternal region of the ventral thorax to the level of the elbow joint on both sides [3,4,29], appears as a half-moon–shaped structure with a smooth contour. It normally has one biphasic contraction per minute. During a 3-minute observation period, three biphasic contractions normally are seen. In cattle with traumatic reticuloperitonitis, inflammatory lesions may be seen on the wall of the reticulum [28]. The most frequently affected area is the caudoventral wall of the reticulum followed by the cranial wall of the craniodorsal blind sac of the rumen. The changes in the contour of the reticulum vary with the severity of the inflammatory changes. Echogenic deposits of fibrin cavitated by hypoechogenic areas of fluid are seen frequently. Adhesions composed solely of fibrin appear echogenic. Reticular abscesses have an echogenic capsule of varying width, which surrounds a central, homogeneously hypoechogenic to moderately echogenic cavity filled with pus. The cavity often contains echogenic fibrinous septa, which compartmentalize the abscess. Abscesses usually are located caudoventral to the reticulum and often are found between the reticulum and spleen, reticulum and liver, or reticulum and omasum or abomasum. Their diameter may range from a few centimeters to more than 15 cm.

In cattle with fibrinosuppurative lesions in the region of the reticulum and craniodorsal blind sac of the rumen (Fig. 1) or between the reticulum and spleen (Fig. 2), antibiotic administration for 5 to 8 days, possibly combined with intraperitoneal oxygen sufflation [30] is recommended. The mode of action of the intraperitoneal oxygen sufflation is still unclear. It is hypothesized that the oxygen helps to destroy anaerobic microorganisms. When a clear response is not observed within 3 days of treatment, exploratory laparotomy may be performed with subsequent rumenotomy if needed. In patients with extensive fibrinous lesions and abscessation involving a large part of the abdomen (Fig. 3), antibiotic and surgical treatment is usually unsuccessful. These animals should be slaughtered or euthanized. Abscesses with a diameter greater than 7 to 10 cm may be lanced. Ideally, lancing is done transcutaneously under ultrasound guidance. This procedure can be used for abscesses situated immediately adjacent to and attached to the abdominal wall (Fig. 4). Abscesses between the reticulum and the spleen (Fig. 5) can be lanced only from within the reticulum [31], and abscesses between the reticulum and the liver or between the reticulum and the omasum preferably are lanced from the right thoracic wall when they are immediately adjacent to the thoracic wall and the intercostal space over the abscess is wide enough. Otherwise, lancing should be attempted from within the reticulum.

Although radiography or ultrasonography alone has diagnostic limitations, the two imaging techniques complement one another well [20]. In most cases, the combined results of radiography and ultrasonography can

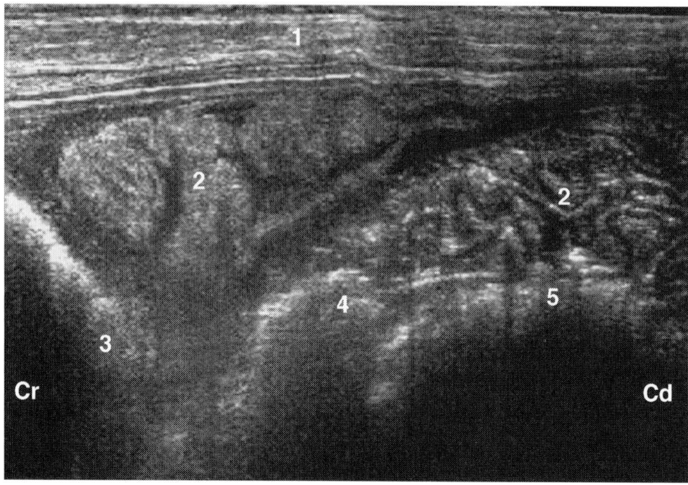

Fig. 1. Ultrasound of the reticulum, craniodorsal blind sac of the rumen, and cranial part of the ventral sac of the rumen of a cow with traumatic reticuloperitonitis. The ultrasound was obtained from the left paramedian side using a 3.5-MHz linear transducer. There are echogenic deposits cavitated by hypoechogenic fluid ventral to the reticulum and craniodorsal blind sac of the rumen. 1, ventral abdominal wall; 2, fibrinous deposits with anechoic inclusions; 3, reticulum; 4, craniodorsal blind sac of the rumen; 5, wall of the cranial part of the ventral sac of the rumen. Cr, cranial; Cd, caudal.

be used to decide whether the patient should be slaughtered, operated, or treated with antibiotics

Left and right displacement of the abomasum

In postpartum cows with reduced appetite, decreased milk production, and recurrent ketosis, left displacement of the abomasum should be considered [32]. In most cases, a characteristic ping is heard during simultaneous swinging and/or percussion and auscultation of the left side of the abdomen, and the diagnosis is straightforward. In cattle with abomasal displacement, both of these tests may be negative, however, and a diagnosis cannot be made clinically. Alternatively, a ping may be heard in animals with ruminal atony, and abomasal displacement may be diagnosed incorrectly. In such cases, ultrasound examination over the last two intercostal spaces on the left side provides a definitive diagnosis. In these intercostal spaces, the wall of the rumen normally is seen [33]. In left abomasal displacement, the abomasum is trapped between the left abdominal wall and the rumen [33]. Reverberation artifacts caused by the gas cap are seen dorsally, and the hypoechogenic-to-echogenic ingesta are observed ventrally (Fig. 6) [33].

In cattle suspected of having left displacement of the abomasum based on clinical findings, such as ketosis or indigestion, but in which simultaneous

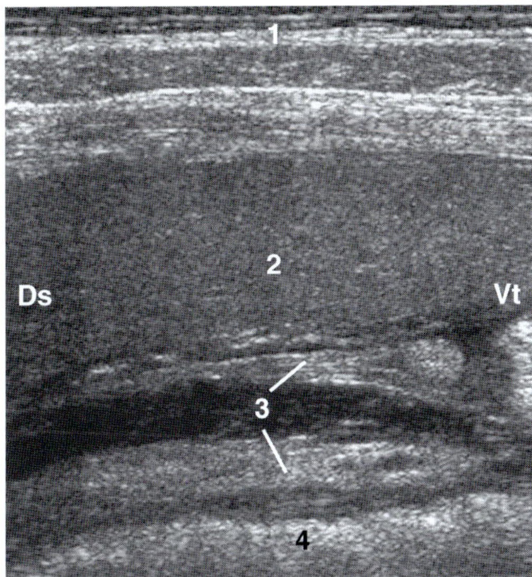

Fig. 2. Ultrasound of the spleen and reticulum of a cow with traumatic reticuloperitonitis. The ultrasound was obtained from the left thoracic wall using a 5-MHz linear transducer. There are echogenic deposits and anechoic fluid accumulations between the reticulum and the spleen. 1, left thoracic wall; 2, spleen; 3, fibrinous deposits and anechoic fluid; 4, reticulum. Ds, dorsal; Vt, ventral.

swinging and/or percussion and auscultation are negative, ultrasound is a valuable diagnostic tool. It allows the clinician to determine whether abomasal displacement has occurred and whether surgical intervention is required. This also is true for right displacement of the abomasum. In unclear cases, ultrasonography performed over the last two or three

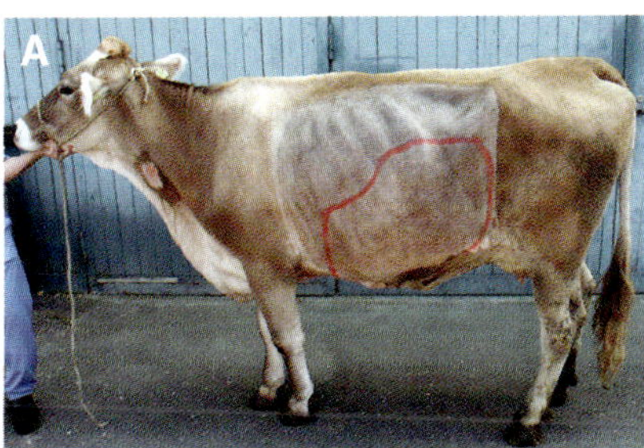

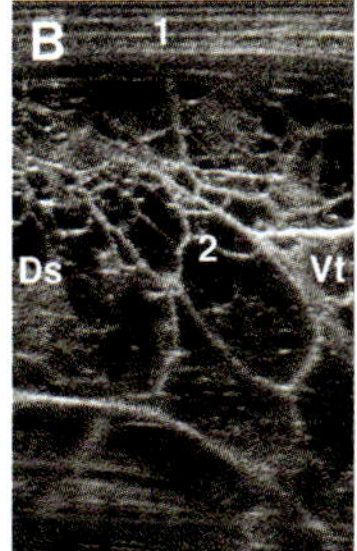

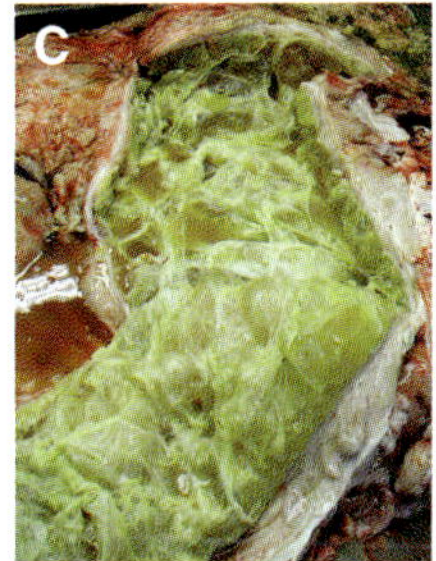

Fig. 3. In this cow with extensive fibrinous lesions involving a large part of the abdomen, antibiotic and surgical treatment would have been unsuccessful. (*A*) The extension of the lesions, determined by ultrasonography, is marked in red. (*B*) Ultrasonogram of the lesions between the lateral abdominal wall and the rumen. The lesions look like a spongiform structure with anechoic fluid inclusions. 1, lateral abdominal wall; 2, spongiform lesions. Ds, dorsal; Vt, ventral. (*C*) Postmortem findings included purulent lesions on the rumen surface.

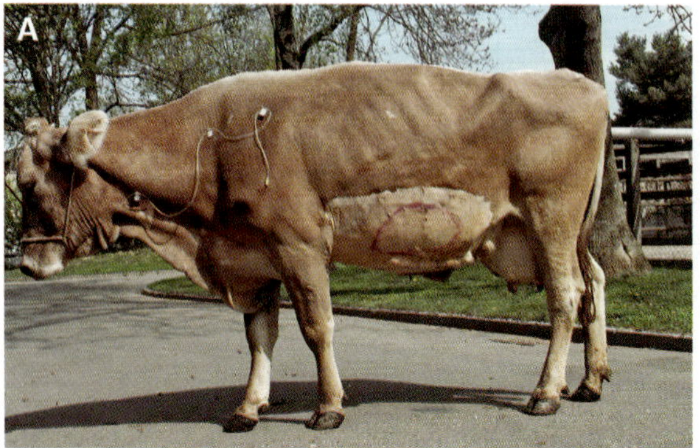

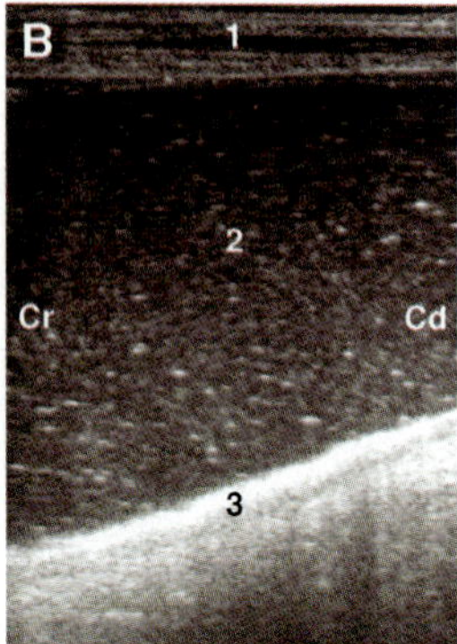

Fig. 4. Large abscess in a cow with traumatic reticuloperitonitis. The abscess is situated immediately adjacent to and attached to the abdominal wall and could be lanced transcutaneously under ultrasound guidance. (*A*) The extension of the abscess, determined by ultrasonography, is marked in violet. (*B*) The ultrasound shows an abscess with an echogenic capsule surrounding a hypoechogenic cavity. 1, lateral abdominal wall; 2, abscess cavity; 3, abscess capsule. Cr, cranial; Cd, caudal.

intercostal spaces on the right side determines whether the abomasum is displaced and whether an operation is necessary. Loops of small intestine normally are seen in the ventral part of the right abdomen [29], and the liver is immediately adjacent to the right abdominal wall further dorsally. In patients with right displacement of the abomasum, the liver is displaced from the abdominal wall and cannot be imaged [29]. Instead the displaced abomasum is seen between the right abdominal wall and liver. The ultrasonographic appearance of the abomasum is the same as that for left displacement of the abomasum.

Ileus of the small intestine

Ileus can involve the small or large intestine. The first step in an ultrasound examination is to determine which part is affected. The small and large intestine can be differentiated via ultrasonography not only by anatomic location, but also by appearance and diameter of the intestine [12,14,15,34].

In cattle, ileus is usually due to a physical problem and only rarely attributable to paralysis [35]. The most important causes of ileus of the small intestine are intussusception [36], obstruction [37], strangulation, incarceration, compression [38], volvulus [39], mesenteric torsion [40], and hemorrhagic bowel syndrome [41]. Ileus may be suspected from the clinical findings. The diagnosis is supported by the transrectal palpation of dilated loops of small intestine; the absence of feces in the rectum; or feces containing blood, mucus, or fibrin. The results of transrectal palpation are important for the diagnosis of ileus, although only about 40% of cases of

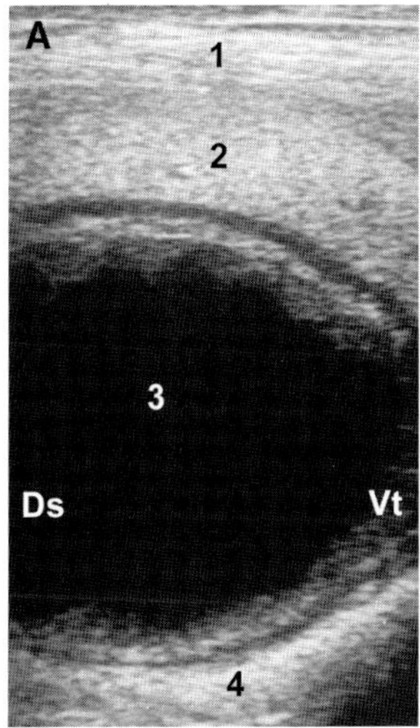

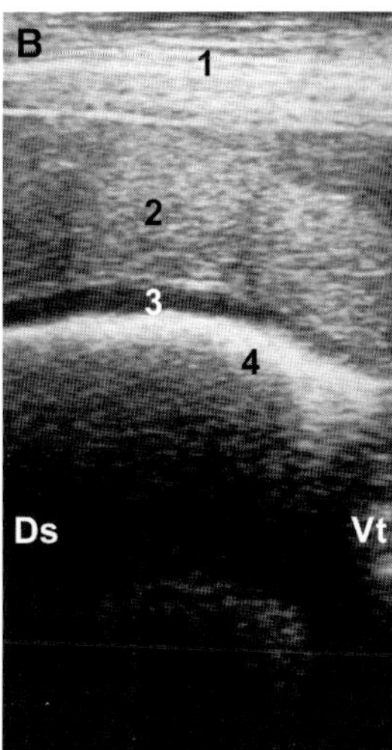

Fig. 5. Ultrasound of an abscess between the reticulum and the spleen imaged from the eighth intercostal space on the left side of a cow with traumatic reticuloperitonitis before (*A*) and 3 days after (*B*) lancing the abscess from within the reticulum. (*A*) The ultrasound shows an abscess with an echogenic capsule and an anechoic cavity. (*B*) The abscess cavity appears as a narrow space 3 days after lancing. 1, left thoracic wall; 2, spleen; 3, abscess; 4, reticulum. Ds, dorsal; Vt, ventral. (*From* Braun U, Iselin U, Lischer C, Fluri E. Ultrasonographic findings in five cows before and after treatment of reticular abscesses. Vet Rec 1998;142:184–9; with permission.)

ileus, in which markedly dilated loops of small intestine are palpated, can be diagnosed correctly [13].

In cattle with severely dilated loops of jejunum, transrectal palpation often reveals no abnormal findings, presumably because the fluid-filled and ingesta-filled intestinal loops sink to the ventral part of the abdomen and out of the examiner's reach. The clinical findings in many cases of ileus are not diagnostic. Such patients often are treated medically rather than surgically, and as a consequence, precious time is lost during which irreparable intestinal damage may occur. Ultrasound examination in these patients is particularly useful because dilated nonmotile loops of intestine are readily identified. The flank, lateral abdominal wall, and 8th to 12th intercostal spaces on the right side are examined from the transverse processes of the vertebrae to the linea alba and from caudal to cranial [34]. The appearance, diameter, content, and motility of the intestine are evaluated. Normal small intestine has a diameter of 2 to 4 cm and a hypoechogenic-to-echogenic content, and there is strong motility.

The most important criteria for diagnosis of ileus are the intestinal diameter and motility [13]. In patients with ileus, the small intestine is dilated with a diameter of greater than 3.5 cm, and motility is reduced or absent. Hypoechogenic fluid resulting from transudation sometimes is seen

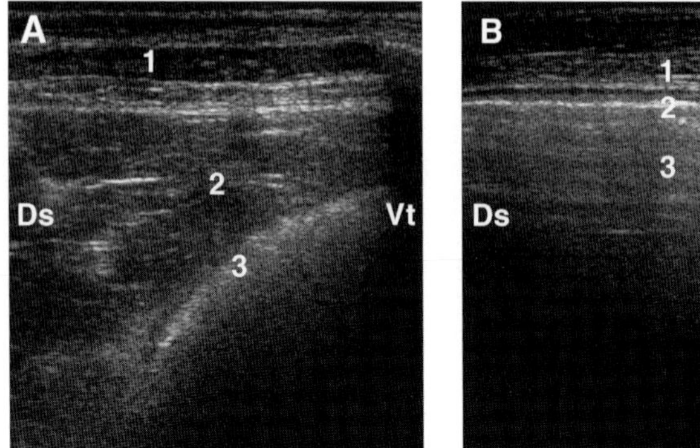

Fig. 6. Ultrasound of left displacement of the abomasum imaged from the ventral (*A*) and from the dorsal (*B*) region of the 12th intercostal space of the left side. (*A*) Ventral region. The abomasum is trapped between the left abdominal wall and the rumen, and the hypoechogenic ingesta can be seen. 1, abdominal wall; 2, abomasum with hypoechogenic ingesta; 3, rumen displaced medially. (*B*) Dorsal region. The abomasal gas cap is not visible because of reverberation artifacts at the abomasal surface. 1, abdominal wall; 2, abomasal wall; 3, reverberation artifacts. Ds, dorsal; Vt, ventral.

between loops of intestine. The number of intestinal loops seen in cross section and longitudinally from the flank or from individual intercostal spaces depends greatly on the location of the ileus. When only one or a few, usually markedly dilated, loops of small intestine are seen, ileus of the duodenum is most likely (Fig. 7). More than five loops of small intestine seen in one area almost always indicates ileus of the jejunum or ileum. The number of dilated loops of small intestine increases if the site of the ileus is more distal (Fig. 8). When the site of the ileus is more proximal, the loops of small intestine are more dilated. The maximal diameter of the intestine when viewed from the 12th intercostal space ranges from 4.4 to 5.5 cm (5 ± 0.4 cm) with ileus of the ileum, from 3.5 to 9.8 cm (5.5 ± 1.7 cm) with ileus of the jejunum, and from 6.5 to 9.9 cm (7.7 ± 1.9 cm) with ileus of the duodenum [13]. Empty intestinal loops that are distal to the ileus often are seen in addition to markedly dilated loops proximally. In addition, the intestinal lumen remains dilated in cases with ileus owing to reduced or absent motility. This situation is in contrast to a healthy animal, in which the intestinal lumen is constantly changing owing to motility.

The actual cause of the ileus seldom is determined via ultrasonography, in part because it usually is located further from the abdominal wall than the penetration capacity of the transducer [13]. Ultrasound examination of the intestine is particularly useful in cattle that are suspected of having ileus but do not have corresponding diagnostic rectal findings. This imaging technique allows one to confirm or rule out ileus and to decide on surgery or slaughter. In cattle with reduced or no fecal output and dilated loops of intestine seen via ultrasonography, a decision of laparotomy or slaughter must be made. In addition to animal welfare considerations, a delay may

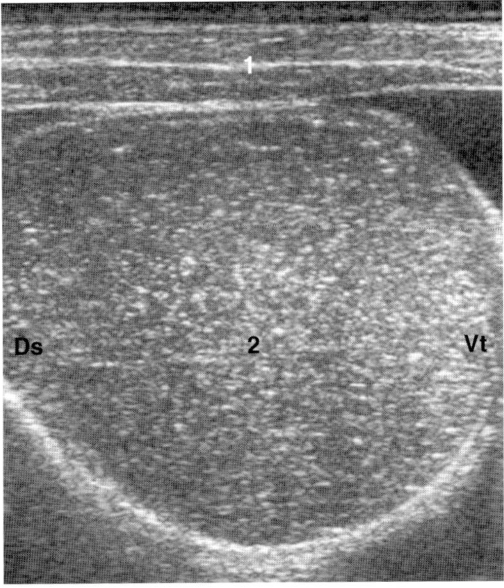

Fig. 7. Ultrasound of a cross section through the dilated duodenum of a cow with duodenal ileus imaged from the 10th intercostal space. 1, abdominal wall; 2, dilated duodenum. Ds, dorsal; Vt, ventral.

result in deterioration of the patient's condition to the point where surgical intervention is no longer feasible or the carcass cannot be used for human consumption.

Cecal dilation

A diagnosis of cecal dilation usually is straightforward when the dilated and caudally displaced cecum can be palpated per rectum [42]. With cranioventral or craniodorsal retroflexion of the cecum, however, a diagnosis may be difficult. The clinician usually runs into difficulty with retroflexion of the cecum when the contour of a distended viscus can be palpated only with the tips of the fingers, or there are no abnormal rectal findings. A differential diagnosis must include right displacement of the abomasum and ileus of the small intestine. In both of these disorders, simultaneous swinging and/or percussion and auscultation can be positive, and ultrasonography is indicated for diagnosis. In healthy cattle, the cecum can be seen only in the midsection or dorsal region of the lateral right abdominal wall [14,15]. In cattle with cecal dilation, the cecum also can be imaged from the ventral part of the abdominal wall and from the 12th, 11th, and 10th intercostal spaces [43].

In healthy cattle, the proximal loop of the colon sometimes can be seen from the dorsal region of the lateral abdominal wall and from the dorsal and

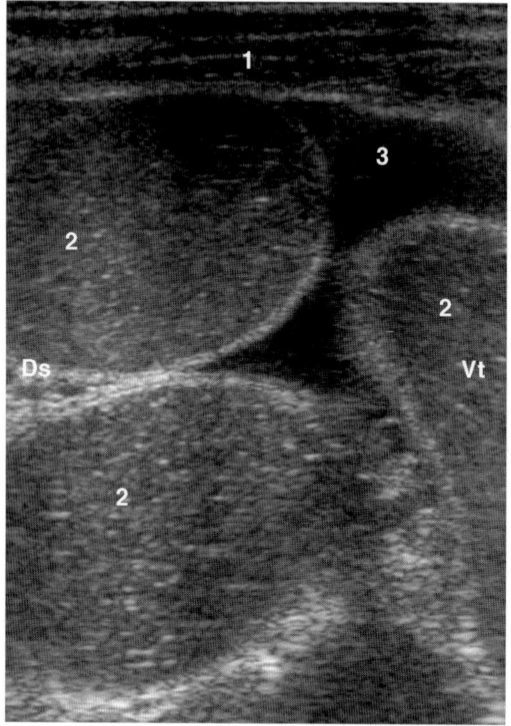

Fig. 8. Ultrasound of cross sections through dilated loops of the jejunum in a cow with ileus imaged from the right flank. The contents of the loops appear echogenic. There is anechoic fluid between the loops. 1, lateral abdominal wall; 2, dilated loops of the jejunum; 3, anechoic fluid between the loops of the jejunum. Ds, dorsal; Vt, ventral.

middle regions of the 12th intercostal space [14,15]. In cattle with cecal dilation, parts of the proximal loop of the colon are seen in all areas examined [43]. In these cattle, the cecum and proximal loop of the colon can be dilated to such an extent that they occupy a major part of the right abdominal wall. The wall of the dilated cecum and proximal loop of the colon closest to the transducer appear as a distinct echogenic semicircular line, immediately adjacent to the peritoneum (Fig. 9) [14,43]. In most cattle, the content of the cecum and the proximal and spiral loops of the colon cannot be visualized because of its gaseous nature. In a few animals, the content appears hypoechogenic to echogenic. In all cattle, the dilated cecum can be imaged from the lateral abdominal wall up to the level of the tuber coxae. In cattle with nondiagnostic rectal findings, ultrasonography can be used to differentiate accurately right displacement of the abomasum, ileus of the small intestine, and cecal dilation. In cattle with cecal retroflexion, immediate laparotomy is indicated; medical treatment alone leads to deterioration in the patient's condition.

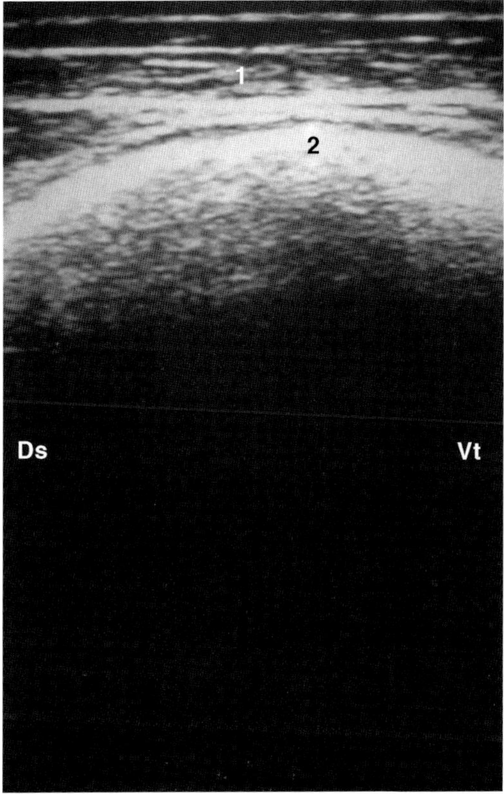

Fig. 9. Ultrasound of a dilated cecum of a cow with cecal dilation imaged from the right flank. The cecal wall closest to the transducer appears as a curved echogenic line. The cecal contents and wall farthest from the transducer are not visible. 1, lateral abdominal wall; 2, cecal wall. Ds, dorsal; Vt, ventral.

Liver disorders

Two liver disorders that often require surgical treatment in cattle are liver abscess [44] and cholestasis [45]. The clinical signs vary greatly between these disorders, and in both, ultrasonography has great diagnostic value because it allows the veterinarian to decide whether and how surgery should be performed.

Liver abscess

The symptoms of a liver abscess are usually nonspecific [46]. Depending on their number, size, and location, liver abscesses can be inapparent or have subacute-to-chronic, nonspecific signs, which often include weight loss and indigestion [29]. Large abscesses between the liver and the reticulum often result in reticulo-omasal stenosis with signs of vagal indigestion.

Similar to the clinical findings, the results of hematologic and biochemical analyses usually are not diagnostic. Sometimes the activities of the liver enzymes, in particular γ-glutamyltransferase, are slightly elevated, and the clotting time of the glutaraldehyde test is reduced [44]. These changes are not specific, however. Liver abscesses generally are diagnosed only after systematic ultrasound examination of the reticulum, liver, and abdomen. In contrast to the clinical and hematologic findings, ultrasonography is useful for the diagnosis of liver abscesses [44,47,48]. Abscesses lead to circumscribed ultrasound changes within the liver, although their appearance can vary greatly. The contents of an abscess vary from anechogenic to hyperechogenic and can be homogeneous or heterogeneous (Fig. 10). The abscess capsule usually is clearly visible as an echogenic line separating the abscess content from the liver parenchyma. With incomplete destruction of the liver parenchyma, the abscess is compartmentalized by multiple echogenic septa. The individual compartments may coalesce during the course of the disease. The diameter of an abscess varies from a few centimeters to more than 20 cm. A liver abscess is seldom visible in only one

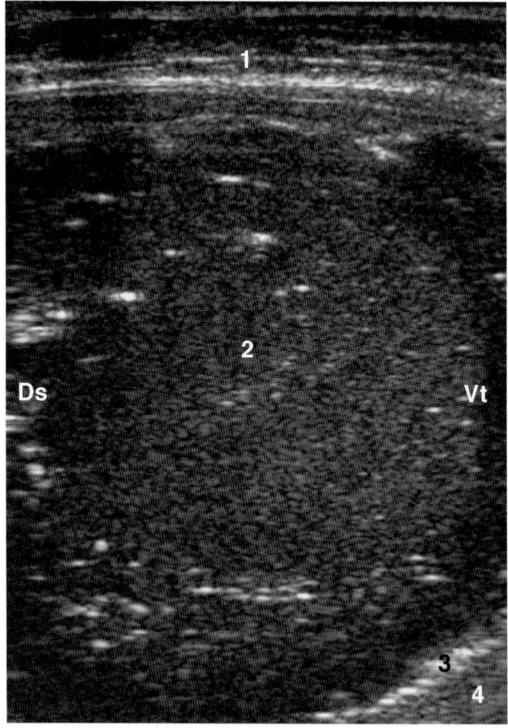

Fig. 10. Ultrasound of a hepatic abscess imaged from the 12th intercosal space of the right side. The abscess content appears echogenic and is surrounded by an echogenic capsule. 1, abdominal wall; 2, hepatic abscess; 3, abscess capsule; 4, liver parenchyma. Ds, dorsal; Vt, ventral.

intercostal space. More often the abscess is seen in two, three, or four adjacent intercostal spaces because of its size. The tentative diagnosis is confirmed by ultrasound-guided transcutaneous centesis using a needle containing a stylet.

Whether and how surgery should be performed depends on the size and location of the abscess and whether other organs are affected. Abscesses that are less than 5 cm in diameter usually cause no symptoms and do not require surgical treatment. In patients with multiple abscesses, with an abscess that has ruptured into the caudal vena cava [49], or with metastatic purulent bronchopneumonia, surgical intervention is not warranted. An operation is recommended in cattle with a single abscess that is more than 5 cm in diameter. Ultrasound-guided transcutaneous lancing and draining is accomplished best in abscesses that are located immediately adjacent to and attached to the abdominal wall. The same is true for abscesses between the reticulum and liver, provided that they are adjacent to the abdominal wall, and the intercostal space over the abscess is wide enough for surgical manipulations. Reticular abscesses can be lanced from within the reticulum. A laparotomy is required to drain abscesses that are not adjacent to the abdominal wall. The site of laparotomy depends on the location of the abscess; a ventral midline or paramedian incision is used for abscesses in the left liver lobe [50,51]. In the author's experience, a right flank laparotomy, perhaps with resection of the last rib, can be used in standing cattle with abscesses in the right liver lobe.

Cholestasis

Cholestasis should be suspected in cattle with colic, bilirubinuria, icterus, or photodermatitis. The diagnosis is supported by hyperbilirubinemia; increased concentrations of bile acids; and increased activities of the liver enzymes, particularly the bile duct enzyme γ-glutamyltransferase. In affected cattle, ultrasonography complements the clinical and biochemical findings and in most cases allows a reliable diagnosis so that a decision regarding the treatment method or slaughter can be made. The cause of cholestasis may be hepatocellular or obstructive in nature [52]. Hepatocellular cholestasis results from severe impairment of liver function, which has a variety of causes. The causes of obstructive cholestasis are mechanical in nature and include mainly fascioliasis, fibrinosuppurative inflammatory products and concretions, and occasionally gallstones or tissue proliferations [53]. Inflammatory products resulting from cholangitis also may lead to impaired bile flow. Compression of the main bile ducts by tumors, abscesses, or peritoneal lesions is a rare cause of impaired bile flow.

In cattle suspected of having cholestasis, the diagnostic workup should include determination of liver enzyme activities, ultrasonography of the liver, histologic examination of a liver biopsy sample, and centesis of the gallbladder with examination of a bile sample [45]. Elevated liver enzyme activities indicate liver disease, the nature of which can be determined by examination of a liver biopsy sample. Ultrasonography can be used to differentiate reliably obstructive and hepatocellular cholestasis [52]. A final diagnosis often is made based on the results of ultrasonography alone [45]. Hepatocellular cholestasis generally is diagnosed when the bile ducts are not dilated. Characteristic changes, such as fatty liver or liver congestion, or uncharacteristic changes often are seen. In most cases, visualization of dilated bile ducts allows the diagnosis of obstructive cholestasis.

The site of obstruction usually is determined by the ultrasonographic pattern of dilated intrahepatic or extrahepatic bile ducts and the appearance of the gallbladder [29,45]; ultrasonography also provides information about adjacent structures, such as liver abscesses. Proximal obstruction in the region of the liver portal is differentiated from distal obstruction near the duodenal papilla. With proximal obstruction, only the intrahepatic bile ducts are dilated (Fig. 11). With distal obstruction, the extrahepatic bile ducts and gallbladder are dilated; with long-standing distal obstruction, the intrahepatic bile ducts, which are not normally seen, also may be dilated. Dilation of the gallbladder alone does not indicate cholestasis. In many anorexic cows, there is no stimulus for gallbladder emptying, and the organ becomes dilated with an increasing volume of bile, without obstruction. Thickening of the gallbladder wall secondary to inflammation and abnormal gallbladder content, such as sediment or concrement, indicates a disease. In such patients, the contents of the gallbladder may appear heterogeneous and include an echogenic sediment and a hypoechogenic supernatant or homogeneous, in which case the contents are usually echogenic. In cattle with a tentative diagnosis of cholestasis, ultrasound-guided centesis of the gallbladder and cytologic and bacteriologic examination of the collected bile is performed. The bile is generally cloudy when there is bacterial infection and suppurative exudate in the bile ducts. A large amount of sediment containing neutrophils and often bacteria collect on the bottom of the collection tube.

Treatment depends on the cause and severity of cholestasis. In cattle with hepatocellular cholestasis resulting from such disorders as hepatic lipidosis, medical treatment alone is indicated [53]. Patients who have clinical signs of cholestasis usually do not respond to treatment, however. Euthanasia or slaughter is recommended in patients with cholestasis attributable to a tumor. In cattle with a single liver abscess, lancing may be performed (see earlier). With obstructive cholestasis secondary to fascioliasis, conservative therapy, including spasmolytics, magnesium sulfate, and antibiotics, can be instituted first, provided that the symptoms are mild [53]. This treatment is used for 24 hours to a maximum of 48 hours; the owner must be advised of the risk of gallbladder rupture [54]. Response to treatment is indicated by resolution of bilirubinuria and normalization of appetite. Surgical intervention is indicated in cattle that do not respond to conservative treatment, that have colic, or in which rupture of the gallbladder is to be avoided. Ideally the concrement in the extrahepatic bile ducts is broken

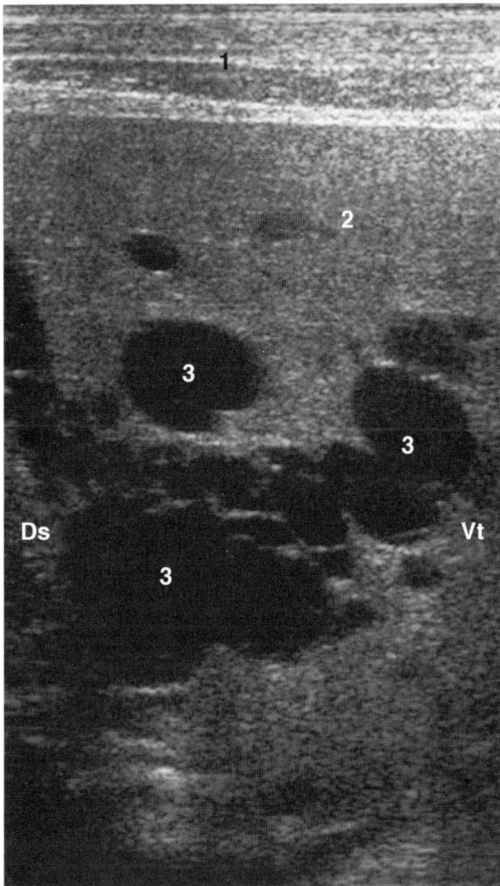

Fig. 11. Ultrasound of dilation of the intrahepatic bile ducts in a cow with cholestasis resulting from compression of the bile ducts by a large liver abscess imaged from the 11th intercostal space of the right side. 1, lateral abdominal wall; 2, liver parenchyma; 3, dilated intrahepatic bile ducts. Ds, dorsal; Vt, ventral.

down manually and massaged toward the intestine [53]. In most cases, a cholecystoduodenostomy must be performed in which a connection between the gallbladder and duodenum is made [53]. In the author's clinic, this operation is performed in standing cattle, and the optimal approach, usually from the region of the 9th to 11th rib, is determined by ultrasonography. Resection of the 9th, 10th, or 11th rib often is required to create enough space for carrying out the operation.

Renal disease

In cattle suspected of having chronic and severe renal disease, the clinician first must determine whether one or both kidneys are affected. Both kidneys usually are affected in suppurative nephritis and nephrosis, and treatment is not warranted. In contrast, with cystic changes or pyelonephritis, usually only one kidney is affected. One or both kidneys may be affected in cattle with urolithiasis. In cattle, both kidneys can be imaged via ultrasonography; the left is visualized transrectally [17] and the right from the right flank [16]. Histologic examination of a kidney biopsy sample provides further information. When one kidney appears ultrasonographically normal and the other markedly abnormal, nephrectomy of the latter may be performed. Nephrectomy is contraindicated in cattle with bilateral kidney disease, and euthanasia or slaughter is advised in patients that do not respond to medical treatment. In the author's experience, rapid improvement in the general condition of the animal usually occurs after unilateral nephrectomy; fever subsides, the urine becomes normal within a few days, and the concentrations of serum creatinine and urea return to normal ranges.

Rupture of the ureter

Severe unilateral dilation of a ureter is a rare and incidental finding during transrectal palpation of cattle with colic. The cause is usually obstruction by urinary calculi and seldom compression (eg, due to dystocia). When the problem is not diagnosed promptly, rupture of the ureter occurs. In such cases, transrectal palpation reveals a diffuse, pillow-like, often gelatinous swelling near the left kidney with rupture of the left ureter and in the region of the right ilial shaft with rupture of the right ureter. The nature of the swelling can be determined via ultrasonography. When dilated, the ureter appears as a hypoechogenic tubular structure. After rupture of the ureter, accumulation of fluid in the retroperitoneal space is seen, and sometimes the ureter can be identified within the fluid. It may be possible to collect fluid and identify urine via transvaginal centesis of the swelling using a needle attached to plastic tubing. With dilation alone, an analgesic can be administered, after which gentle massage transrectally may dislodge the obstruction. The affected kidney and part of the ureter may be removed surgically, however, as in the case of rupture of the ureter. Before surgery is done, the other kidney must be examined ultrasonographically; when lesions are seen, particularly when the kidney contains concrement, surgery is not advised, and the fate of the animal must be decided.

Rupture of the urinary bladder

Rupture of the urinary bladder results from obstructive urolithiasis in male cattle and from trauma in female cattle. Diagnosis is based on the results of ultrasound examination of the abdomen and by determination of the concentration of creatinine in serum and abdominal fluid. Cattle with a ruptured urinary bladder have uroperitoneum. On ultrasound, there is

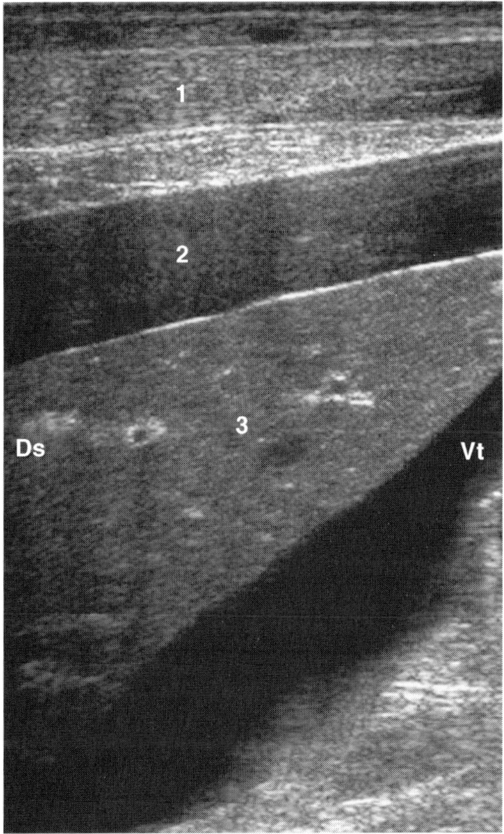

Fig. 12. Ultrasound of noninflammatory ascites in a cow with right heart insufficiency imaged from the 10th intercostal space of the right side. The liver is swimming in an anechoic fluid accumulation. 1, lateral abdominal wall; 2, fluid accumulation; 3, liver. Ds, dorsal; Vt, ventral.

hypoechogenic fluid in which the abdominal organs appear to be floating. Abdominocentesis yields light yellow fluid with concentrations of creatinine and urea that are higher than serum concentrations [55]. An immediate decision regarding laparotomy, euthanasia, or slaughter must be made in cases with rupture of the urinary bladder. Laparotomy is performed in the caudal region of the right flank, the rent in the urinary bladder is closed, and the urine is removed from the abdominal cavity. In the author's experience, the prognosis after this procedure is good.

Ascites

Ultrasonography is useful for identifying fluid within the abdomen. Analysis of the fluid collected via abdominocentesis allows differentiation of inflammatory and noninflammatory ascites.

Noninflammatory ascites is characterized on ultrasound by a varying amount of hypoechogenic fluid in the abdomen [29]. The most common causes are chronic cardiac disease and severe liver disease with portal hypertension (Fig. 12). Other causes include renal disease (eg, amyloidosis), intestinal disease (eg, ileus), peritoneal disease (eg, neoplasia), and vascular disorders (eg, thrombosis of the caudal vena cava). Surgical treatment is indicated only when noninflammatory ascites is due to ileus or portal hypertension resulting from a liver abscess. Ascites attributable to severe fascioliasis can be treated accordingly. For long-term resolution of symptoms, the cause of the ascites must be removed first, after which the ascites resolves relatively quickly. All other causes of noninflammatory ascites have a poor prognosis, and euthanasia or slaughter is indicated.

Inflammatory ascites results from peritonitis, caused most commonly by a perforating reticular foreign body or perforating abomasal ulcer. Ultrasonography reveals anechoic-to-hypoechogenic fluid within the abdomen. Echogenic bands of fibrin are seen frequently floating in the fluid, and echogenic fibrinous deposits are seen on the peritoneum or internal organs (Fig. 13). Differentiation of transudate secondary to noninflammatory ascites and exudate secondary to peritonitis cannot always be accomplished reliably via ultrasonography, and abdominocentesis and analysis of a fluid

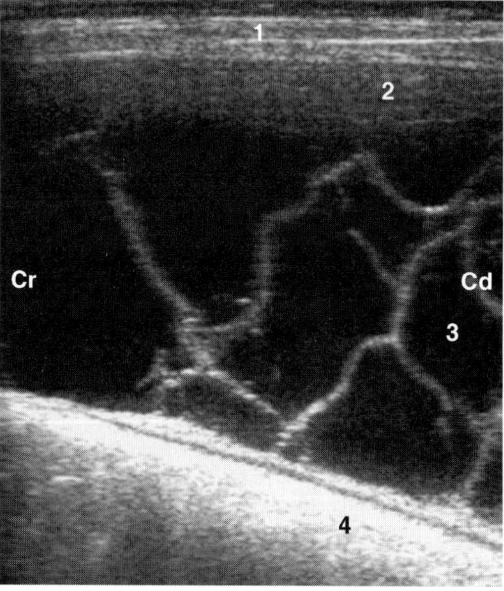

Fig. 13. Ultrasound of inflammatory ascites in a cow with generalized peritonitis imaged from the right paramedian side of the ventral abdomen. A fluid accumulation with fibrin deposits on the peritoneum of the ventral abdominal wall and echogenic fibrin bands between the abdominal wall and the rumen are visible. 1, ventral abdominal wall; 2, fibrin deposits on the peritoneum; 3, anechoic fluid with echogenic fibrin bands between the abdominal wall and the rumen; 4, rumen wall. Cr, cranial; Cd, caudal.

sample is recommended. In cattle with generalized peritonitis of unknown cause, laparotomy almost always is contraindicated.

Abdominal wall swelling

Ultrasonography is useful for investigating swellings of the abdominal wall [29,56]. Hernias and abscesses are diagnosed easily. Diagnosis of hematomas, cellulites, and tumors is not always straightforward using ultrasonography, and ultrasound-guided centesis or biopsy of the swelling may be necessary. Depending on the diagnosis, the patient may undergo surgery (hernia, tumor), undergo abscess lancing or local treatment with a hyperemic salve, receive anti-inflammatory drugs parenterally (cellulitis), or be slaughtered at the owner's request.

Summary

In many patients, abdominal ultrasonography is an excellent diagnostic and prognostic tool. It aids in deciding whether the animal should undergo surgical or medical treatment or be slaughtered. This is particularly true in cattle with traumatic reticuloperitonitis (in combination with radiography of the reticulum) or with a tentative diagnosis of left or right displacement of the abomasum. Ultrasound also is an excellent aid for identification of ileus of the small and large intestine, liver abscesses, cholestasis, various urinary tract disorders, and the different forms of ascites.

References

[1] Doll K, Schillinger D, Klee W. Der Glutaraldehyd-Test beim Rind—seine Brauchbarkeit für Diagnose und Prognose innerer Entzündungen. Zbl Vet Med A 1985;32:581–93.
[2] Breukink HJ, Kuiper R. Abomasal reflux in cattle with various gastrointestinal disorders. 9th Congr. Internat. sur les Maladies du Bétail, Paris, France, rapports et résumés; 1976. p. 439–45.
[3] Götz M. Sonographische Untersuchungen an der Haube des Rindes. Dissertation, Faculty of Veterinary Medicine, University of Zurich, Zurich; 1992.
[4] Braun U, Götz M. Ultrasonography of the reticulum in cows. Am J Vet Res 1994;55:325–32.
[5] Sicher D. Sonographische Untersuchungen an Lunge, Mediastinum und Milz des Rindes. Dissertation, Faculty of Veterinary Medicine, University of Zurich, Zurich; 1995.
[6] Wild K. Sonographische Untersuchungen am Labmagen des Rindes. Dissertation, Faculty of Veterinary Medicine, University of Zurich, Zurich; 1995.
[7] Braun U, Wild K, Guscetti F. Ultrasonographic examination of the abomasum of 50 cows. Vet Rec 1997;140:93–8.
[8] Braun U. Ultrasonographic examination of the liver in cows. Am J Vet Res 1990;51:1522–6.
[9] Gerber D. Sonographische Befunde an der Leber des Rindes. Dissertation, Faculty of Veterinary Medicine, University of Zurich, Zurich; 1993.
[10] Braun U, Gerber D. Influence of age, breed, and stage of pregnancy on hepatic ultrasonographic findings in cows. Am J Vet Res 1994;55:1201–5.
[11] Blessing S. Sonographische Untersuchungen am Psalter des Rindes. Dissertation, Faculty of Veterinary Medicine, University of Zurich, Zurich; 2004.

[12] Marmier O. Sonographische Untersuchungen am Darm des Rindes. Dissertation, Faculty of Veterinary Medicine, University of Zurich, Zurich; 1993.
[13] Braun U, Marmier O, Pusterla N. Ultrasonographic examination of the small intestine of cows with ileus of the duodenum, jejunum or ileum. Vet Rec 1995;137:209–15.
[14] Amrein EM. Ultraschalluntersuchungen bei Kühen mit Blinddarmdilatation. Dissertation, Faculty of Veterinary Medicine, University of Zurich, Zurich; 1999.
[15] Braun U, Amrein E. Ultrasonographic examination of the caecum and proximal and spiral ansa of the colon of cattle. Vet Rec 2001;149:45–8.
[16] Braun U. Ultrasonographic examination of the right kidney in cows. Am J Vet Res 1991;52: 1933–9.
[17] Braun U. Ultrasonography of the left kidney, the urinary bladder, and the urethra in cows. J Vet Med A 1993;40:1–9.
[18] Radostits OM, Gay CC, Blood DC, Hinchcliff KW. Traumatic reticuloperitonitis. In: Radostits OM, Gay CC, Blood DC, Hinchcliff KW, editors. Veterinary medicine: a textbook of the diseases of cattle, sheep, pigs, goats and horses. 9th edition. London: WB Saunders; 2000. p. 303–11.
[19] Dirksen G. Krankheiten von Haube und Pansen beim ruminanten Rind. In: Dirksen G, Gründer HD, Stöber M, editors. Innere Medizin und Chirurgie des Rindes. 4th edition. Berlin: Paul Parey; 2002. p. 397–455.
[20] Braun U, Flückiger M, Götz M. Comparison of ultrasonographic and radiographic findings in cows with traumatic reticuloperitonitis. Vet Rec 1994;135:470–8.
[21] Bargai U, Pharr JW, Morgan JP. Traumatic reticulitis/reticuloperitonitis. In: Bovine radiology. Ames (IA): Iowa State University Press; 1989. p. 175–8.
[22] Fubini SL, Yeager AE, Mohammed HO, Smith DF. Accuracy of radiography of the reticulum for predicting surgical findings in adult dairy cattle with traumatic reticuloperitonitis: 132 cases (1981–1987). J Am Vet Med Assoc 1990;197:1060–4.
[23] Nägeli F. Die Röntgendiagnostik bei der Reticuloperitonitis traumatica des Rindes: Technik, Befunde, Interpretation und diagnostische Bedeutung. Dissertation, Faculty of Veterinary Medicine, University of Zurich, Zurich; 1991.
[24] Partington BP, Biller DS. Radiography of the bovine cranioventral abdomen. Vet Radiol 1991;32:155–68.
[25] Braun U, Flückiger M, Nägeli F. Radiography as an aid in the diagnosis of traumatic reticuloperitonitis in cattle. Vet Rec 1993;132:103–9.
[26] Braun U, Gansohr B, Flückiger M. Radiographic findings before and after oral administration of a magnet in cows with traumatic reticuloperitonitis. Am J Vet Res 2003; 64:115–20.
[27] Gansohr B. Untersuchungen zur Eingabe von Fremdkörper-Nacktmagneten beim Rind. Dissertation, Faculty of Veterinary Medicine, University of Zurich, Zurich; 2001.
[28] Braun U, Götz M, Marmier O. Ultrasonographic findings in cows with traumatic reticuloperitonitis. Vet Rec 1993;133:416–22.
[29] Braun U. Atlas und Lehrbuch der Ultraschalldiagnostik beim Rind. Berlin: Parey Buchverlag; 1997.
[30] Blaser E. Intraperitoneale Sauerstoffanwendung in der Buiatrik: Indikationen und Resultate. Tierärztl Umsch 1986;41:56–62.
[31] Braun U, Iselin U, Lischer C, Fluri E. Ultrasonographic findings in five cows before and after treatment of reticular abscesses. Vet Rec 1998;142:184–9.
[32] Dirksen G. Linksseitige Labmagenverlagerung. In: Dirksen G, Gründer HD, Stöber M, editors. Innere Medizin und Chirurgie des Rindes. 4th edition. Berlin: Paul Parey; 2002. p. 473–87.
[33] Braun U, Pusterla N, Schönmann M. Ultrasonographic findings in cows with left displacement of the abomasum. Vet Rec 1997;141:331–5.
[34] Braun U, Marmier O. Ultrasonographic examination of the small intestine of cows. Vet Rec 1995;136:239–44.

[35] Dirksen G. Ileus beim Rind. In: Dirksen G, Gründer HD, Stöber M, editors. Innere Medizin und Chirurgie des Rindes. 4th edition. Berlin: Paul Parey; 2002. p. 514–7.
[36] Dirksen G, Doll K. Darminvagination. In: Dirksen G, Gründer HD, Stöber M, editors. Innere Medizin und Chirurgie des Rindes. 4th edition. Berlin: Paul Parey; 2002. p. 517–25.
[37] Dirksen G, Doll K. Innere Darmverlegung, Verstopfungsileus. In: Dirksen G, Gründer HD, Stöber M, editors. Innere Medizin und Chirurgie des Rindes. 4th edition. Berlin: Paul Parey; 2002. p. 531–3.
[38] Dirksen G, Doll K. Einklemmung, Abschnürung, Kompression des Darmes. In: Dirksen G, Gründer HD, Stöber M, editors. Innere Medizin und Chirurgie des Rindes. 4th edition. Berlin: Paul Parey; 2002. p. 530–1.
[39] Dirksen G, Doll K. Dünndarmverschlingung. In: Dirksen G, Gründer HD, Stöber M, editors. Innere Medizin und Chirurgie des Rindes. 4th edition. Berlin: Paul Parey; 2002. p. 525–7.
[40] Rademacher G. Darmscheibendrehung. In: Dirksen G, Gründer HD, Stöber M, editors. Innere Medizin und Chirurgie des Rindes. 4th edition. Berlin: Paul Parey; 2002. p. 527–30.
[41] Dennison AC, Vanmetre DC, Callan RJ, Dinsmore P, Mason GL, Ellis RP. Hemorrhagic bowel syndrome in dairy cattle: 22 cases (1997–2000). J Am Vet Med Assoc 2002;221:686–9.
[42] Braun U, Eicher R, Hausammann K. Clinical findings in cattle with dilatation and torsion of the caecum. Vet Rec 1989;125:265–7.
[43] Braun U, Amrein E, Koller U, Lischer C. Ultrasonographic findings in cows with dilatation, torsion and retroflexion of the caecum. Vet Rec 2002;150:75–9.
[44] Braun U, Pusterla N, Wild K. Ultrasonographic findings in 11 cows with a hepatic abscess. Vet Rec 1995;137:284–90.
[45] Braun U, Pospischil A, Pusterla N, Winder C. Ultrasonographic findings in cows with cholestasis. Vet Rec 1995;137:537–43.
[46] Liberg P, Jönsson G. Ultrasonography and determination of proteins and enzymes in blood for the diagnosis of liver abscesses in intensively fed beef cattle. Acta Vet Scand 1993;34:21–8.
[47] Itabisashi T, Yamamoto R, Satoh M. Ultrasonogram of hepatic abscess in cattle inoculated with *Fusobacterium necrophorum*. Jpn J Vet Sci 1987;49:585–92.
[48] Lechtenberg KF, Nagaraja TG. Hepatic ultrasonography and blood changes in cattle with experimentally induced hepatic abscesses. Am J Vet Res 1991;52:803–9.
[49] Braun U, Flückiger M, Feige K, Pospischil A. Diagnosis by ultrasonography of congestion of the caudal vena cava secondary to thrombosis in 12 cows. Vet Rec 2002;150:209–13.
[50] Fubini SL, Ducharme NG, Murphy JP, Smith DF. Vagus indigestion syndrome resulting from a liver abscess in dairy cows. J Am Vet Med Assoc 1985;186:1297–300.
[51] Dirksen G. Bakteriell bedingte Lebernekrosen und–abszesse. In: Dirksen G, Gründer HD, Stöber M, editors. Innere Medizin und Chirurgie des Rindes. 4th edition. Berlin: Paul Parey; 2002. p. 631–4.
[52] Banholzer P, Weigold B. Gallenwege. In: Kremer H, Dobrinski W, editors. Sonographische Diagnostik, Innere Medizin und angrenzende Gebiete. 4th edition. München: Urban & Schwarzenberg; 1993. p. 113–21.
[53] Dirksen G. Gallengangs- und Gallenblasenentzündung. In: Dirksen G, Gründer HD, Stöber M, editors. Innere Medizin und Chirurgie des Rindes. 4th edition. Berlin: Paul Parey; 2002. p. 634–9.
[54] Braun U, Schweizer G, Pospischil A. Clinical and ultrasonographic findings in three cows with rupture of the gallbladder. Vet Rec, in press.
[55] Radostits OM, Gay CC, Blood DC, Hinchcliff KW. Rupture of the bladder (uroperitoneum). In: Radostits OM, Gay CC, Blood DC, Hinchcliff KW, editors. Veterinary medicine: a textbook of the diseases of cattle, sheep, pigs, goats and horses. 9th edition. London: WB Saunders; 2000. p. 493.
[56] Braun U, Bleul U, Schweizer G, Nuss K. Ultrasonographic findings in three cows with cellulites. Vet Rec, in press.

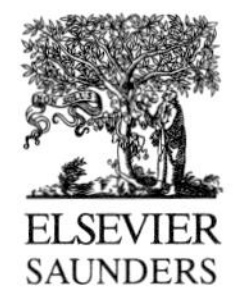

ELSEVIER
SAUNDERS

Vet Clin Food Anim 21 (2005) 55–72

VETERINARY
CLINICS
Food Animal Practice

Routine Surgical Procedures in Dairy Cattle Under Field Conditions: Abomasal Surgery, Dehorning, and Tail Docking

Pascale Aubry, DMV

Department of Clinical Sciences, Faculté de Médecine Vétérinaire, Université de Montréal, C.P. 5000, Saint-Hyacinthe, Québec J2S 7C6, Canada

Dairy cattle veterinarians routinely perform, or educate their clients on how to perform properly, many surgical procedures on the farm. Among the most common are correction of abomasal displacement, dehorning, tail docking, cesarean section, hernia repair in calves, and teat laceration repairs. The last three procedures are discussed elsewhere in this issue. This article first discusses the decision-making process in the correction of left displaced abomasums (LDA). Next, pain management during and after dehorning is addressed. Finally, the tail docking of dairy cows is discussed.

Left displaced abomasum

Dilation or displacement of the abomasum is probably the most common surgical condition of the bovine patient. Three different diseases are described: left-side displacement of the abomasum (LDA), right-side dilation of the abomasum (RDA), and abomasal volvulus. Of the total cases of displacement or volvulus, 85% to 95.8% are left-side displacements [1,2]. Left displacement of the abomasum first was described in dairy cattle in the early 1950s [3,4]. Since then, it has become one of the most common and costly diseases to the dairy industry. In a study of dairy herds in Michigan, the lactational incidence rate for displacement of the abomasum was 6% for primiparous and 7% for multiparous cows [5]. In New York State, a sample of dairy farms had a lactational incidence risk for displacement of the abomasum of 6.3% [6]. In Ontario dairy herds, the lactational incidence risk

E-mail address: pascale.aubry@umontreal.ca

doi:10.1016/j.cvfa.2004.11.002 *vetfood.theclinics.com*

for LDA is about 2% [7]. The cost of an LDA has been estimated to be $312 per case, or $2184 per 100 cows per lactation, for medium to large commercial dairy herds in New York State. This is assuming that 90% of the LDA were corrected by a closed technique and 10% by open surgery (Charles L. Guard, DVM, Ithaca, NY, unpublished data, May 2004). Another study of Holstein dairy farms in central Michigan estimated the cost at $256.50 for LDA corrected by a closed technique or $406.40 when corrected surgically [8].

Three open surgical approaches have been described to correct the condition: right paralumbar fossa omentopexy (RPFO) [9–15] or right paralumbar fossa pyloropexy [15,16], left paralumbar fossa abomasopexy (LPFA) [13–15,17] or left paralumbar fossa omentopexy (LPFO) [13,14,18], and right paramedian abomasopexy (RPA) [13–15,19–22]. More recently, a left paramedian abomasopexy has been described [23]. Two closed surgical techniques also have been described. The blind stitch (BS) technique was introduced in the early 1970s [24], and the toggle pin (bar) suture (TPS) technique was described in 1982 [25]. These two techniques initially were proposed as a cheaper alternative for older commercial animals or for cows with concurrent diseases that do not justify a more expensive open surgical procedure. There is now a good amount of evidence in the literature, however, showing that the TPS might be a reasonable and economical choice for most animals. A laparoscopic repositioning and fixation of the LDA also has been described and is gaining popularity among practitioners in Europe [26,27]. Finally, a nonsurgical method of rolling the cow was described, but it has a high rate of recurrence: In a study of 100 cows with LDAs corrected by rolling, 70% recurred, usually within 1 to 2 days [22].

Diagnosing an LDA is usually straightforward with the use of simultaneous percussion and auscultation [28], but deciding which technique should be used to correct the displaced abomasum is more complex. The veterinarian and the dairy producer must take many factors into account: the value of the animal and cost of replacement; the immediate and long-term efficacy of the different techniques; the cost; the limitations and potential risks; and the presence or absence of concurrent diseases, which are likely to worsen the prognosis significantly. Also, the importance of the veterinarian's familiarity with the different techniques cannot be overlooked. The focus of this discussion is on helping the practicing veterinarian make a sound decision when choosing which technique will be used to correct an LDA. Although part of the discussion also could apply to the correction of a RDA or abomasal volvulus, it mainly focuses on LDAs because they are more common, and all the techniques mentioned can be used to correct them, which is not true for RDAs. Also, the prognosis for abomasal volvulus is different than for LDA. First, the advantages and disadvantages of each technique are reviewed, followed by discussion of the success rates for these techniques, the most common complications, and what to do when the technique used has failed.

The advantages and disadvantages of the different techniques are summarized in Table 1. In general, the open surgical techniques have the advantage that the surgeon can identify positively the structure to be fixed (omentum, abomasum, or pyloric part), and he or she can explore the abdomen and assess possible complicating factors, such as perforating abomasal ulcers and adhesions, fatty liver, and traumatic reticuloperitonitis. Also, complications following flank approach surgery (recurrence, incisional abscess) are rarely fatal to the cow, whereas fatal peritonitis or pyloric outflow obstruction is more likely to occur after a closed technique. To the author's knowledge, the incidence of these complications is not known for the surgical correction of abomasal displacement by laparotomy or for the closed suturing techniques. The advantages and disadvantages are exactly the same for both closed techniques, but the TPS has the undeniable advantage over the BS that the surgeon can ensure placement of the sutures in the abomasum. One of the advantages of the TPS mentioned in Table 1 is that it is simple to perform. Although it is true that TPS is a simple and highly successful procedure in the hands of an experienced surgeon, it might be different for a beginner. Becoming proficient at the TPS procedure probably requires almost as much practice as for the open surgical techniques.

An excellent website [29] presents some useful strategies that ultimately result in the successful outcome of LDA repair by the TPS technique. The website includes a step-by-step method that provides many practical tips and pictures of each step of the procedure. The front and rear legs of the cow can be tied to an immovable object. That might not be practical in every situation, but for the veterinarian and his assistants' safety, at least the rear legs need to be tied. At the Ambulatory Clinic of the New York State College of Veterinary Medicine, clinicians use the casting rope itself to tie the cow's legs. After the cow has been cast on her right side, a knot is tied in the rope (Fig. 1). The cow is rolled onto her back, and her rear legs are inserted in the rope in front of the udder (Fig. 2). This method allows the procedure to be undertaken even in areas where immovable objects are not available to tie the legs to, such as a green patch of grass. The authors of the website and inventors of the TPS method of LDA fixation strongly recommend the use of preoperative and postoperative antibiotics, but many practitioners choose not to use antibiotics to avoid having to discard milk. A nonrandomized study [30] found no effect of the use of antibiotics for either the RPFO or the TPS. A randomized clinical trial is needed to address the issue. Other postoperative care after a TPS procedure includes the administration of calcium because a large percentage of cows with LDAs are hypocalcemic [31]. Finally, the treatment of any concurrent disease, such as ketosis, metritis, or mastitis, is of foremost importance.

Table 2 summarizes the short-term cull, death, and recurrence rates after correction of an LDA by different procedures. There is no randomized study comparing these parameters between an open and a closed technique. The postsurgical combined death or cull rate is 4.5% to 22% for the first month

Table 1
Advantages and disadvantages of different techniques used for correction of a left displaced abomasum

Advantages	Disadvantages
Right paralumbar fossa omentopexy	
Animal is standing	Recurrence
Surgeon can work alone	Requires long arms in large cows
Most thorough examination of the abdomen	Adhesion to the left body wall cannot be visualized
Allows prophylactic correction of displacement	Position of the abomasum anatomically less correct
Left paralumbar fossa abomasopexy or omentopexy	
Animal is standing	Cannot be used for right displacement or volvulus
Best technique for cows in late pregnancy (≥7 mo)	Requires an assistant
Apparent ulcers can be oversown	Requires long arms in large cows
Adhesions can be visualized more thoroughly and dissected	
Right paramedian abomasopexy	
Strong adhesion between abomasum and body wall	More than one person necessary for positioning the animal
Abomasum returns in near-normal position	Physically more demanding for the surgeon
Approach of choice for surgical treatment of abomasal ulcers and impaction (allows the most complete exteriorization of the abomasum)	Risk of bloat, regurgitation, and aspiration of ruminal contents
	Does not allow thorough exploration of abdomen
	Ventral incision more difficult to keep clean
	Udder edema precludes the use of a paramedian incision
Blind stitch	
Quick and inexpensive	Surgeon cannot be certain the needle has penetrated the abomasum
	Two or three assistants required to cast and position the animal
	Dorsal recumbency
	Can be used only to correct uncomplicated left-sided displacements
Toggle pin suture	
Quick and inexpensive	Two or three assistants required to cast and position the animal
Allows surgeon to ensure placement of sutures in the abomasum (by smelling distinctive odor of abomasal gas or measuring pH)	Dorsal recumbency
	Can be used only to correct uncomplicated left-sided displacements

Data from Saint Jean GD, Hull BL, Hoffsis GF, Rings MD. Comparison of the different surgical techniques for correction of abomasal problems. Compend Cont Educ Pract Vet 1987;9:F377–82.

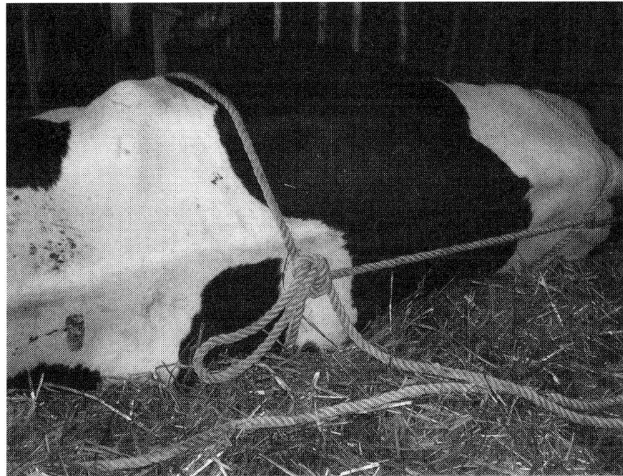

Fig. 1. The cow is cast with a rope onto her right side, and a quick release knot is made just cranial to the hip bones.

after the LDA correction. The recurrence rate for the first 2 weeks to 1 month varies between 1.4% and 10%. Table 3 reports the long-term cull, death, and recurrence rates after correction of an LDA by different procedures. The data reported exclude the lost-to-follow-up cows and include the short-term data. Because necropsies were not performed in all cows, death rates in both tables include deaths related and unrelated to the surgical procedures. The long-term death or cull rate ranges between 6.1%, for an unknown period after the repair of an LDA, and 87%, for more than 270 days into the second lactation after the LDA correction. The few

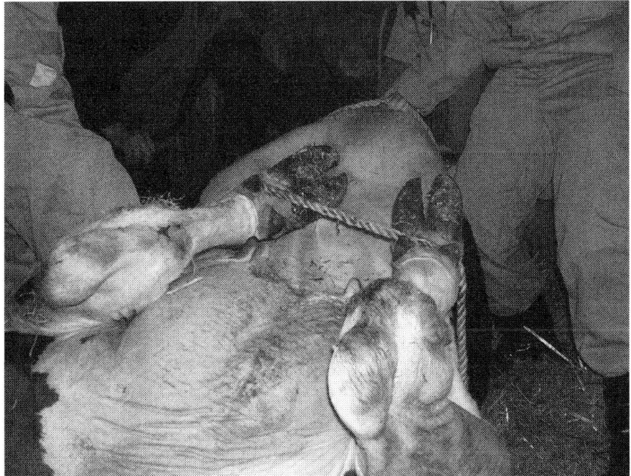

Fig. 2. The cow is rolled onto her back, and the two rear legs are inserted into the rope, which is placed between the feet and the dewclaws.

Table 2
Short-term cull, death, and recurrence rate after correction of a left displaced abomasum by different procedures

Reference	Technique	No. animals	Postsurgical cull rate % (time postsurgery)	Postsurgical death rate % (time postsurgery)	Postsurgical death or cull rate % (time postsurgery)	Recurrence % (time postsurgery)
Gabel, 1969 [9]	RPFO	147	UNK	5.4 (2 wk)	UNK	1.4 (2 wk)
Hull, 1972 [63]	BS	44	2.4 (UNK)	9.8 (UNK)	12.2 (UNK)	UNK
Grymer, 1982 [25]	TPS	27	UNK	14.8 (approx 2 wk)	UNK	3.7 (approx 2 wk)
Fubini, 1992 [64]	RPFO	50	UNK	UNK	6 (1 mo)	UNK
	RPA	44	UNK	UNK	4.5 (1 mo)	UNK
Vlaminck, 1998 [65]	LPFO	53	1.9 (1 wk)	7.5 (1 wk)	9.4 (1 wk)	1.9 (1 wk)
Des Coteaux, 2001 [30]	TPS[a]	108	UNK	UNK	22 (30–35 d)	5–10 (<1 mo)
	RPFO[a]	80	UNK	UNK	13.7 (30–35 d)	UNK
Raizman, 2002 [66]	TPS	188	UNK	UNK	14.9 (1st DHI test) 20 (20 d)	UNK

Abbreviations: DHI, Dairy Health Improvement; UNK, unknown.
[a] Not randomized.

Table 3
Long-term cull, death, and recurrence rate after correction of a left displaced abomasum by different procedures

Reference	Technique	No. animals	Postsurgical cull rate % (time postsurgery)	Postsurgical death rate % (time postsurgery)	Postsurgical death or cull rate % (time postsurgery)	Recurrence % (time postsurgery)
Foster Mather, 1966 [67]	RPA	82	1.2 (UNK)	4.9 (UNK)	6.1 (UNK)	2.4 (UNK)
Gabel, 1969 [9]	RPFO	143	6.3 (17 mo)	5.6 (17 mo)	11.9 (17 mo)	2.1 (17 mo)
Wallace, 1975[68]	RPFO	312	UNK	10.6 (UNK)	UNK	3.7 (UNK)
Petty, 1981 [69]	RPA	143	9.1 (3 mo)	8.4 (3 mo)	17.5 (3 mo)	UNK
Kelton, 1988 [70]	TPS	31	29 (2 mo into next lact)	12.9 (2 mo into next lact)	41.9 (2 mo into next lact)	3.2 (2 mo into next lact)
	RPA	28	46.4 (2 mo into next lact)	0 (2 mo into next lact)	46.4 (2 mo into next lact)	3.6 (2 mo into next lact)
Fubini, 1992 [64]	RPFO	44	UNK	UNK	66.7 (1–2 years)	UNK
	RPA	48	UNK	UNK	59.1 (1–2 years)	UNK
Bartlett, 1995 [8]	RPFPO	35	5.7 (4 mo)	28.6 (4 mo)	34.3 (4 mo)	UNK
	TPS	37	13.5 (4 mo)	2.7 (4 mo)	16.2 (4 mo)	UNK
Bartlett, 1997 [71]	TPS	26	3.8 (6 mo)	3.8 (6 mo)	7.6 (6 mo)	UNK
Grymer, 1997 [72]	TPS	74	29.7 (1 y)	10.8 (1 year)	40.5 (1 y)	UNK
Vlaminck, 1998 [65]	LPFO	53	7.7 (6 mo)	7.7 (6 mo)	15.4 (6 mo)	5.8 (6 mo)
			18.4 (1 y)	8.2 (1 year)	26.6 (1 y)	8.2 (1 y)
Geishauser, [73]	Any	135[a]	UNK	UNK	41 (> 270 d)	UNK
			UNK	UNK	76 (> 270 d into next lact)	UNK
			UNK	UNK	87 (> 270 d into 2nd next lact)	13 (2nd next lact)
Raizman, 2002 [66]	TPS	188	UNK	UNK	23.4 (70 DIM) 35.6 (320 DIM)	UNK

Abbreviations: DIM, days in milk; lact, lactation; UNK, unknown.
[a] Includes cows diagnosed with left displaced abomasum (90%) and right displaced abomasum (10%).

randomized studies that compared open surgery versus TPS could not show a significant difference in death, cull, or recurrence rate. There seems to be a trend, however, toward a higher cull rate after an open surgery and a higher death rate after a TPS. The combined death or cull rate seems to be higher for open surgeries. The TPS procedure should be considered a good choice of repair for most cows diagnosed with an LDA. The exception would be cows of extremely high economic and genetic value, for which the slight risk of fatal complications would not be acceptable. Also, pregnant cows beyond 5 months of gestation, cows with severe ventral edema, cows with fatty liver, or cows with severe respiratory problems would not be good candidates for the TPS repair [29].

Because all the procedures seem to be equally successful at correcting an LDA, it is important to weigh the economics into the decision. A decision-tree analysis was used in one study to evaluate three treatment possibilities [32]: open surgery (RPFO, LPFA, or RPA), closed surgical techniques (BS and TPS), and simply rolling the cow. This study concluded that the expected monetary value of an animal after an open surgery was only $26 more than after a closed technique. Rolling the cow had an expected monetary value, however, of approximately $884 less than for the surgical techniques. In their analysis, the authors assumed a lesser probability of recovery for the closed techniques versus open surgery. That might be true for the BS technique, but according to Table 3, the TPS technique can be considered equally successful to the open surgical techniques. Assuming that the only closed technique used is the TPS, and assuming the same probability of recovery as for open surgeries, the expected monetary value would be approximately $50 more for the TPS than for open surgery. In a randomized study, an economic comparison of the RPFO and TPS was conducted [8]. Cows treated with RPFO had significantly more economic loss ($150 more) than cows treated with the TPS procedure. The authors concluded that the TPS procedure may be a reasonable alternative to the open-surgical approach in some herds, but the rate of complications after the TPS procedure need to be determined and compared with other techniques.

Recurrence is probably one of the most common complications after the correction of a displaced abomasum. According to Tables 2 and 3, the prevalence of recurrence after omentopexy is 1.4% to 8.2%, whereas is it 2.4% to 3.6% for abomasopexy and 3.2% to 10% for TPS. The most common reasons for recurrence include incorrect placement of an omentopexy or abomasopexy and stretching or disruption of the omentopexy [33]. In one study of 40 cows in which a second laparotomy was performed at least 1 day after the first surgery to correct a displaced abomasum, 80% were discharged from the hospital, and 70% of the 20 animals discharged and available for follow-up were productive [33]. Animals presented with left and right displacement of the abomasum and abomasal volvulus in either the first or repeat laparotomy were included in the study.

The authors concluded that surgery for recurrence of displacement of the abomasum is economically warranted.

As discussed earlier, the complications after a closed surgery have the potential to be far more severe than the complications described for laparotomy. The BS technique carries even more risks than the TPS fixation because of the inability to identify definitively and suture the abomasum. A retrospective study of 20 cases of complications of BS abomasopexy mentions the following findings [34]: 14 cows had a relapse (12 LDAs and 2 RDAs), 2 had an abomasal fistula, 1 had a mammary thrombophlebitis, and 1 had an abomasal rupture with localized peritonitis. Of the two cows presented for necropsy, one had a pyloric obstruction, and one had a blind suture placed into the rumen and acute peritonitis. Of the 18 animals presented to the hospital, 12 recovered, 3 were slaughtered because of the presence of extensive adhesions and generalized peritonitis, and 3 were euthanized. In 6 of the 12 cows that had a recurrence of displaced abomasum, the suture had penetrated only the omentum. This problem usually can be avoided with the TPS because the surgeon can smell and hear the gas coming out of the abomasum, which would not happen if the trochar were in the omentum. Another complication that usually can be avoided is mammary thrombophlebitis. If the mammary vein is marked before the cow is cast on her back, the surgeon will be aware of the position of the vein even if it collapses when the cow is on her back. It is also possible to avoid placing the sutures in the rumen with the TPS procedure. Most experienced surgeons are able to differentiate rumen from abomasal smell, but when in doubt, it is possible to collect a small amount of fluid via a small-diameter plastic tubing inserted through the trocar and check it for low pH. This can be accomplished easily using pH paper; most turn blue in the presence of high (rumen) pH and yellow-orange under low (abomasum) pH. Alternatively, the push rod can be inserted in the trocar, and its tip can be applied to the pH paper.

Being aware that most of these possible serious complications of the BS technique can be avoided using the TPS procedure, which is equally fast and inexpensive, it is difficult to justify the use of the BS technique. Pyloric outflow obstruction is a complication that can happen with the BS and the TPS because this technique does not provide a good opportunity to determine the anatomic location of the sutures within the abomasum. For the four cows mentioned in one clinical report [35], however, the clinical signs of obstruction developed within 72 hours of TPS fixation, and the two cows that had the external knot that secured the TPS cut 48 hours after the procedure recovered without recurrence. It is recommended that cows that have had an LDA corrected by TPS be observed closely for the first 48 hours after the procedure. A cow not showing signs of improvement or deteriorating should be reexamined, and the external knot should be cut. Another study showed that one of the factors associated with the success of a TPS was the number of trocar perforations [30]. Six percent, 14%, and

50% of cows had a culling decision taken by days 4 to 7 when two, three, or four perforations were done. It is advisable to abort the TPS procedure after three perforations have failed to introduce the two toggle pins into the abomasum, and the cow should undergo open surgery to correct the abomasal displacement.

If an RPFO approach is chosen as the open surgical procedure, the surgeon often finds that the surgical time is reduced because rolling the cow usually replaces the abomasum in its normal anatomic position. In such a case, it is usually unnecessary to deflate and reposition the abomasum, and the pylorus is readily visible. For the same reason, an LPFA would not be the approach of choice after an aborted TPS procedure because the abomasum usually would have returned to its normal location, making it impossible for the surgeon to perform an abomasopexy. One retrospective study looked at the prognosis for survival after an open surgery after an unsuccessful TPS fixation [36]. The cows that had open surgery immediately after an aborted TPS procedure were not included in that study. The records of 53 cows that had a failed TPS during their present lactation were reviewed. Most were presented to the hospital within the week after the unsuccessful TPS. Sixty-two percent of the cows were discharged alive from the hospital, but only 41% were still in their herd 60 days postdischarge. Using a probabilistic model, the authors estimated an expected monetary loss of $982 for surgical repair versus $888 for immediate culling. In the long run, an average cow should be culled after a failed TPS, when making this decision on a cash basis, so as to minimize financial losses.

Dehorning

Dehorning dairy calves has become a routine practice in modern cattle husbandry. The purpose of this practice is to reduce the risk of injury to farm personnel and other animals. In addition, cattle with horns are harder to handle in chutes and require three times more space at feed bunkers and during transport [37]. Horn buds of young calves less than 3 months of age typically are removed with a caustic paste or burned with a hot iron (electric or butane). In older calves, the horns have to be removed surgically by various techniques: scoop (tube dehorner), guillotine shears (Barnes and Keystone dehorner), saw, or embryotomy wire. A preliminary study has been published on the use of cryosurgery for dehorning calves, but the technique does not seem to be a realistic alternative to hot iron dehorning [38]. In the United Kingdom, the various Codes of Practice for farm animals stipulate that disbudding of calves is permitted using a caustic paste without anesthesia if the calf is less than 1 week of age, but local anesthesia must be used if any other method of dehorning is used in older calves (The Protection of Animals [Anaesthetics] Act, 1964). The Canadian code of practice recommends using local anesthetic for dehorning [39], but it is a common practice in North America to perform the procedure without analgesics or anesthetics. In Sweden, the 1992 animal rights law states that dehorning by cautery should be done under anesthesia and sedation [38]. In Denmark, calves 4 weeks old can be dehorned without local anesthesia [40].

Until the mid-1980s, pain-induced distress after dehorning had been given little attention. The first study on the subject found no effect on plasma cortisol levels, but this was probably due to the design of the study and the few samples taken [41]. Later studies indicated that dehorning with a conventional hot iron without anesthesia had no effect on feed intake or growth of 8-week-old calves, but the cortisol concentration in plasma was elevated for 4 hours after dehorning [42,43].

Wohlt et al [44] compared the use of a conventional hot iron with the Buddex dehorner (Jenrik Marketing Group Inc, Scandia, MN), which operates at a higher temperature and requires only 10 seconds of application. They found that handling of the 3- to 4-week-old calves increased plasma cortisol twofold, and dehorning increased it fourfold to fivefold. There was no effect of the type of dehorner used. The authors also found that the peak cortisol concentrations in plasma were always less when the right horn bud was removed versus the left. Asymmetry in human pain perception has been described for several sensory modalities, and this asymmetry frequently produces greater sensitivity to pain on the left side of the body [45]. The study of Wohlt et al [44] suggests a pattern of cerebral organization of emotional function in cattle similar to that in humans.

Petrie et al [46] compared dehorning of 6- to 8-week-old calves with a dehorning scoop (Barnes Dehorner, Moore Maker Inc., Matador, TX) or gas-heated dehorning iron, with or without local anesthesia. They concluded that although cautery causes some moderate distress for a short time, it should be used in preference to scoop dehorning in 6-week-old calves. Local anesthesia is of only little benefit in reducing the overall distress caused by scoop dehorning, but it does reduce the distress experienced during the first 2 hours after dehorning. As the anesthetic wears off, however, a sharp increase in plasma cortisol can be noted, the magnitude of which is similar to that elicited by dehorning without local anesthesia; this explains why the integrated cortisol response is the same with or without the use of local anesthesia. The authors suggest that the use of analgesics be considered to alleviate the distress that appears after the local anesthetic wears off. Finally, there are marginal benefits in the prior administration of local anesthetic to calves disbudded by cautery.

A study by McMeekan et al [47] provides a better understanding of the two phases of the cortisol response after dehorning (Fig. 3). The first phase is the initial cortisol peak that is due to the amputation itself. It is followed by a second plateau phase and subsequent decline to baseline levels. This plateau phase is due to the inflammation occurring in the dehorning wound. Ketoprofen is an analgesic whose action is primarily anti-inflammatory. Given alone to 3- to 4-month-old calves before dehorning, it only slightly

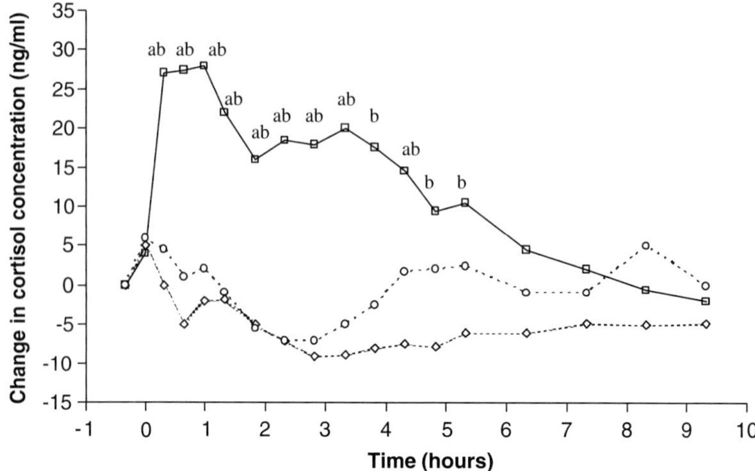

Fig. 3. Changes in the plasma cortisol concentration in calves. Vertical bars represent standard errors. Time 0 represents time of dehorning. ◇, lignocaine plus ketoprofen control; ○, lignocaine plus ketoprofen plus dehorning; □, dehorning. a, dehorning significantly greater ($P < .01$) than lignocaine plus ketoprofen plus dehorning; b, dehorning significantly greater ($P < .05$) than lignocaine plus ketoprofen control. (*Adapted from* McMeekan CM, Stafford KJ, Mellor DJ, Bruce RA, Ward RN, Gregory NG. Effects of regional analgesia and/or a non-steroidal anti-inflammatory analgesic on acute cortisol response to dehorning in calves. Res Vet Sci 1998;64:149; with permission.)

reduced the initial cortisol peak, but it completely abolished the plateau response. The authors recommended that if a local anesthetic is to be administered to calves before dehorning, an anti-inflammatory drug also should be used to eliminate the delayed pain-induced distress caused by inflammation. The same authors came to a similar conclusion in a different study evaluating the behavioral response of calves to dehorning [48], in which they found that dual administration of a local anesthetic and an anti-inflammatory drug is an effective way of alleviating scoop dehorning pain in 3- to 4-month-old calves. A later study by the same group of researchers showed, that ketoprofen, but not phenylbutazone, combined with local anesthesia significantly reduced but did not eliminate the delayed cortisol response [49]. The authors did not know the reasons for this difference between the studies.

Using behavioral and cardiac response in addition to cortisol levels, Grøndahl-Nielsen et al [40] concluded that the dehorning of 4- to 6-week-old calves using a hot iron without any analgesia was unacceptably painful. The difference in plasma cortisol concentration between animals dehorned without anesthesia and the other groups was statistically significant during the first 30 minutes after the procedure. The findings in this study and others were contradicted by studies by Sutherland et al [50] and Sylvester et al [51], which showed that cauterizing the amputation wound under local anesthesia almost abolished the cortisol response to dehorning. Finally, a study showed that ketoprofen administration resulted only in a slight, short-lived reduction in cortisol concentration after butane dehorning of dairy calves less than 2 weeks of age [52]. Ketoprofen administration did not result in a reduction of behavioral indicators of pain. The authors hypothesized that dehorning calves at a younger age minimizes the amount of tissue damage and inflammatory pain because the horn buds are smaller than in older calves.

Surgical amputation of the horns seems to be more painful than hot iron dehorning. In addition, surgical amputation of the horns can lead to the transmission of bovine leukemia virus. Veterinarians should encourage producers to dehorn calves as young as possible with the use of a hot iron. When the size of the horns precludes the use of a hot iron, surgical amputation can be performed, but the wound should be cauterized to minimize blood loss and reduce the cortisol response to dehorning. Local anesthesia should be performed before any dehorning procedure. The routine administration of ketoprofen might not be justified, however, when calves less than 2 weeks of age are dehorned with a hot iron. Ketoprofen would be more beneficial in alleviating pain in older calves and calves dehorned with methods other than a hot iron. Although most people agree that the use of a sedative such as xylazine before the dehorning of calves facilitates the administration of local anesthesia and eliminates the need for physical restraint during dehorning, it does not provide sufficient analgesia to eliminate the initial pain of horn amputation [40,53,54]. When the xylazine is reversed by tolazoline after dehorning, it elicits a marked cortisol response within the first 2 hours after treatment, even in calves that were not dehorned [53]. This cortisol response must be balanced against the benefits of providing early reversal of sedation.

Tail docking

Another practice that is becoming more of a routine in cattle husbandry, and especially in free stall barns, is tail docking. The procedure is usually done by the producers by applying a round latex castration ring (Ideal Instruments, Schiller Park, IL) 7 to 8 cm below the level of the vulva in young calves, often at the time of dehorning. The necrotic tails are usually left to fall by themselves, or they can be removed a few weeks later. In purchased pregnant heifers, the elastic band is placed 5 to 6 cm below the vulva. The procedure was introduced in New Zealand in an attempt to reduce the transmission of leptospirosis to farm workers who may come into contact with cows' tails during milking [55]. In North America, many farmers now use the procedure because they believe that tail docking results in increased cow cleanliness and milk quality. Milker comfort also would be improved, especially in parlors in which milking occurs between the hind limbs. Several European countries, including Norway, Sweden, the Netherlands, the United Kingdom, and Switzerland, have prohibited tail docking of dairy cattle [56]. There is now a good body of evidence that shows the absence of benefits of tail docking and the possible concerns for animal welfare. Possible disadvantages for the cow include pain, impaired social communication, and impaired fly control [57].

Eicher et al [58] studied tail docking influences on behavioral, immunologic, and endocrine responses in 21 dairy heifers housed in box stalls, 1 month before calving. Tail banding had little effect on cortisol responses, immune measures, and behavior of primiparous heifers.

The effects of tail docking with or without anesthetic on behavior and production of 64 lactating cows housed in tie stalls were determined by Tom et al [59]. The authors concluded that the application of a rubber ring to the tail of lactating cows causes only mild discomfort, and the amputation of the tail below the ring 6 days later also may cause some mild discomfort. There is no advantage to using an epidural anesthetic before the procedure.

Indicators of acute pain and fly avoidance behavior in 3-week-old calves housed in hutches after tail docking were examined by Eicher and Dailey [60]. They found that the behavior of calves after banding was in contrast with the lack of response of primiparous heifers or lactating cows in the two previously mentioned studies. An increase in agitation was evidenced, and the specific pain indicator movement (head-to-tail movement) was almost eight times more frequent in the banded calves than in controls. Afternoon fly counts were greater on the rear legs of docked calves than control calves. Ear twitching was more frequent in the docked calves than in the control calves at the morning and noon observations. Tail swings were more frequent for control calves at the noon and afternoon observations. This study raises the possibility of learned helplessness, which is a lack of behavioral responses seen in animals after being exposed to inescapable aversive stimuli. The calves may have quit using their tails, having not experienced a benefit of tail swings. Mature heifers that had used their tails for 2 years before tail docking continued to use the tail to dislodge flies [61]. Licking, which could be an attempt by the calves to alleviate the fly annoyance, was more frequent in docked calves. The authors concluded that tail docking calves by banding at the age of 3 weeks during fly season temporarily reduced calf well-being.

Another study examined the effect of tail docking on fly numbers and fly avoidance behaviors of 16 primiparous heifers housed in a tie-stall barn [61]. The effect of tail docking on cleanliness also was evaluated. Docked cows' rear quarters, but not udders, were cleaner. They had almost twice as many flies on their rear legs as the intact cows, showing that it is not true that cleaner cows result in fewer flies. Ability to swat flies would be more important than cleanliness in keeping fly counts low. Other fly avoidance behaviors, such as tail swings and feed tossing, were greatest in docked cows. They also stood more than intact cows, which could indicate that they were uncomfortable. The authors concluded that if it is necessary to dock cows' tails, it is essential to pay particular attention to fly control.

Two more studies showed the lack of influence of tail docking on milk quality and cow cleanliness. Tucker et al [57] found that tail docking did not provide cleanliness or udder health benefits because no significant differences were found in either somatic cell count or udder cleanliness of 487 cows housed in a barn with free stalls. Also, the variation in cleanliness between cows within treatment groups supports the idea that some cows simply tend to get dirtier regardless of management practices. Cow behavior, appropriate use of stalls, and general cleanliness of the cows' environment might be more important. Finally, Schreiner and Ruegg [62] published the first report on the effect of tail docking on the rate of intramammary infections. They were unable to identify a significant difference in somatic cell count or prevalence of intramammary infections in 1250 cows housed in free-stall housing. Tail docking made no consistent difference on animal cleanliness.

Tail docking seems to have minimal adverse effects on mature dairy cows, but might cause slightly more distress to young calves, especially during fly season. No positive benefits to the cows have been identified, and fly control must be put in place in farms where cows' tails are docked. With the ever-increasing public concerns regarding food-producing animal welfare, the dairy industry might be well advised to refrain from the practice of routine tail docking. Alternatives such as switch trimming should be considered, and research needs to be done to assess comfort and cleanliness of farm personnel as a reason for tail docking of cows.

References

[1] Grymer J. Displaced abomasum—a disease often associated with concurrent diseases. Compend Cont Educ Pract Vet 1980;11:S290–5.

[2] Markusfeld O. The association of displaced abomasum with various periparturient factors in dairy cows: a retrospective study. Prev Vet Med 1986;4:172–83.

[3] Begg H. Diseases of the stomach of the adult ruminant. Vet Rec 1950;62:797–808.

[4] Ford EJ. A case of displacement of the bovine abomasum. Vet Rec 1950;62:763–4.

[5] Cameron REB, Dyk PB, Herdt TH, et al. Dry cow diet, management, and energy balance as risk factors for displaced abomasum in high producing dairy herds. J Dairy Sci 1998;81:132–9.

[6] Gröhn YT, Eicker SW, Hertl JA. The association between previous 305-milk yield and disease in New York State dairy cows. J Dairy Sci 1995;78:1693–702.

[7] Kelton DF. Monitoring and investigating the relationships among health, management, productivity and profitability on Ontario dairy farms. PhD dissertation. University of Guelph, Guelph, ON, Canada; 1995.

[8] Bartlett PC, Kopcha M, Coe PH, Ames NK, Ruegg PL, Erskine RG. Economic comparison of the pyloro-omentopexy versus the roll-and-toggle procedure for treatment of left displacement of the abomasum in dairy cattle. J Am Vet Med Assoc 1995;206:1156–62.

[9] Gabel AA, Heath BR. Correction and right-sided omentopexy in treatment of left-sided displacement of the abomasum in dairy cattle. Can Vet J 1978;19:3–9.

[10] Hoffsis GF. Right paralumbar omentopexy for correction of left displaced abomasum. In: Proceedings of the 4th AABP Annual Conference, Denver; 1971. p. 179–85.
[11] Robertson JT. Right-sided torsion of the abomasum in the cow. Comp Cont Educ Pract Vet 1980;2:S105–9.
[12] Gertsen KE. Right-sided omentopexy for correction of left-sided displacement of the abomasum. Vet Med Sm Anim Clin 1969;63:867–71.
[13] Horney FD, Wallace CE. Surgery of the bovine digestive tract. In: Jennings PB, editor. The practice of large animal surgery. Vol. I. Philadelphia: WB Saunders; 1984. p. 523–40.
[14] Hofmeyr CFB. The digestive system. In: Oehme FW, editor. Textbook of large animal surgery. Baltimore: Williams & Wilkins; 1974. p. 416–21.
[15] Trent AM. Surgery of the abomasum. In: Fubini SL, Ducharme NG, editors. Farm animal surgery. St. Louis: WB Saunders; 2004. p. 196–219.
[16] Baker JS. Diagnosis and surgery of right displacement of the abomasum in the bovine. In: Proceedings of the 14th World Congress on Diseases of Cattle, Dublin; 1986. p. 30–5.
[17] Gertsen KE. Surgical correction of the displaced abomasum. Vet Med Sm Anim Clin 1967; 62:679–82.
[18] Steenhaut M, DeMoor A, VerSchooten F, et al. Surgical treatment of left abomasal displacement. Vet Med Sm Anim Clin 1974;69:161–5.
[19] St. Pierre H, Lamothe P, Ménard L. Les affections de la caillette chez la vache laitière au Québec: revue de littérature, diagnostic différentiel et correction chirurgicale. Can Vet J 1978;19:3–9.
[20] Robertson JM, Boucher WB. Treatment of left displacement of the bovine abomasum. J Am Vet Med Assoc 1966;149:1423–9.
[21] Lowe JE, Loomis WK, Kramer LL. Abomasopexy for repair of left abomasal displacement in dairy cattle. J Am Vet Med Assoc 1965;147:389–93.
[22] Smith DF. Treatment of left displacement of abomasums: Part 1. Compend Cont Educ Pract Vet 1981;3:S415–23.
[23] Lee I, Yamagishi N, Obosho K, Yamada H. Left paramedian abomasopexy in cattle. J Vet Sci 2002;3:59–60.
[24] Walton JF, Muir RM, Turbok JL, Schroeder DL, Sears PM, Williamson FH. Roll-and-suture technic for displaced abomasum. Mod Vet Pract 1973;54:31–2.
[25] Grymer J, Sterner KE. Percutaneous fixation of left displaced abomasum, using a bar suture. J Am Vet Med Assoc 1982;180:1458–61.
[26] Janowitz H. Laparoskopishe reposition und fixation des nach links verlagerten labmagens beim rind. Tierãrztl Prax Ausq G Grosstiere Nutztiere 1998;26:308–13.
[27] Babkine M. La laparoscopie chez les bovins. In: Proceedings of the 62e Congrès annuel de l'Ordre des médecins vétérinaires du Québec, Saint-Hyacinthe; 2003. p. 329–35.
[28] Richmond DH. The use of percussion and auscultation as a diagnostic aid in abomasal displacement of dairy cows. Can Vet J 1964;5:5–7.
[29] Grymer J, Sterner KE. Grymer/Sterner toggle suture. repair of left displaced abomasum (LDA) in the bovine. Available at: http://www.ldatogglesuture.com/.
[30] DesCôteaux L, Woods-Lavoie E, Cécyre A, Larouche Y, Rioux R, Dubreuil P. Left displaced abomasum: to toggle or not to toggle, that is the question! In: Proceedings of the 34th AABP Annual Conference, Vancouver; 2001. p. 167.
[31] Delgado-Lecaroz R, Warnick LD, Guard CL, Smith MC, Barry DA. Cross-sectional study of the association of abomasal displacement or volvulus with serum electrolyte and mineral concentrations in dairy cows. Can Vet J 2000;41:301–5.
[32] Ruegg PL, Carpenter TE. Decision-tree analysis of treatment alternatives for left displaced abomasum. J Am Vet Med Assoc 1989;195:464–7.
[33] Bliksalger AT, Anderson KL, Bristol DG, Fubini SL, Anderson DE. Repeat laparotomy for gastrointestinal disorders in cattle: 57 cases (1968–1992). J Am Vet Med Assoc 1995;207: 939–43.

[34] Tithof PK, Rebhun WC. Complications of blind-stitch abomasopexy: 20 cases (1980–1985). J Am Vet Med Assoc 1986;189:1489–90.
[35] Kelton DF, Fubini SL. Pyloric obstruction after toggle-pin fixation of left displaced abomasum in a cow. J Am Vet Med Assoc 1989;194:677–8.
[36] Perkins GA, Nydam DV, Kimball SA, Fubini SL. Prognosis for survival after an open surgical surgery following an unsuccessful toggle-pin fixation in dairy cows. In: Proceedings of the AABP 36th Annual Conference, Columbus; 2003. p. 176–7.
[37] Faulkner PM, Weary DM. Reducing pain after dehorning in dairy calves. J Dairy Sci 2000; 83:2037–41.
[38] Bengtsson B, Menzel A, Holteniun P, Jacobsson SO. Cryosurgical dehorning of calves: a preliminary study. Vet Rec 1996;138:234–7.
[39] Agriculture Canada. Recommended code of practice for the care and handling of dairy cattle. Ottawa: Agriculture Canada; 1990.
[40] Grøndahl-Nielsen C, Simonsen HB, Damkjer Lund J, Hesselholt M. Behavioural, endocrine and cardiac responses in young calves undergoing dehorning without and with use of sedation and analgesia. Vet J 1999;158:14–20.
[41] Johnston JD, Buckland RB. Response of male Holstein calves from seven sires to four management stresses as measured by plasma corticoid levels. Can J Anim Sci 1976;56: 727–32.
[42] Boandl KE, Wohlt JE, Carsia RV. Effects of handling, administration of a local anesthetic and electrical dehorning on plasma cortisol in Holstein calves. J Dairy Sci 1989;72:2193–7.
[43] Ladden SA, Wohlt JE, Zajac PK, Carsia RV. Effects of stress from electrical dehorning on feed intake, growth and blood constituents in Holstein heifer calves. J Dairy Sci 1985;68: 3062–6.
[44] Wohlt JE, Allyn ME, Zajac PK, Katz LS. Cortisol increases in plasma of Holstein heifer calves from handling and method of electrical dehorning. J Dairy Sci 1994;77:3725–9.
[45] Chandramouli R, Kanchan BR, Ambodevi B. Right-left asymmetry in tonic pain perception and its modification by simultaneous contralateral noxious stimulation. Neuropsychologia 1993;31:687–94.
[46] Petrie NJ, Mellor DJ, Stafford KJ, Bruce RA, Ward RN. Cortisol response of calves to two methods of disbudding used with or without local anaesthetic. N Z Vet J 1995;44:9–14.
[47] McMeekan CM, Stafford KJ, Mellor DJ, Bruce RA, Ward RN, Gregory NG. Effects of regional analgesia and/or a non-steroidal anti-inflammatory analgesic on acute cortisol response to dehorning in calves. Res Vet Sci 1998;64:147–50.
[48] McMeekan CM, Stafford KJ, Mellor DJ, Bruce RA, Ward RN, Gregory NG. Effects of a local analgesic and a non-steroidal anti-inflammatory analgesic on the behavioural responses of calves to dehorning. N Z Vet J 1999;47:92–6.
[49] Sutherland MA, Mellor DJ, Stafford KJ, Gregory NG, Bruce RA, Ward RN. Cortisol response to dehorning of calves given a 5-h local anesthetic regimen plus phenylbutazone, ketoprofen or adrenocorticotropic hormone prior to dehorning. Res Vet Sci 2003;73:115–23.
[50] Sutherland MA, Mellor DJ, Stafford KJ, Gregory NG, Bruce RA, Ward RN. Effect of local anaesthetic combined with wound cauterization on the cortisol response to dehorning in calves. Aust Vet J 2002;80:165–7.
[51] Sylvester SP, Mellor DJ, Stafford KJ, Bruce RA, Ward RN, Gregory NG. Acute cortisol responses of calves to four methods of dehorning by amputation. Aust Vet J 1998;76:123–6.
[52] Milligan BN, Duffield T, Lissemore K. The utility of ketoprofen for alleviating pain following dehorning in young dairy calves. Can Vet J 2004;45:140–3.
[53] Stafford KJ, Mellor DJ, Todd SE, Ward RN, McMeekan CM. The effect of different combinations of lignocaine, ketoprofen, xylazine and tolazoline on the acute cortisol response to dehorning in calves. N Z Vet J 2003;51:219–26.
[54] Faulkner PM, Weary DM. Reducing pain after dehorning in dairy calves. J Dairy Sci 2000; 83:2037–41.

[55] Stookey J. Is intensive dairy production compatible with animal welfare? In: Proceedings of the 1994 Western Canadian Dairy Seminar, Red Deer, Alberta; 1994. p. 209–19.

[56] Tucker CB, Weary DM. Tail docking in dairy cattle. Animal Welfare Information Center Bulletin 2002;11:1–3. Available at: http://www.nal.usda.gov/awic/newsletters/v11n3/11n3tuck.htm.

[57] Tucker CB, Fraser D, Weary DM. Tail docking dairy cattle: effects on cow cleanliness and udder health. J Dairy Sci 2001;84:84–7.

[58] Eicher SD, Morrow-Tesch JL, Albright JL, Dailey JW, Young CR, Stanker LH. Tail-docking influences on behavioural, immunological and endocrine responses in dairy heifers. J Dairy Sci 2000;83:1456–62.

[59] Tom EM, Duncan IJH, Widowski TM, Bateman KG, Leslie KE. Effects of tail docking using a rubber ring with or without anesthetic on behaviour and production of lactating cows. J Dairy Sci 2002;85:2257–65.

[60] Eicher SD, Dailey JW. Indicators of acute pain and fly avoidance behaviors in Holstein calves following tail-docking. J Dairy Sci 2002;85:2850–8.

[61] Eicher SD, Morrow-Tesch JL, Albright JL, Williams RE. Tail-docking alters fly numbers, fly-avoidance behaviours and cleanliness, but not physiological measures. J Dairy Sci 2001; 84:1822–8.

[62] Schreiner DA, Ruegg PL. Effects of tail docking on milk quality and cow cleanliness. J Dairy Sci 2002;85:2503–11.

[63] Hull BL. Closed suturing technique for correction of left abomasal displacement. Iowa State Univ Vet 1972;34:142–4.

[64] Fubini SL, Ducharme NG, Erb HN Sheils RL. A comparison in 101 dairy cows of right paralumbar fossa omentopexy and right paramedian abomasopexy for treatment of left displacement of the abomasum. Can Vet J 1992;33:318–24.

[65] Vlaminck L, Steenhaut M, Gasthuis F, et al. Omentopexy for correction of left displaced abomasum: outcome results in 53 cattle. Vlaams Diergeneeskundig Tijdschrift 1998;67: 118–22.

[66] Raizman EA, Santos GEP. The effect of left displacement of the abomasum corrected by toggle-pin suture on lactation, reproduction, and health of Holstein dairy cows. J Dairy Sci 2002;85:1157–63.

[67] Foster Mather M, Dedrick RS. Displacement of the abomasum. Cornell Vet 1966;56: 323–44.

[68] Wallace CE. Left abomasal displacement—a retrospective study of 315 cases. Bovine Practitioner 1975;10:50–8.

[69] Petty RD. Surgical correction of left displacement abomasum in cattle: a retrospective study of 143 cases. J Am Vet Med Assoc 1981;178:1274–6.

[70] Kelton DF, Garcia G, Guard CL, et al. Bar suture (toggle pin) versus open surgical abomasopexy for treatment of left displaced abomasum in dairy cattle. J Am Vet Med Assoc 1988;193:557–9.

[71] Bartlett PC, Grymer J, Houe H, Sterner KE. Cohort study of milk production and days to first insemination following roll-and-toggle LDA correction. Bovine Practitioner 1997;31: 83–5.

[72] Grymer J, Bartlett PC, Houe H, Sterner KE. One-year survival of cows with left displacement of the abomasum corrected with the roll-and-toggle procedure. Bovine Practitioner 1997;31:80–2.

[73] Geishauser T, Shoukri M, Kelton D, Leslie K. Analysis of survivorship after displaced abomasum is diagnosed in dairy cows. J Dairy Sci 1998;81:2346–53.

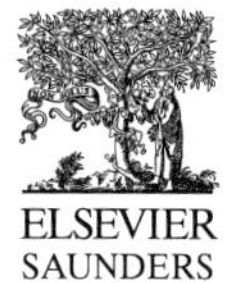

ELSEVIER
SAUNDERS

Vet Clin Food Anim 21 (2005) 73–100

VETERINARY
CLINICS
Food Animal Practice

Cesarean Section in Cows

Kenneth D. Newman, DVM*,
David E. Anderson, DVM, MS

Food Animal Medicine and Surgery, Department of Veterinary Clinical Studies, College of Veterinary Medicine, The Ohio State University, Columbus, OH 43210, USA

Cesarean section is one of the oldest surgical procedures in human and veterinary medicine. In veterinary medicine, species, productive use, and experience tend to influence the frequency, ease, and success of this procedure. Dairy practices perform fewer cesarean sections, but these occur year round. In contrast, cesarean sections in beef practice are numerous and heavily concentrated during the late winter and early spring. Adverse weather conditions associated with beef calving practices requires appropriate in-clinic or farm facilities for performing cesarean sections. Nevertheless, the basic goals of performing a cesarean section are independent of practice type: preservation of the dam and the calf and the future reproductive efficiency of the dam.

Numerous variables determine whether the procedure is successful. The most important is the health status of the dam and calf at the time of surgery. For this reason, it is worthwhile to categorize cesarean section as elective, emergency (nonemphysematous), or emphysematous procedures. This article briefly discusses the indications, approaches, anesthesia, and surgical techniques for cesarean section. Complications, especially complications arising from emergency and emphysematous procedures, are discussed in more detail.

Indications

There are maternal and fetal indications for performing a cesarean section. Maternal indications include immature heifers, pelvic deformities, failure of cervical dilation, uncorrectable uterine torsion, uterine tear, hydrops, and prepartum paralysis [1]. Beef breeds that have double muscling

* Corresponding author.
E-mail address: newman.258@osu.edu (K.D. Newman).

0749-0720/05/$ - see front matter
doi:10.1016/j.cvfa.2004.12.001

such as Charolais, Limousin, and Belgian Blue breeds, often require cesarean sections [2,3]. Risk factors in cattle are increased by heifer's age less than 2 years (odds ratio 3.09 compared with multiparous cows), long gestation period, preceding long interval from first service to conception, long dry period, double-muscled (odds ratio 10.85) or Piedmont (odds ratio 4.26) sire, and previous cesarean section calving (odds ratio 18.89 compared with dams having a previous normal calving) [4].

Fetal indicators include normal and pathologic fetal conditions. Normal fetal conditions consist of absolute fetal oversize (relative to a normal maternal pelvis size) and malposition. A high-value calf, such as an embryo transfer or clone, may be an indication for an elective cesarean section. Pathologic fetal conditions include fetal anasarca, schistosomus reflexus, hydrocephalus, conjoined twins, emphysematous, mummification, and prolonged gestation [1]. Depending on the circumstances, including the availability of a fetotome and the practitioner's experience, a fetotomy is not always a viable option. Attempting a fetotomy on an emphysematous fetus when the uterus is tightly contracted, little uterine fluid is present, cervix is incompletely dilated, or uterus is friable is inadvisable [1]. Fetotomy also is not recommended on a downer cow, necessitating a cesarean section.

Approach

The traditional approaches have been well described in the literature [1, 5–7]. Restraint (appropriately based on the breed); space; light; help available; location; and the veterinarian's training, experience, and confidence [1] are issues that need to be considered, in conjunction with the underlying reason for performing the cesarean section because this can determine the surgical approach [1,5,7]. The two main options are whether to do a cesarean section on a standing or on a recumbent cow. Depending on the demeanor of the dam, a recumbent approached using sedation and tying the legs forward and back may be more appropriate in cases when no chute is present. If the cow may not remain standing for duration of the surgery, it may easier to start with her recumbent rather than having her fall down during the operation. The recumbent approach, because it facilitates exteriorization of the uterus, especially when an oversized fetus is present, reduces the opportunity to contaminate the abdominal cavity [5]. The recumbent approach can be midline or over the pregnant horn using a paramedian, low-flank [5], or paramammary approach (Fig. 1) [5]. The paramammary approach, located between the udder and the fold of the flank, is useful in dairy cows because it is more likely to avoid the caudal epigastic veins and ventral edema located on the paramedian and midline areas. The midline approach likely requires the longest incision because the linea alba is relatively inflexible.

The standing flank approach may be done from either the left or the right; it is more commonly performed from the left [1,5,7,8]. The primary

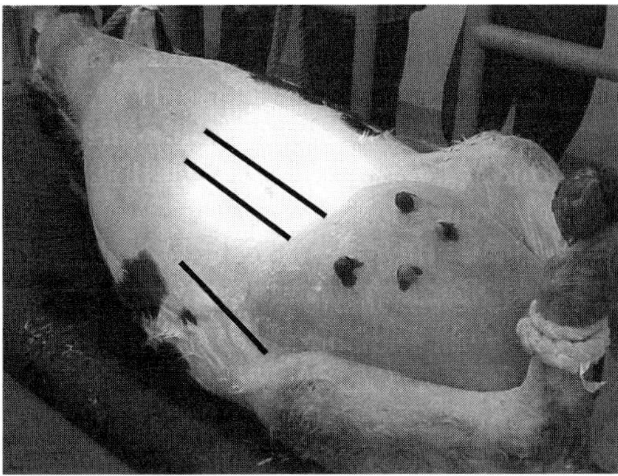

Fig. 1. Preoperative ventral view shows the locations of the midline (*top line*), right paramedian (*middle line*), and right low oblique or paramammary approaches (*bottom line*).

advantage of the left approach is that the rumen prevents evisceration of the small intestines, but rumen prolapse may occur if straining during surgery. When the pregnancy is located in the right horn, some practitioners find it easier to use the right approach especially if the calf is big (clone, double muscles, extended pregnancy). The primary disadvantage of this approach is retaining the small intestines within the abdominal cavity. In cases in which the left approach has been used exclusively to perform several cesarean sections over time in the same cow, the practitioner may find it easier to use the right approach.

More recently, a left oblique flank approach in standing cows has been described (Fig. 2) [9]. An incision is started 10 cm cranial and 8 to 10 cm ventral to the cranial aspect of the tuber coxae. The incision is extended cranioventrally at a 45° angle, ending 3 cm caudal to the last rib. The apex of the uterine horn is more readily accessible, facilitating manipulation and exteriorization of the uterus. This incision is larger and extends more cranioventrally compared with the traditional vertical flank incision. This technique may be useful to remove large calves or when the uterine contents are contaminated. The internal abdominal oblique muscle is incised parallel to the muscle fibers; the abdominal viscera apply tension to this muscle, facilitating apposition during closure.

Anesthesia

Sedation may be required in anxious cows. Although xylazine hydrochloride (Rompum), 0.03 to 0.1 mg/kg intravenously [10], is the most widely used sedative in bovine practice, it also increases uterine tone, making manipulation and exteriorization of the gravid uterus more difficult [7,11,12]. A study using endoscopy showed that xylazine alters laryngeal and pharyngeal anatomy and impairs sensation in adult dairy cattle [13], which likely increase

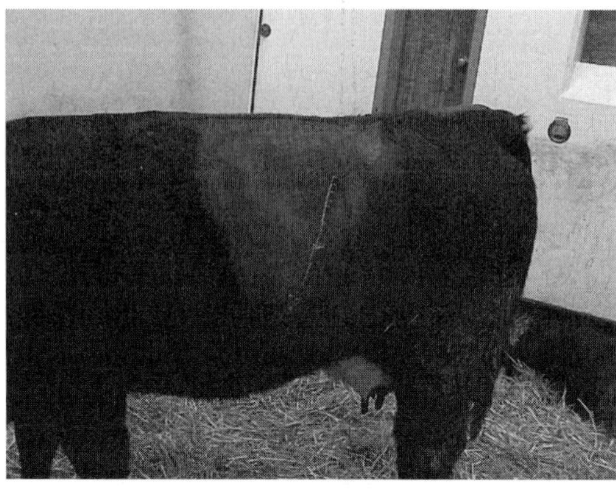

Fig. 2. Postoperative photograph shows the location of the left oblique approach for cesarean section. (Courtesy of Dr. Matt Miesner, The Ohio State University, Columbus, OH.)

the risk of aspiration pneumonia if the cow is positioned in either lateral or dorsal recumbency. Xylazine also may induce ataxia—an undesirable effect while doing a standing cesarean section. When a halter is the sole means of restraint in dairy heifers, the authors have found that the combination of 7.5 mg of acepromazine maleate (Acepromazine maleate) and 10 mg of butorphanol tartrate (Torbugesic) administered intravenously provides adequate sedation (unless the cow is already in a highly excitable state) for standing surgery without causing either ataxia or increased uterine tone.

Surgical approach determines which local anesthesia technique is used. Techniques for local anesthesia using 2% lidocaine hydrochloride are well documented in the literature [7,14–16]. The most common techniques are the proximal paravertebral and distal paravertebral, inverted "L," and line blocks. The technique used reflects the surgeon's preference. The proximal paravertebral block is technically more challenging because the needle is inserted just adjacent to the vertebral body, and the tip of the needle should be close to the nerve roots exiting the vertebral foramen, requiring more restraint and a long needle (18G, 10 cm long). Extremely muscular or fat beef cows may require a longer needle. An easier technique is the "modified" proximal paravertebral block, in which the needle is inserted midway between the spinous process and the tip of the transverse process (Fig. 3). This block uses the smallest dose of local anesthetic, provides the maximal anesthetic region, and induces maximal relaxation of flank musculature. The distal block requires less skill and may be performed using an 18G, 3.75-cm needle (Fig. 4). This block works well, provided that the local anesthetic injections are fanned above and below the edge of the transverse processes (see Fig. 4). Although the line block is the least technically challenging, it requires the greatest amount of local anesthetic [14–16]. Lidocaine is available with or without epinephrine. Epinephrine reportedly increases the duration of the local anesthesia by causing vasoconstriction; however,

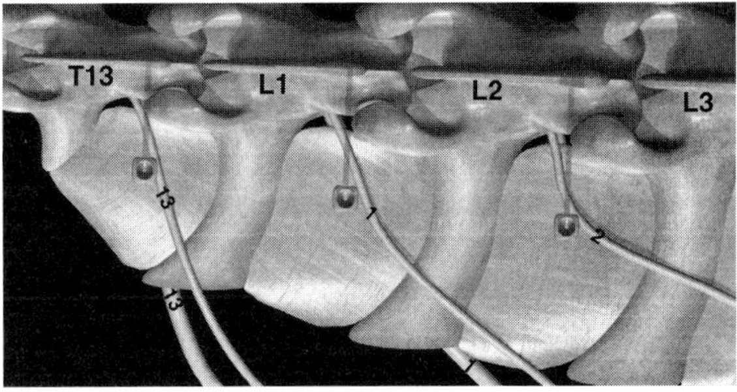

Fig. 3. The modified proximal paravertebral block, shown on this dorsal view of the left lateral aspect. T13, L1, L2, and L3 are the spinous processes of the last thoracic and first, second, and third lumbar vertebrae. Note location of T13 (13), L1 (1), and L2 (2) nerves and the placement of needles.

incisional complications, such as delayed healing and skin slough, have been associated with the use of lidocaine with epinephrine for line blocks.

A caudal epidural anesthesia, which desensitizes the caudal nerve roots as they emerge from the dura, often is indicated if the calf or obstetric manipulations have initiated strong abdominal contractions (Ferguson's reflex). An 18G, 1.5-inch needle can be used to give 2% lidocaine hydrochloride (Lidocaine 2% Injection), 0.2 to 0.4 mg/kg [14–16]. Provided that the recommended maximal volume of 0.5 mL/50 kg is not exceeded, the caudal epidural should not affect motor control of the hind limbs. The onset of a properly placed epidural is usually within minutes. An anterior epidural anesthesia can be used as an alternative that provides flank anesthesia and may be administered using one of three techniques: at the lumbosacral (L6–S1) position (1 mL/4.5 kg) or at either the sacral-coccygeal (S5–Co1) or the first intercoccygeal (Co1–2) space (40–150 mL for an adult cow) [15]. In contrast to the caudal epidural, the anterior epidural does affect motor control of the hind limbs. A modified dorsolumbar epidural anesthesia was described for flank surgery in 40 adult cattle [17]. A 16G, 120-mm-long Tuohy needle

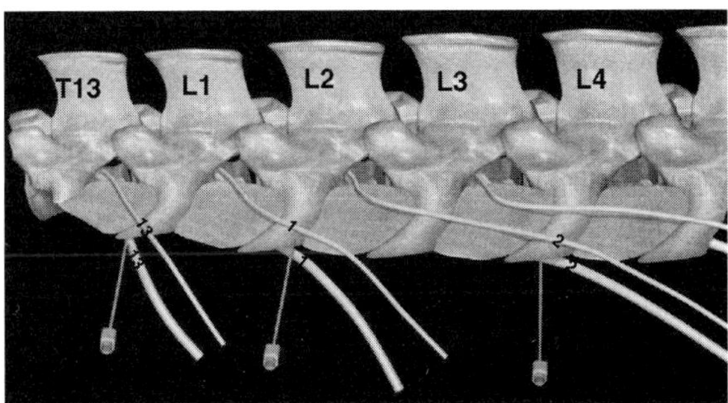

Fig. 4. The distal paravertebral block, shown on the left lateral aspect. T13, L1, L2, L3, and L4 are the spinous processes of the last thoracic and first, second, third, and fourth lumbar vertebrae. Note location of T13 (13), L1 (1), and L2 (2) nerves and the placement of needles.

was inserted into the first interlumbar epidural space. A maximal volume of 5 mL containing 0.025 mg/kg of xylazine and 0.1 mg/kg of lidocaine in 0.9% sodium chloride was used successfully for standing laparotomy in cattle without either adverse effects or requiring additional local anesthesia.

A xylazine caudal epidural has been described in the literature [18–20]. Xylazine, (0.05–0.07 mg/kg) is diluted with 0.9% sodium chloride (0.9% Sodium Chloride) to provide a final volume of 5 to 7.5 mL. Excessive systemic effects, such as low head carriage, partially closed eyes, drooping lower lip, excessive salivation with drooling, low moaning, and partial ruminal atomy with moderate ruminal distention, were observed when volumes of 10 mL or greater were used [18]. Sedation, in addition to paralumbar anesthesia for at least 2 hours [19], was achieved by a single epidural administration. Cows became mildly ataxic (but remained standing) in 80% of the cases. Xylazine epidural has a delayed onset of approximately 30 minutes. Additional local anesthetic was required in 15% to 20% of the cows [20]. Consequently, this technique may not be the most efficient in field situations. Other systemic effects of xylazine with this technique have been observed in healthy cows: heart rate, respiratory rate, ruminal contraction rate, arterial blood pressure, alveolar oxygen partial pressure, packed cell volume (PVC), and total solids were significantly ($P < .05$) decreased, whereas alveolar carbon dioxide partial pressure, base excess, and bicarbonate concentrations were significantly ($P < .05$) increased [19]. This study cautions that the use of the xylazine epidural should be restricted to healthy cows. This technique can be used in conjunction with local techniques to enhance sedation and analgesia in uncooperative patients and to decrease straining if indicated. Provided that the maximal 7.5-mL volume is not exceeded, a portion of the 0.9% sodium chloride volume can be substituted with 2% lidocaine for a more complete caudal epidural anesthesia without inducing ataxia [16].

When performing local anesthesia with small ruminants, accumulation of a toxic dose of lidocaine (>5 mg/kg) [14] should be avoided. The clinical signs of systemic toxicity are predominantly central nervous system signs, including drowsiness, convulsions, respiratory depression, and cardiovascular collapse potentially leading to death [14–16]. Toxicity is treated with intravenous fluids and supportive care. The volume of 2% lidocaine required to elicit systemic toxicity is approximately 0.2 mL/kg or 9 mL/45kg. In small ruminants, the authors find it safest first to draw up the maximal lidocaine dose for the patient in a syringe and dilute the lidocaine with 0.9% sodium chloride to achieve a final concentration of 1% lidocaine before administering the local block.

Surgical preparation

Hair removal by clipping alone has been reported to incite fewer skin reactions with no significant difference in incisional infections compared with clipping and shaving [21]. No significant difference was observed between chlorhexidine gluconate and povidone-iodine. When isopropyl alcohol was used after washing, there were significantly fewer colony-forming units and more negative cultures when chlorhexidine gluconate was used compared with povidone-iodine [22]. Nevertheless, both disinfectants were equally effective in preventing surgical wound infection. Povidone-iodine creates more foam compared with chlorhexidine; there is a tendency to apply more disinfectant and to scrub more when using chlorhexidine. Chlorhexidine gluconate is less likely to mask the degree of cleanliness because its use likely facilitates observing when the skin surface is sufficiently clean.

Surgical technique

Details of the surgical techniques for performing a cesarean section are well described in the literature [1,7,14]. The abdominal wall incision should be sufficiently large to remove the fetus safely through the abdominal wall. A small abdominal incision tends to increase the level of difficulty in removing the fetus and increases the risk of subcutaneous emphysema or seroma formation or both. After identifying the uterus, the portion of the uterus containing a hind leg is pulled up into the abdominal incision. Placing one hand under the hock or hocks and the other on the dorsal aspect of the pastern facilitates "locking" the foot into the abdominal incision (Figs. 5 and 6). With breech or posterior presentations, the front limb is grasped. This presentation increases the level of difficulty exteriorizing the uterus and may require a larger incision. During ventral approaches, the greater

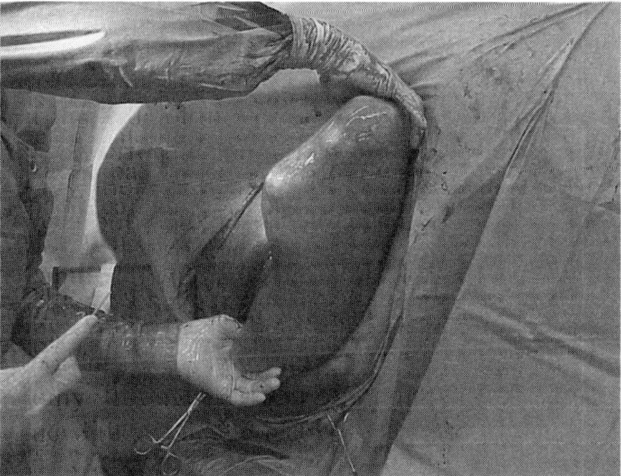

Fig. 5. By grasping the hock and the fetlock, the uterus may be manipulated up to the incision and exteriorized. (Courtesy of Matt Miesner, DVM, MS, The Ohio State University, Columbus, OH.)

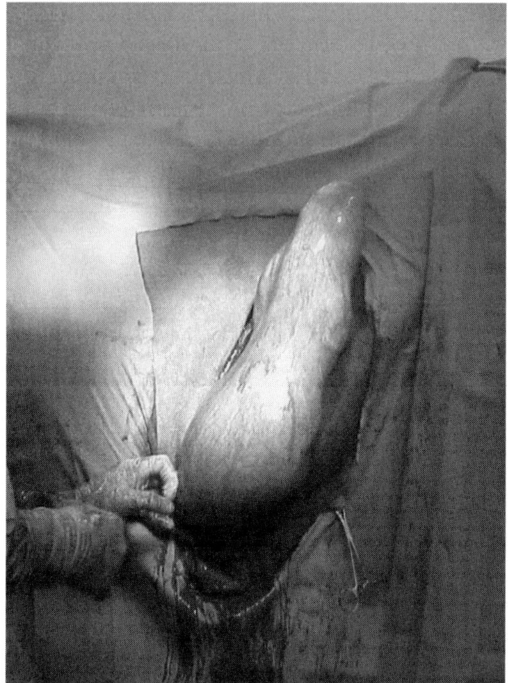

Fig. 6. The uterus locked into the incision. (Courtesy of Matt Miesner, DVM, MS, The Ohio State University, Columbus, OH.)

omentum often must be retracted cranially when the uterus is located within the omental sling. The greater curvature of the uterus should be partially exteriorized and an incision made along the greater curvature of the uterus. This incision avoids most blood vessels and caruncles. A small uterine incision increases the risk of tearing the uterus during fetal extraction. Uterine tears most often occur at angles to the uterine incision; this increases the difficulty in closing the uterus.

Under ideal circumstances, spillage of uterine contents into the abdomen should be avoided. When both legs are exteriorized (and sometimes the head if dealing with a posterior presentation), calving chains can be placed on the calf's legs to facilitate fetal extraction. While the calf is being extracted, the uterus needs to be held in place to prevent spillage of uterine contents into the abdomen. This process can be facilitated using bovine uterine grasping forceps. Large beef calves often are extracted without uterine exteriorization without affected morbidity or mortality in the cows because obstetric manipulations have been minimized and the calf is usually alive. Although dairy clients likely observe their calving cows more frequently compared with beef clients, the higher calf and cow survival likely represents client and breed economic bias. In beef cattle, the calf is the primary return on investment compared with dairy cattle, in which the cow's milk production is often valued greater than calf survival. Beef clients may be more likely to seek veterinary attention sooner compared with dairy clients. For these reasons, it is the authors' impression that more positive outcomes occur with beef cattle cesarean sections compared with dairy cattle cesarean sections.

The umbilical cord should be stretched and ruptured in a controlled fashion by holding it adjacent to the abdominal wall. Normal retraction and contraction of the umbilical arteries may be impaired by surgical excision of the umbilical cord. If elective cesarean section is performed, careful attention is paid to the umbilical vessels, as there is increased likelihood of excess hemorrhage because the umbilical vessels are not prepared for spontaneous rupture. Temporary clamping of the umbilical arteries and vein may be required. In the authors' experience, umbilical complications are seen in 30% of calves delivered by cesarean section; most infections occurred in calves that required either umbilical clamping or suturing. Clone calves tend to be especially prone because their umbilicus tends to be larger and their body walls thinner compared with normal calves. After the calf is removed, the veterinarian *always* should check for a second calf. The authors' preferred technique is to use an arm in a sweeping motion around the uterus to maximize uterine exteriorization and facilitate suturing the uterus incision. If the placenta readily detaches from the caruncles, it should be removed; otherwise the veterinarian should trim the portion that is hanging outside the uterus to prevent its inclusion into the closure of the uterus.

If the calf is alive and the uterus is healthy (ie, an elective procedure), one layer of closure with absorbable suture material, such as 2 chromic catgut (Chromicgut USP 2), using a swaged-on needle is sufficient. Two-layer closure is recommended if the calf is dead or contaminated uterine fluids are suspected to be present (ie, an emergency or emphysematous procedure), or the uterine wall is compromised or torn during fetal extraction. Closing the uterus can be facilitated by having an assistant hold the uterine horn dorsal to the uterine incision and permitting the uterus to hang down vertically—the two sides of the uterine incision are more closely opposed, facilitating suturing. Continuous inverting suture patterns, such as the Cushing (Fig. 7), Utrecht (Figs. 8–12), and Lembert (Fig. 13), should be used because they provide a tight seal, minimize suture exposure, and promote healing, as the uterus heals initially by serosal-to-serosal contact. The blood clots should be teased away gently using irrigation and a gloved hand because these clots may give rise to adhesions that can affect future fertility adversely. Gauze sponges should not be used to wipe the uterus clean because this causes serosal abrasion, which increases the likelihood of detrimental uterine adhesions. Changing to new surgical gloves after the uterus is closed potentially reduces the risk of abdominal contamination.

The abdominal wall usually requires two to three layers of closure. The peritoneum and transversus are usually closed in one layer, using absorbable suture material (eg, 3 chromic catgut) in a simple continuous pattern. When

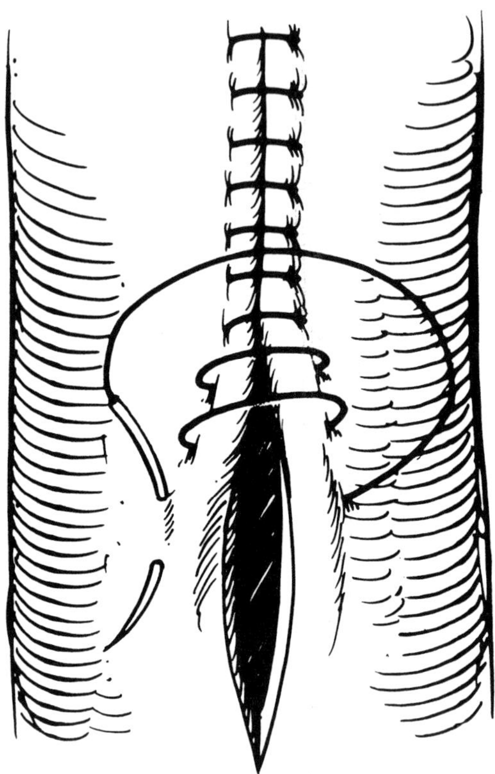

Fig. 7. Continuous Cushing suture pattern. The knots should be buried. Suture placement is well away from the incision margin and parallel to the incision. (*From* Turner AS, McIlwraith CW. Cesarean section in the cow. In: Techniques in large animal surgery. 2nd edition. Philadelphia: Lea & Febiger; 1989:101; with permission.)

the first layer is almost closed, an assistant (usually the client) should push on the opposite abdominal wall to push out the extra air inside the abdominal cavity. The internal and external abdominal oblique muscles are closed together using absorbable suture material (eg, 3 chromic gut) in a simple continuous pattern. The internal abdominal oblique may be incorporated to the first layer when peritoneum and transversus are tearing in thin or excessively straining cows; the external abdominal oblique is then sutured alone. Excessive straining may be minimized using sedation, using an epidural, and or placing a nasotracheal tube. A nasotracheal tube prevents closure of the glottis, preventing positive thoracic pressure against the diaphragm, which restricts abdominal straining. To reduce dead space and potential seroma formation, the layers can be periodically tacked down to the preceding layer. The skin can be closed using either a continuous ford interlocking, simple interrupted cruciate, or simple interrupted sutures using 3 polyamide (Braunamid USP 3). If the ford interlocking pattern is used, the

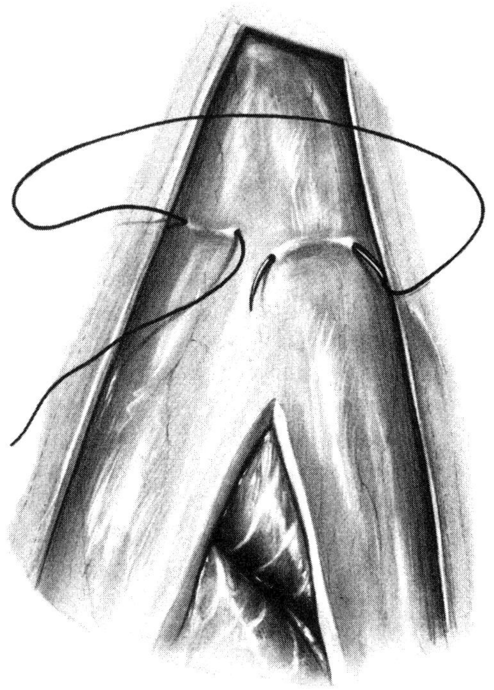

Fig. 8. The Utrecht suture pattern is started by burying the knot. Placement of the knot is well above the incision. This technique of burying the knot also may be used to start the continuous Cushing and Lembert suture patterns. (*From* Turner AS, McIlwraith CW. Cesarean section in the cow. In: Techniques in large animal surgery. 2nd edition. Philadelphia: Lea & Febiger; 1989:277–83; with permission.)

current recommendation is to place several simple interrupted sutures at the base of the incision. These sutures could be removed to facilitate drainage in the event of an incisional infection.

In cases of uncorrected uterine torsions, there is some debate whether the uterus should be detorsed before or after removal of the calf. Uterine torsions in the bovine are most often counterclockwise (63%) rotation [23] when viewed from behind the dam, with the right gravid horn rotated over the left nongravid horn. Of 164 hospital referral cases, cesarean section was required in 62% of the cows [23]. If the calf is removed first, the incision is in the horn opposite the body wall incision, which may make suturing the uterine incision more difficult. To exteriorize the uterus, the uterus must be manipulated to the abdominal incision. First, the veterinarian reaches with both arms under the gravid uterus and locks the hands around the dorsal aspect of the gravid uterine horn. Second, the veterinarian pulls down and toward himself or herself with both hands to complete the rotation. This technique can be used whenever the gravid horn is located away from the

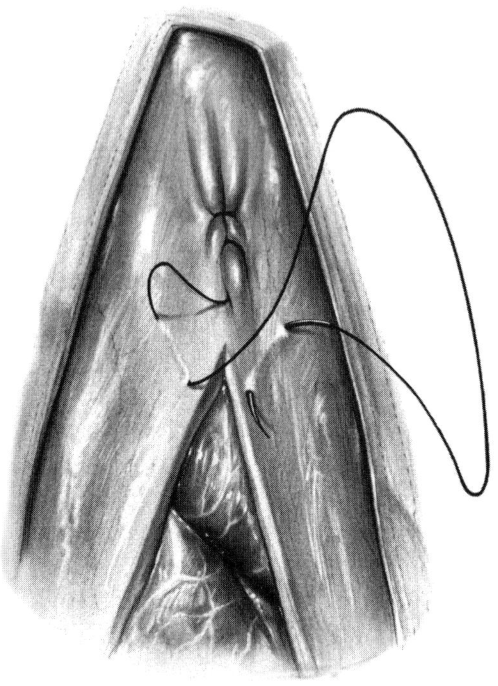

Fig. 9. Utrecht suture pattern. Note suture placement is angled 45° toward the incision. The knot is buried when the suture line is tightened. (*From* Turner AS, McIlwraith CW. Cesarean section in the cow. In: Techniques in large animal surgery. 2nd edition. Philadelphia: Lea & Febiger; 1989:277–83; with permission.)

abdominal incision. Occasionally during a left paralumbar fossa approach, the cow's abdominal strains prolapse the rumen through the incision, preventing exteriorization of the uterus. Using a stomach tube as a nasotracheal tube inhibits the cow from building up positive abdominal pressures, reducing rumen prolapse. The cow's position and the rumen may prevent manipulation and exteriorization of the uterus under rare circumstances, especially during a left paralumbar approach. In the most extreme cases, a rumenotomy before the hysterotomy is performed to remove sufficient rumen contents to permit completion of the cesarean section. This option is considered as a last resort.

Suture materials

Tensile strength is defined as the force required to break the suture divided by the cross-sectional area of the suture material. In using this formula, suture material of differing sizes can be compared objectively (Table 1). Despite having the highest initial tensile strength compared with

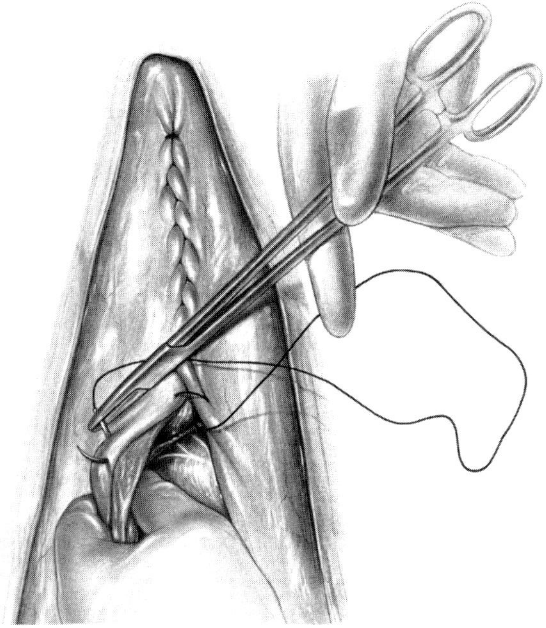

Fig. 10. Continuation of the Utrecht suture pattern. Suture placement is well away from the incision margin. (*From* Turner AS, McIlwraith CW. Cesarean section in the cow. In: Techniques in large animal surgery. 2nd edition. Philadelphia: Lea & Febiger; 1989:277–83; with permission.)

other suture materials, polyglecaprone 25 (Monocryl) also has rapid loss of tensile strength and rapid absorption characteristics. Polyglecaprone 25 should not be used for muscle or linea alba closure. Because of growing concerns regarding the transmission of bovine spongiform encephalopathy, the use of catgut in certain affected countries is prohibited [24].

Postoperative care

The use, type, and frequency of antibiotics vary on a case-by-case basis. The most commonly used antibiotics are penicillin G procaine (US Vet Hanford's US Vet Products Sterile penicillin G procaine; 22,000 U/kg intramuscularly every 24 hours for 3–5 days), oxytetracycline (Oxycure 200; 19.8 mg/kg intravenously, intramuscularly, or subcutaneously every 1–3 days), or ceftiofur (Naxcel or Excenel) (1 mg/kg intravenously, intramuscularly, or subcutaneously every 12–24 hours for 3–5 days). In beef cattle, florfenicol (Nuflor) (20 mg/kg intramuscularly every 48 hours or 40 mg/kg subcutaneously every 96 hours) has been used. The appropriate milk and meat withdrawals need to be followed. If required, off-label use of antibiotics should be done cautiously and with close attention to preventing

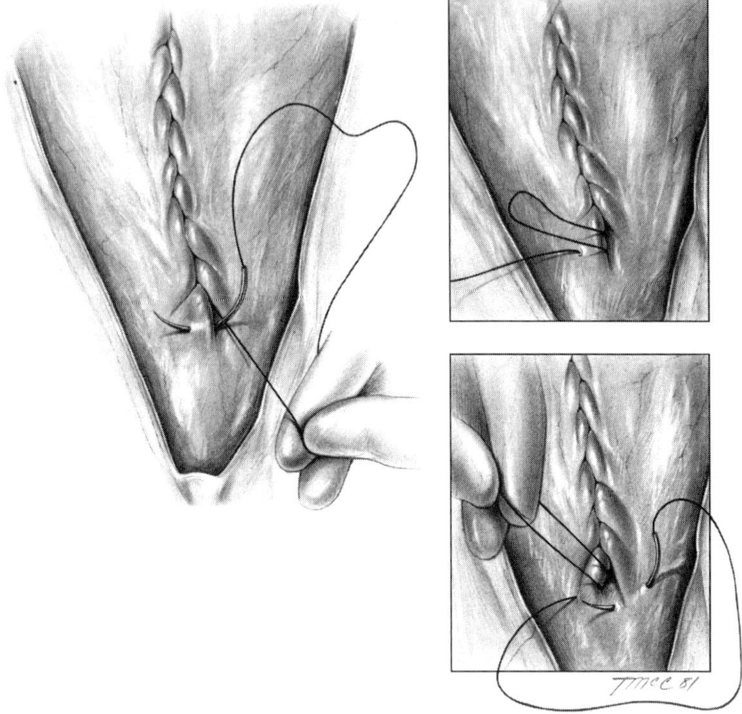

Fig. 11. The Utrecht suture pattern is ended by burying the knot. This technique of burying the knot also may be used to complete the continuous Cushing and Lembert suture patterns. (*From* Turner AS, McIlwraith CW. Cesarean section in the cow. In: Techniques in large animal surgery. 2nd edition. Philadelphia: Lea & Febiger; 1989:277–83; with permission.)

residue violations. Flunixin meglumine (Banamine) (1 mg/kg intravenously or intramuscularly every 12 hours for 2 days) may be useful to prevent abdominal adhesion formation.

Elective or uncomplicated cesarean sections in which there is a live calf, healthy cow, healthy uterus, minimal obstetric manipulation preoperatively, and minimal abdominal contamination during calf extraction likely do not require antibiotics. Antibiotics are indicated when the calf is dead, when there is a prolonged dystocia, when there is a compromised uterus, when extensive obstetric manipulations occurred preoperatively, and when abdominal contamination has occurred. In the authors' experience, intravenous oxytetracycline for 5 to 7 days is the antibiotic of choice when the concern for postoperative peritonitis is high (ie, an emphysematous fetus).

Standing flank incisions require little postoperative care and attention compared with ventral approaches. Cows with flank incisions often do not require stall rest that provides restricted activity and can be rebred using a bull without undue concern regarding abdominal wall herniation. In contrast, ventral approaches require strict stall rest for 6 weeks. Although

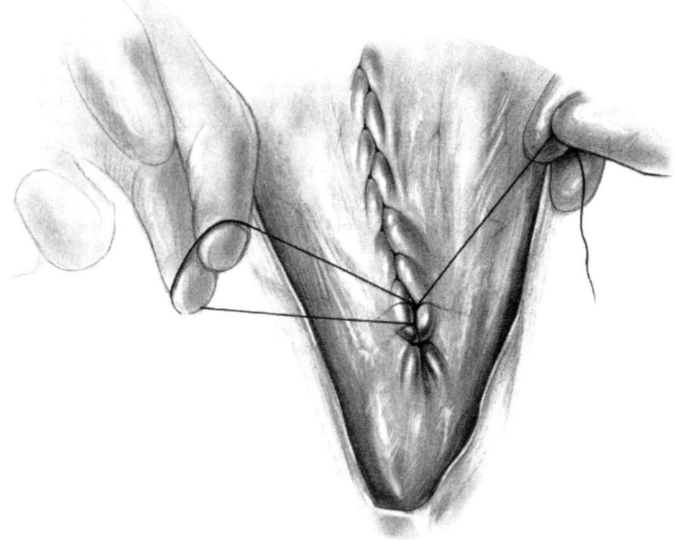

Fig. 12. Completing the Utrecht suture pattern. Pulling the suture ends parallel to the incision ensures the knot is buried. This technique of burying the knot also may be used to complete the continuous Cushing and Lembert suture patterns. (*From* Turner AS, McIlwraith CW. Cesarean section in the cow. In: Techniques in large animal surgery. 2nd edition. Philadelphia: Lea & Febiger; 1989:277–83; with permission.)

these cows may be rebred using artificial insemination at 6 weeks, they should not be mounted by either their herd mates or the bull until 8 weeks after surgery, the time required to allow the ventral incisions to reach maximal holding strength.

Complications

An extensive list of preoperative, operative, postoperative, and long-term complications has been reported previously [25]. Preoperative complications include delayed delivery, anorexia, fetal death, emphysematous fetus, forced extraction, fetal abnormalities, fetal limb fractures, uterine inertia, uterine trauma, uterine rupture, obturator/sciatic nerve damage, and severe trauma during manipulation. Operative complications include excessive uterine trauma, peritoneal cavity contamination, gastrointestinal trauma, excessive trauma to abdominal wall, and inadequate uterine closure. Postoperative complications include peritonitis, seroma formation, retained placenta, metritis, endometritis, skin suture dehiscence, subcutaneous emphysema, adhesions, mastitis, straining cow, and calf death. Long-term complications include downer cow, debilitated cows, production losses, increased calving-service intervals, increased services per conception, spontaneous abortions,

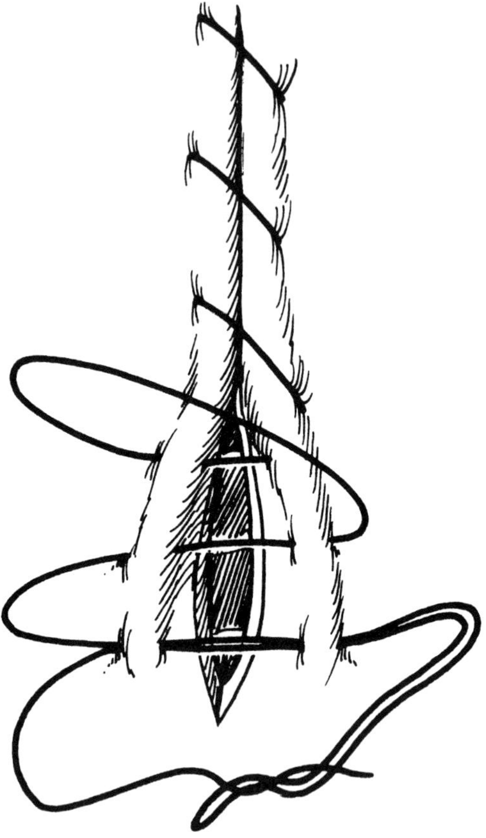

Fig. 13. Continuous Lembert suture pattern. Suture placement is well away from the incision margin and perpendicular to the incision. The knot should be buried, as shown in Figs. 11 and 12. (*From* Turner AS, McIlwraith CW. Cesarean section in the cow. In: Techniques in large animal surgery. 2nd edition. Philadelphia: Lea & Febiger; 1989:101; with permission.)

and infertility. One study observed that 30% of the cows had poor appetite, fever, metritis, or diarrhea after cesarean section [26].

Case selection

Case selection may be the most easily overlooked issue by clients and veterinarians. A cesarean section tends to be a self-fulfilling prophecy [7,26,27]. When a cesarean section is considered an option of last resort, a negative outcome is more likely. When a cesarean section is chosen early in dystocia cases, the procedure is more rewarding, and clients are more agreeable to future cesarean sections. Categorizing the procedure as an elective, emergency (nonemphysematous), or emphysematous procedure is worthwhile because the expected outcomes and anticipated complications are

Table 1
Absorbable suture materials, handling, absorption and tensile strength characteristics, and uses

Suture type	Material	Material handling characteristics	Absorption characteristics	Tensile strength remaining	Use
Chromic catgut	Submucosa of cow/sheep, braided	Easy to handle, poor knot security, rapid breakdown when infection present	Phagocytosis by cell and tissue proteases	50% at 7 d 30% at 14 d 0% at 21 d	Uterus, muscle layers
Vicryl	Polyglactin 910, braided	Easy to handle, poor knot security, capillary action	Hydrolysis[a], in 60–90 d	75% at 14 d 50% at 21 d 8% at 28 d 0% at 35 d	Uterus, muscle layers, linea alba
PDS II	Polydioxanone, monofilament	Difficult to handle, has memory	Hydrolysis, in 180 d	70% at 14 d 25% at 42 d 0% at 90 d	Uterus, muscle layers, linea alba
Monocryl	Polyglecaprone 25, monofilament	Good knot security	Hydrolysis, in 110 d	40% at 14 d 0% at 28 d	Uterus only

[a] Hydrolysis is the process by which the suture material is degraded by the addition of water and metabolized.

Data from Desrochers A, Harvey D. Surgeries of the abomasum in cattle. Montreal: University of Montreal; 2002 and Blackford LW, Blackford JT. Suture materials and patterns. In: Auer JA, Stick JA, editors. Equine surgery, second edition. Philadelphia: WB Saunders; 1999. p. 91–103.

dramatically different for these three situations. It generally is accepted that the condition of the cow at the time of surgery is a major determining factor deciding outcome [7,25,26]. Cows undergoing elective cesarean sections are less likely to encounter intraoperative and postoperative complications. Cows having an emergency cesarean section are more likely to encounter intraoperative and postoperative complications (ie, peritonitis) and are less likely to survive compared with cows that had an elective cesarean.

The ideal emergency case is a dam that has been in labor briefly, with a live calf, and the decision to perform a cesarean section is made quickly without prolonged obstetric manipulation by either the client or the attending veterinarian. A survey conducted in Ireland revealed that 12.7 minutes was the average (range 0–60 minutes) time spent trying to deliver a calf before deciding on surgery [8]. Another practitioner survey revealed that rapid clinical assessment was associated with improved successful outcomes [27]. Excessive manipulations by the owner and veterinarian alike were associated with higher postoperative complications. If the legs and the head cannot be manipulated into the birth canal, the decision to perform a cesarean section should be immediate. In beef breeds, there should be sufficient room in the pelvic canal for the calf's head and legs with space remaining to sweep an arm around the calf's shoulders to extract the fetus safely through the birth canal.

Exteriorizing the uterus

A bovine cesarean section is considered a clean-contaminated procedure. Exteriorizing the uterus and avoiding abdominal contamination is most important when dealing with a dead calf and after extensive obstetric manipulations. The most common intraoperative complication observed in a study of 1000 cesarean sections was exteriorizing the uterus (20.8% difficult, 5.8% impossible) [28]. More experienced surgeons seemed to have less difficulty in exteriorizing the uterus. The study found that increased parity, increased uterine contractions, posterior presentations, and abdominal adhesions were associated with increasing significance with the degree of difficulty in exteriorizing the uterus [28]. Overall, cows in which the uterus was exteriorized during the surgery were more likely to survive. When the uterus was not exteriorized, improved survival was noted in cows that had a live fetus. Improved survival was observed in cows in which the uterus was exteriorized to remove a dead fetus compared with when the uterus was not exteriorized.

Retained fetal membranes

The bovine placenta typically is shed within 24 hours after surgery [27]; a retained fetal membrane is failure to shed the placenta within this time period. In one study of 133 cases, the placenta was removed easily during surgery in 6% of cows, and 59% shed the placenta within 12 hours [26]. The occurrence of retained fetal membranes was 35% to 40.8% [26,29]. These rates generally are accepted as being higher compared with unassisted calvings.

In cases when the placenta was not removed during surgery, low doses (20–40 IU) of oxytocin (Oxytocin Injection) frequently may be administered intramuscularly postoperatively, provided that the cervix is open [7]. Administering oxytocin when the cervix is closed increases the pressure on the suture line [7] and likely would increase the risk of uterine incisional dehiscence. If the fetal membranes have not been shed by 24 hours postoperatively, oxytocin may be continued on days 2 and 3 postcalving at 20 USP every 3 hours, then increasing the dose and frequency of oxytocin to 30 USP every 2 hours on day 4 [30]. Smaller doses administered more frequently are recommended rather than high doses administered less frequently. Smaller doses induce productive uterine contractions in a tubulo-cervical manner, whereas high doses seem to cause tetanic-like spasms, which can last 6 to 10 minutes [30].

Uterine relaxants

In three European practitioner surveys, uterine relaxants at the time of surgery are used frequently (50–100%) [8,26,27]. The use of uterine relaxants may be a confounding variable not accounted for in the European studies. When the uterus has contracted tightly on the fetus, it is more difficult either to correct malpresentations or to exteriorize the uterus during a cesarean section. Clenbuterol and isoxsuprine have been available to bovine practitioners as aids in obstetric manipulation [31,32]. Presently, these drugs are not permitted for use in food-producing animals in North America. Isoxsuprine has sympathomimetic properties, with structural similarities to epinephrine [31]. Epinephrine (Epinephrine Injection) may have inherent tocolytic pharmacologic properties. An empirical dose of 10 mL of 1:1000 epinephrine, diluted in isotonic fluid, administered intravenously 10 minutes preoperatively seems to relax the uterus, facilitating exteriorizing the uterus. Ritodrine, another β_2-adrenergic agonist, has been administered experimentally in dairy cows, providing effective relaxation of the myometrium [33]. The authors have noted the uterine wall tends to thin secondary to the relaxed myometrium, which makes closing the uterine incision more challenging. A small tapered needle is required to avoid full-thickness bites, and the sutures need to be placed more closely together to ensure proper closure of the uterus.

Uterine tears

Tearing the uterus during surgery accounted for 6.8% of complications [28], which is comparable to the authors' experience. No difference was observed in cow survival with uterine tears and whether the calf was alive or dead at the time of surgery. Only cows with uterine tears and emphysematous fetuses at the time of surgery were killed. The impact of uterine tears on adhesion formation and reproductive efficiency is not known.

Recumbency

Cows may become recumbent during surgery (14.8%) [28]. It is believed that cows are more likely to become recumbent during attempts to exteriorize the uterus. Falling down during surgery is believed to a consequence of pain that arises from traction on the broad ligament during difficult uterine manipulations. Administration of xylazine epidural preoperatively or butorphanol tartrate intraoperatively may reduce painful stimuli. The authors have observed that these cows were more likely to develop peritonitis and experienced greater postoperative mortality compared with cows that remained standing during the surgery. Cows that remain standing during the procedure have a better chance of survival, with reports of 91% to 94% cow survival rate and a 95% to 100% calf survival rate [26]. Another study observed a 94% cow survival rate, and that 100% of the calves alive at the start of surgery survived.

Mortality

A retrospective study that looked at 159 dairy cow cesarean sections found a strong correlation between cow survival and calf viability at the time of surgery [29]. Cow survival decreased from 86% with a live calf, to 79% with a dead calf, to 33% with an emphysematous fetus. Surgery time greater than 1 hour reduced the dam survival rate from 96% to 86% [27]. The most common complications associated with maternal death are peritonitis, toxemia, metritis, uterine rupture, and fatty liver [25]. Infection by *Clostridium chauvoei* distant to the surgery site is reportedly rare (0.5%) and has been associated with sudden death of the cow within 24 hours of surgery [25].

Peritonitis

Clinical signs of peritonitis are expected to occur 3 to 4 days after surgery [1,7,11]. One practitioner survey [8] in 1993 (381 respondents, representing an estimated 60,195 deliveries/year and 10,457 cesareans), observed that the leading cause of mortality (mortality rate not reported) associated with cesarean sections was peritonitis (70.3%), followed by shock (18.1%). Five percent of the respondents did not routinely disinfect the surgical site.

Peritonitis may be caused by compromise of the uterine wall, even before surgery [25]. Peritonitis can be caused by either exogenous (through the abdominal incision) or endogenous bacterial flora [34]. Fetal fluids can become contaminated by obligate, anaerobic vaginal bacterial flora, especially after either rupturing the amniotic sac or extensive obstetric manipulations. Bacteria can be cultured from uterine fluids before amniotic sac rupture; however, their numbers increase significantly after the sac is ruptured. During cesarean section, the uterine fluids are found to be heavily contaminated 83% of the time by a polymicrobial population; this validates the classification of this surgery as a clean-contaminated procedure, warranting the use of antibiotics in most cows. Traditionally the appropriate antibiotic selection is directed toward the anticipated bacteria of the postpartum uterus. Fifty percent of cows that had a normal calving on two hygienically contrasting farms were positive on uterine culture. *Arcanobacterium pyogenes* (formerly known as *Actinomyces pyogenes*) was the most common isolate, followed by *Escherichia coli*, *Fusobacterium nucleatum*, *Proteus mirabilis*, and *Bacteroides melanogenicus* [35]. Enterobacteriaceae, *Clostridium,* and *Actinomyces* have been cultured from peritonitis and incisional infections [28]. This study also observed that despite the apparent bacterial contamination, the incidence of peritonitis was relatively low at 10.5%.

Adhesions

An imbalance between fibrin formation and fibrinolysis is thought to result in adhesion formation. Adhesions can be clinically irrelevant, beneficial, or detrimental. Detrimental effects of adhesions include partial and complete intestinal obstruction, pain, and infertility. The significance of adhesions is determined by their degree and location. Detrimental adhesions in the bovine abdomen after cesarean section are associated primarily with elements of the reproductive tract; the ovary, infundibulum, oviduct, and uterus in descending order are the most crucial elements with respect to future fertility. Preexisting uterine adhesions were found in 9.4% of cows compared with 31% of cows that had had a previous cesarean section [28]. Other studies observed rates of uterine adhesions of 20% to 60% [34]. Halsted's principles of surgery have been viewed as the mainstay of adhesion prevention [36,37]. One study that looked at the complications associated with standing cesarean sections observed a significant difference between surgeons and adhesion formation [34].

Suture type has been the subject of great debate with regard to adhesion formation. Although no advantage was observed using polyglactin 910 compared with plain catgut [38], synthetic materials have significant advantages over biologic material. Advantages of polyglactin 910 include uniform material quality, less readily damaged by surgical instruments, superior handling qualities (ie, less stiff, knot tying, less fraying), and a mild inflammatory reaction compared with plain catgut. It is not known whether polyglactin 910 induces less scar formation within the myometrium, which could have a positive effect on future fertility. The disadvantages of polyglactin 910 are increased drag (because it is braided) and cost. It generally is accepted that suture exposure (especially at the knots) rather than the type of suture material is thought to be the most significant cause of adhesions along the uterine incision. It is likely beneficial to bury knots while closing the uterine incision (see Figs. 8 and 11).

Continuous inverting patterns that do not take full-thickness bites, such as the Lembert, Cushing, or Utrecht, are preferred because these patterns provide an excellent seal and minimize suture exposure. According to two European practitioner surveys [8,26], the Lembert was most commonly used (73–88.2%) compared with the Cushing (5.8%) or Utrecht (6%), using either chromic (87.2%) or plain (10.6%) suture. A third European study used the Lembert pattern exclusively [27]. No difference between the Lembert and Utrecht suture patterns and adhesion formation was noted [34]. Instead, this study revealed a dramatic difference between surgeons and adhesion formation. This study illustrates the basic principle of good surgical technical skill and how this can affect adhesion formation. The primary disadvantages of the Lembert pattern are it requires more suture material, has more suture material exposed, and, in the authors' experience, takes more time to complete. When the uterus is closed, blood clots and debris from the serosal surface of the uterus must be removed. The ovarian bursa should be examined because blood clots can lodge there, cause adhesions, and affect future fertility adversely. Gauze squares used to help remove blood clots should be avoided because the gauze mechanically removes the thin mesothelial layer on the serosal surface of the uterus, which can predispose to the likelihood of adhesion formation and affect fertility adversely. Provided that the uterus is kept moist, sterile physiologic saline or lactated Ringer's solution is sufficient to rinse off blood clots adhered to the uterus. After rinsing, the uterus is replaced inside the abdomen.

The authors believe that the prerequisites for adhesion formation are (1) tissue trauma, (2) bacteria, and (3) inflammation. Adhesion prevention includes good surgical technique, antibiotics, and nonsteroidal anti-inflammatory drugs. When appropriate, nonsteroidal anti-inflammatory drugs (ie, flunixin meglumine or ketoprofen) and antibiotics are administered for 48 to 72 hours postoperatively.

Abdominal lavage and, depending on the surgeon, a combination of heparin (40 U/kg) and potassium penicillin G (22,000 U/kg), ceftiofur (1 mg/kg), or oxytetracycline hydrochloride (200 mg/kg) mixed in 500 mL of 0.9% sodium chloride irrigation solution and instilled into the abdomen is used empirically to reduce adhesion formation. Postoperatively, flunixin meglumine is administered (1 mg/kg intravenously or intramuscularly every 12 hours) for 3 days to reduce adhesion formation. In addition, there may some scientific merit to administering flunixin meglumine (1 mg/kg IV) before surgery, applying 1% sodium carboxymethyl cellulose (CSMC) on the uterine incision and administering heparin (40 USP/kg intravenously) intraoperatively, and administering heparin (40 USP/kg subcutaneously every 12 hours for 2 days) postoperatively [39].

Incisional complications

Disadvantages of the recumbent approaches include increased surgical time and increased risks of intraoperative hemorrhage, postoperative seroma formation, and incisional herniations. The increased vascularity and muscle tissues associated with the paramedian approach were thought to enhance healing and reduce incisional herniation [5]. The advantage of the midline approach is that the linea alba provides a stronger holding layer compared with the paramedian or the low oblique approach. The thin facial layers with interposed muscle layers may be why the lateral approaches are more likely to herniate. There are fewer layers of closure compared with the paramedian or the low oblique approach, which reduces surgery time. Adhesions between the uterus and the body wall incision tend to be more dramatic with the ventral approaches.

There are few reports in the literature of paralumbar incisional complications. Two practitioner surveys reported infection rates of 1.3% to 8.2% and dehiscence rates of 3.8% [27]. One study reported an incisional infection rate of 15% [3] caused by *Actinobacillus lignieresii*. It is believed the veterinarian spreads this infection by either poor aseptic technique or inadequately sterilized equipment. Subcutaneous emphysema rates have been reported to be 0% to 41% [11,26,27]. Subcutaneous emphysema can be avoided by closing the peritoneum along with the transversus, sealing the abdomen. These numbers are fraught with confounding variables. Differences in surgical site preparation; local anesthetic technique; length of incision; difficulty removing the calf through the incision; time of surgery; and the use, type, and duration of postoperative antibiotics make it difficult to make clear inferences. Applying pressure to the opposite abdominal wall to expel intra-abdominal air during closure of the first layer also has been suggested as a means to reduce subcutaneous emphysema [25].

Fertility

Cesarean section in dairy cattle did not change the interval to first service or subsequent gestation length [40]. The calving to first service was 81 ± 29 days in dairy cattle [26]. Cows having a cesarean section had an increase in services per conception and days open [1,25]. The number of services per conception was 2.1 ± 1.4 for dairy cows and 1.2 ± 0.4 for beef cows [26]. The calving to conception interval was 110 ± 43 days in dairy cattle and 99 ± 18 days in beef cattle. No difference in the rate of abortion between cesarean sections and normal deliveries was observed [40]. The overall pregnancy rate in dairy and beef cows that had had cesarean sections has been shown to be 72% and 91% [26]. These rates seem reasonable for routine cases. The lower pregnancy rates in the dairy cattle could be attributed to confounding variables, such as culling for nonreproductive reasons (eg, lameness). It is possible the apparent culling for reproductive reasons is an overestimation of the true rate. It is generally accepted that beef cows likely tolerate surgery better with better outcomes because they are usually in better body condition and have significantly lower metabolic demands compared with high producing dairy cows. In beef cows, infertility increased as the level of calving assistance was required, especially when a cesarean section was performed (odds ratio = 6 of a cow being infertile after cesarean section) [41]. The effect of body condition was not considered in this study and may have been a confounding variable in the pregnancy rates. Poorly conditioned and overly conditioned cows are well known to be difficult to get pregnant.

Production

The effect of a cesarean section on milk production is difficult to elucidate because of numerous confounding variables. In dairy cattle, milk production and lactation after a cesarean section is thought to be reduced by 80 to 1500 L compared with their previous lactation [26,28]. When the effects of herd, year, parity, calving season, and abortion were corrected, cows that had a cesarean section produced were less likely to reach 100 days in milk (DIM) and produced on average 79.9 kg less milk in the first 100 DIM compared with controls [40]. A second study confirmed that the entire milk reduction occurs during the first 100 DIM [42]. No difference was observed between groups between 100 DIM and 240 DIM [40].

In the Netherlands, dairy cattle frequently are crossbred to beef sires. A risk-benefit economic study considered the extra income received by Dutch dairies compared with the increased costs associated with cesarean sections. Based on the extra return from crossbred calve sales, the odds ratio would have to increase to 26 before being economically unjustifiable in Dutch dairies [40]. The overall risk of being culled is higher for cows with cesarean sections compared with controls [42].

Emphysematous fetus

Removing an emphysematous fetus by fetotomy is not always a viable option. Of 159 dairy cows referred to the veterinary hospital for cesarean section, 16 cows had emphysematous fetuses—6 cows (33%) survived and were released from the hospital [29]. A paramammary approach was used to remove these calves. Not only are these results not surprising, but also they are not encouraging for either the client or the veterinarian. In the authors' experience, cows with emphysematous fetuses can be managed successfully with intensive medical treatment, achieving 80% success rate in our hospital. One possible explanation is the intense perioperative patient management. Typically, these cows are toxic, pyrexic, hypotensive, and in shock. A minimal database is collected containing a packed cell volume and total protein. Fluid therapy is initiated usually at shock rates (80 mL/kg/h) [15], using either Ringer's solution or 0.9% sodium chloride. Oxytetracycline, 200 mg/mL (19.8 mg/kg every 24 hours intravenously), and flunixin meglumine, 50 mg/mL (1 mg/kg every 12 hours intravenously), are administered preoperatively. When the cardiovascular system is sufficiently stabilized, the cow either is sedated and a local anesthetic block is performed or is induced, intubated, and maintained on gas anesthetic.

Fluids are continued during surgery. The cow is positioned in right lateral recumbency, with the upper hind leg tied up and back, which facilitates exteriorizing of the uterus. Depending on the surgeon's preference, either a ventral midline or a paramammary approach is used. The ventral midline approach usually is started 10 cm cranial to the umbilicus and is extended just cranial to the udder, avoiding the numerous veins that drain the udder. A Mayo Stand Cover may be used to envelop the exteriorized uterine horn, placing the ends of the cover as deep as possible within the abdominal cavity. The cover effectively isolates the uterus from the abdominal cavity and surgical field. The end of the cover is cut open to reveal the exteriorized uterine horn. The surgical instruments required for the hysterotomy are partitioned on the table, to ensure proper aseptic technique. "Clean" instruments are used to close the body wall. The uterus is exteriorized as much as possible to prevent contamination of the abdominal cavity.

The uterus is incised, the fetus is removed, and the uterus is closed in two inverting layers by a simple continuous Cushing pattern using 2 chromic catgut. The uterus is extensively lavaged to remove blood clots and contaminated fluids, and the cover is removed. Changing to new gloves and, if necessary, new gowns and drapes may reduce abdominal contamination. The clean instruments are used to close the linea alba, subcutaneous layer, and skin. If the cow is in lateral recumbency, the authors find it easier to close the linea alba if the cow is slightly repositioned intraoperatively after closing the uterus, by rotating the hindquarters more into dorsal recumbency. The linea alba is closed using 2 polyglactin 910 in a simple cruciate pattern. The subcutaneous layer is closed using 2 polyglactin 910 in a simple continuous pattern. Careful attention in closing the dead space associated with the subcutaneous layer prevents significant postoperative seroma formation. The skin is closed using 3 polyamide (Braunamid) in a continuous ford interlocking pattern. A few simple interrupted sutures are placed at the cranial portion of the incision because this would be the most dependent portion of the incision when the cow is standing. If necessary, these sutures can be cut to facilitate drainage.

Postoperatively the cow is kept on fluids for 24 hours at a maintenance rate (2 mL/kg/h) [16]. Antibiotics are continued for a minimum of 3 to 7 days. Anti-inflammatories are continued every 12 hours for 3 days, then reduced to every 24 hours for 3 more days. The cow is kept separated in a pen for 4 weeks. Skin sutures are removed after 3 weeks.

Economic analysis questions if it is cost-effective to remove an emphysematous calf surgically. Cow survival represents only a portion of a successful outcome of surgery, and the future reproductive efficiency of the cow is equally important. In the authors' experience, fertility seems to be poor (ie, <25%). An earlier study did not stratify which cows were bred back successfully [29].

Summary

The goals of the cesarean section are preservation of the dam and calf and the future reproductive efficiency of the dam. The outcome of the cesarean section is a self-fulfilling prophecy. Numerous variables may affect the successful outcome of this procedure. Case selection is the most important and often overlooked variable. In addition, skin preparation, surgical technique, calf viability at the time of surgery, and exteriorizing the uterus can affect outcome. Minimizing excessive adhesion formation is equally important because it may affect reproductive efficiency adversely. Good surgical technique, including gentle tissue handling, appropriate suture materials and patterns, and adequate infolding of the uterine incision to prevent leakage, combined with antibiotics and anti-inflammatories when indicated can help minimize detrimental adhesions that may affect adversely the future reproductive efficiency of the cow. When dealing with an emphysematous fetus, intensive medical management perioperatively is a crucial determining factor of cow survival. Anti-inflammatories, high doses of intravenous antibiotics, and a ventral midline approach that permits adequate uterine exteriorization and reduces abdominal contamination also are likely key elements that contribute to the high survival rates of cows with emphysematous fetuses.

References

[1] Campbell M, Fubini S. Indications and surgical approaches for cesarean section in cattle. Compend Cont Educ 1990;12:285–91.

[2] Walker D, Vaughan J. Bovine and equine urogenital surgery. Philadelphia: Lea & Febiger; 1980. p. 85–98.

[3] de Kruif A, Mijten P, Haesebrouck F, Hoorens J, Devriese L. Actinobacillosis in bovine caesarean sections. Vet Rec 1992;131:414–5.

[4] Barkema H, Schukken Y, Guard C, Brand A, van der Weygen G. Cesarean section in dairy cattle: a study of risk factors. Theriogenology 1992;37:489–506.
[5] Noorsdy JL. Selection of an incision site for cesarean section in the cow. Vet Med Small Anim Clin 1979;74:530–7.
[6] Oehme FW. The ventro-lateral cesarean section in the cow. Vet Med Small Anim Clin 1967; 62:889–94.
[7] Frazer GS, Perkins NR. Cesarean section. Vet Clin North Am Food Anim Pract 1995;11: 19–35.
[8] Vaughan L, Mulville P. A survey of bovine cesarean sections in Ireland. Ir Vet J 1995;48: 411–5.
[9] Parish SM, Tyler JW, Ginsky JV. Left oblique celiotomy approach for cesarean section in standing cows. J Am Vet Med Assoc 1995;207:751–2.
[10] Knight AP. Xylazine. J Am Vet Med Assoc 1980;176:454–5.
[11] Sloss V, Dufty JH. Elective caesarean operation in Hereford cattle. Aust Vet J 1977;53: 420–4.
[12] LeBlanc M, Hubbell J, Smith H. The effects of xylazine hydrochloride on uterine pressure in the cow. Theriogenology 1984;21:681–90.
[13] Anderson D, Gaughan E, DeBowes R, Lowry S, Yvorchuck K, St. Jean G. Affects of chemical restraint on the endoscopic appearance of laryngeal and pharyngeal anatomy and sensation in adult cattle. Am J Vet Res 1994;55:1196–200.
[14] Turner S, McIlwraith C. Techniques in large animal surgery. Philadelphia: Lea & Febiger; 1989.
[15] Skarda RT. Local and regional anesthetic techniques: ruminants and swine. In: Thurman J, Tranquilli W, Benson G, editors. Lumb and Jones' Veterinary Anesthesia, third edition. Baltimore: Lippincott Williams & Wilkins; 1996. p. 486–96.
[16] Muir WW, Hubbell J, Skarda RT, Bednarski R. Handbook of veterinary anesthesia, third edition. St. Louis: Mosby; 2000. p. 57–71.
[17] Lee I, Yamagishi N, Oboshi K, Ayukawa Y, Sasaki N, Yamada H. Clinical use of modified dorsolumbar epidural anesthesia in cattle. 23rd World Buiatrics Congress. Quebec City, Quebec, Canada. Med Vet Q 2004;34:156.
[18] Zuagg J, Nussbaum M. Epidural injection of xylazine: a new option for surgical anesthesia of the bovine abdomen and udder. Vet Med 1990;85:1043–6.
[19] St. Jean G, Skarda RT, Muir WW, Hoffis G. Caudal epidural analgesia induced by xylazine administration in cows. Am J Vet Res 1990;8:1232–6.
[20] Caulkett N, Cribb P, Duke D. Xylazine epidural analgesia for cesarean section in cattle. Can Vet J 1993;34:674–6.
[21] Bedard S, Desrochers A, Fecteau G, Higgins R. [Comparison of four protocols for pre-operative preparation in cattle]. Can Vet J 2001;42:199–203.
[22] Desrochers A, St. Jean G, Anderson D, Rogers D, Chengappa M. Comparative evaluation of two surgical scrub preparations in cattle. Vet Surg 1996;25:336–41.
[23] Frazer GS, Perkins NR, Constable PD. Bovine uterine torsion: 164 hospital referral cases. Theriogenology 1996;46:739–58.
[24] Desrochers A, Harvey D. Surgeries of the abomasum in cattle. Montreal: University of Montreal; 2002.
[25] Dehghani S, Ferguson J. Cesarean section in cattle: complications. Compend Cont Educ 1982;4:s387–92.
[26] Cattell JH, Dobson H. A survey of caesarean operations on cattle in general veterinary practice. Vet Rec 1990;127:395–9.
[27] Dawson JC, Murray R. Caesarean sections in cattle attended by a practice in Cheshire. Vet Rec 1992;131:525–7.
[28] Hoeben D, Mijten P, de Kruif A. Factors influencing complications during caesarean section on the standing cow. Vet Q 1997;19:88–92.

[29] Bouchard E, Daignault D, Belanger D, Couture Y. [Cesareans on dairy cows: 159 cases]. Can Vet J 1994;35:770–4.
[30] Frazer G. Hormonal therapy in the postpartum cow—days 1 to 10—fact or fiction. American Association of Bovine Practitioners 2001;34:109–30.
[31] Menard L. Tocolytic drugs for use in veterinary obstetrics. Can Vet J 1984;25:389–93.
[32] Menard L. The use of clenbuterol in large animal obstetrics: manual correction of bovine dystocias. Can Vet J 1994;35:289–92.
[33] Boileau M, Babkine M, Desrochers A. Effet de la ritodine sur le myomètre lors de manipulations obstétricales chez la vache. Med Vet Q 2001;31:191.
[34] Mijten P, van den Bogaard A, Hazen M, de Kruif A. Bacterial contamination of fetal fluids at the time of cesarean section in the cow. Theriogenology 1997;48:513–21.
[35] Noakes D, Wallace L, Smith G. Bacterial flora of uterus of cows after calving on two hygienically contrasting farms. Vet Rec 1991;128:440–2.
[36] Daly WR. Wound infections. In: Slatter D, editor. Textbook of veterinary surgery, second edition. Philadelphia: WB Saunders; 1985. p. 42.
[37] Southwood LL, Baxter GM. Current concepts in management of abdominal adhesions. Vet Clin North Am Equine Pract 1997;13:415–35.
[38] Mijten P, de Kruif A, Van der Weyden GC, Deluyker H. Comparison of catgut and polyglactin 910 for uterine sutures during bovine caesarean sections. Vet Rec 1997;140: 458–9.
[39] Hague BA, Honnas CM, Berridge BR, Easter JL. Evaluation of postoperative peritoneal lavage in standing horses for prevention of experimentally induced abdominal adhesions. Vet Surg 1998;27:122–6.
[40] Barkema H, Schukken Y, Guard C, Brand A, van de Weygen G. Fertility, production and culling following cesarean section in dairy cattle. Theriogenology 1992;38:589–99.
[41] Ducrot C, Cimarosti I, Bugnard F, Schukken Y. Calving effect on French beef-cow fertility. Prev Vet Med 1994;19:126–36.
[42] Rougoor C, Dijkhuizen A, Barkema H, Schukken Y. The economics of caesarian section in dairy cattle. Prev Vet Med 1994;19:27–37.

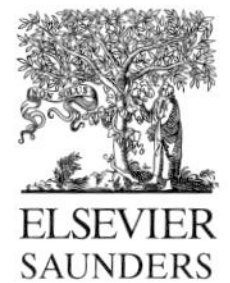
ELSEVIER
SAUNDERS

Vet Clin Food Anim 21 (2005) 101–132

VETERINARY
CLINICS
Food Animal Practice

Surgical Abdomen of the Calf

Pierre-Yves Mulon, DMV*,
André Desrochers, DMV, MS

Department of Clinical Sciences, Université de Montréal, Faculté de Médecine Vétérinaire, 3200, Sicotte, St Hyacinthe, Québec, J2S 6K9, Canada

The calf should adapt quickly to its new environment in the first months of life. Major physiologic and anatomic changes occur in a stressful environment. The important events are adaptation to aerial life, umbilical structure regression, immunologic maturity, and changing from a milk-fed monogastric to a ruminant. Although all the forestomachs are present, the abomasum represents for the newborn calf the main digestive organ. Development of the forestomachs begins during the first weeks of life, but they are not fully functional until 4 months of age. The full ruminant volume proportion between sizes of the reticulorumen and the abomasum is obtained at 9 to 12 months. During the preruminant period, the reticular groove allows the bypass of the rumen and direct passage of milk into the abomasum [1,2]. Because of the specific topography of the abdomen in calves, good anatomic knowledge is a prerequisite before performing surgeries.

Although diarrhea and pneumonia are the most frequent diagnoses on a daily basis in calves, specific surgical abdominal diseases can occur. Clinical presentation may be different from adult cattle, ranging from sudden death to chronic bloating. A good knowledge of common conditions and a thorough clinical evaluation of the animal lead the veterinarian to take proper action. Some conditions are treatable in a field practice environment, but others necessitate hauling the animal to a clinic or a referral center for immediate care.

Special considerations have to be taken before going into surgery with sick calves in regard to concomitant diseases affecting lungs, immunity status, and pH/electrolyte imbalances. Some of these concomitant diseases

* Corresponding author.
E-mail address: pierre-yves.mulon@umontreal.ca (P.-Y. Mulon).

doi:10.1016/j.cvfa.2004.12.004

are more life-threatening than the abdominal surgical conditions. The clinician should not be blinded by evident abdominal abnormalities and always should perform a complete physical examination.

This article focuses on the clinical presentation and physical examination of the calf affected by acute abdominal conditions and patient preparation for the surgery. Specific surgical conditions of the abdomen that are frequently encountered are described.

Clinical assessment

History and physical examination

A complete history should be taken first with emphasis on duration of the clinical signs, colostrum intake for neonates, feeding management, and drugs used, particularly nonsteroidal anti-inflammatory drugs (NSAIDs). NSAIDs can cause abomasal ulcers [3] if the drug regimen is not adapted to the abnormal physiologic state of the animal. Supplementation with vitamin E/selenium should be ascertained. Calves with myositis may show signs of discomfort similar to colic signs [4].

The physical examination starts with a distance examination of the animal: state of alertness, standing or recumbent, abdominal pain, and abdominal distention. Abdominal distention is helpful to localize the involved underlying structure. Abdominal pain is easier to recognize in calves than in adult cows. The calf could be kicking at its belly, going up and down, and looking at its flank [5–7]. In some peracute abdominal conditions, such as perforated abomasal ulcer, the calf may be found dead or moribund [6]. Temperature, heart rate, and respiratory rate are valuable signs of health that can change quickly. Thoracic auscultation is crucial. Auscultation findings do not explain colic signs; however, diaphragmatic hernia should be suspected if digestive sounds are audible at the thoracic auscultation [8]. Lung auscultation is more important as a presurgical evaluation. Young calves are susceptible to pneumonia, which could be problematic during anesthesia. In contrast to surgery on adult animals, calves always are positioned in lateral or dorsal recumbency, predisposing themselves to poor oxygenation, which is worsened with a concomitant pneumonia.

Abdominal auscultation, percussion, and ballottement should be performed. A metallic sound ("ping") when percussion is performed on the right flank is often a sign of a distended gastrointestinal organ, most likely the small intestines, or abomasal distention (dilation or volvulus). At this point, surgical intervention should be considered. Splashing sounds when succussion is performed can be associated with fluid in the forestomachs, fluid in the intestines (eg, diarrhea), or free abdominal fluid (eg, peritonitis). Rarely, calves with a large umbilical abscess may have a ping if there is liquid and gas in it. This presentation easily can be mistaken for an abomasal displacement.

Excessive bloating compromising normal breathing should be corrected rapidly even if physical examination or diagnostic procedures are not finished. A stomach tube is passed orally down the forestomachs until gas is coming out. The authors have operated on calves that chewed on stomach tubes and swallowed a portion of it. An oral speculum made of a 60-mL syringe case or a roll of tape is placed in the mouth before passing the tube. Depending on the amount of fluid in the forestomachs and the origin of bloat, efficacy of orogastric tubing decompression varies [9]; if it fails, percutaneous decompression should be performed [9]. Left-sided percutaneous decompression goes in either the rumen or the abomasum. The clinician should withhold from doing right-sided percutaneous decompression if the origin of the dilation is unknown. The authors have seen general peritonitis and lacerated small intestine after repeated percutaneous decompression on the right side. If decompression is not effective after one needle puncture on the right side, additional punctures should not be performed until a final diagnosis is made.

Palpation of the umbilical structures should be performed routinely even if the history precludes it. The same holds true for palpation of the joints. Any existing infections in those structures may affect the prognosis.

Ultrasound

Ultrasound examination is becoming more available in field practice. Ultrasound is useful to determine which structure is dilated and if there is free fluid in the abdomen compatible with peritonitis [10]. The authors use a sectorial 3.5-MHz probe for transabdominal ultrasound in calves. Umbilicus examination is part of the routine ultrasound examination even if it does not look abnormal. Specific imaging results can be obtained, which are discussed further for each diagnosis.

Laboratory studies

Electrolytes and acid-base abnormalities are frequent in calves. Although not always readily available in practice, biochemistry profile and complete blood count are helpful before performing abdominal surgery. As in adults, proximal gastrointestinal obstruction has been associated with an hypochloremic, hypokalemic metabolic alkalosis [11–13]. These imbalances return to normal after correction of the obstruction [11]. Laboratory findings generally reflect the calf's hydration and metabolic status, but are not usually diagnostic [5]. High blood urea nitrogen, creatinine, and phosphorus concentrations are frequent in dehydrated calves and can be compatible with prerenal failure. Renal failure should be considered if the values are not back to a normal range after 48 hours of fluid administration.

Acid-base imbalance is evaluated by measuring the pH via a venous sample. Calves with nonspecific gastrointestinal obstruction are generally in metabolic alkalosis, but they may become acidotic quickly if the obstruction is caused by a torsion or volvulus secondary to hypoperfusion and ischemia [13,14]. The pH value can be considered as a part of the presurgical prognosis; severe acidosis (pH <7.3) has been associated with a poor prognosis [15]. In a retrospective study of 66 calves with atresia coli, a trend to predict mortality was obtained with an anion gap greater than 24 mEq/L [16].

The packed cell volume and the total plasma proteins give valuable information about the hydration status of the calf and its immunologic status. In the absence of dehydration, a serum protein concentration greater than 50 g/L is considered adequate for the passive transfer of immunity [17]. Mild-to-severe leukocytosis associated with a neutrophilia and a left shift usually is observed in obstructed calves [14,16]. Long-term duration of the condition is associated with a hyperfibrinogenemia in accordance with the associated peritonitis [12].

Heart rate, hydration status, suckling reflex, and blood work analysis should help the clinician in starting fluid therapy before a surgical procedure. If the calf is in critical condition, the surgery should be postponed and scheduled as soon as the animal is stable. Isotonic fluids are administered during the operation to avoid further loss of fluids and maintain a good blood pressure. Administration of plasma or whole blood is necessary if the calf has low plasmatic protein concentration because of passive transfer failure or severe peritonitis [13,18].

Broad-spectrum antibiotics need to be administered before surgery; duration of treatment depends on the condition and may be modified based on surgical findings. NSAIDs may be administered as needed before surgery to reduce inflammation and pain during the recovery period. Repeated administration of NSAIDs should not be done routinely in all animals [13]. Clinicians should be cautious if the calf has poor hydration status, insufficient urine output, and anorexia.

Choice of surgical approach

The choice of surgical approach depends on the disease. Ventral midline laparotomy is the only solution to perform an umbilical surgery or to repair a ruptured bladder. Approaches are more controversial in cases of abomasal displacements or intestinal obstruction, and the surgeon's choice is often based on his or her personal experience with all approaches. Routine preparation of the surgical site is needed, including a large clipping and a scrub with either povidone-iodine or chlorhexidine gluconate soaps [19]. Appropriate preparation is planned if the initial incision could be extended with in situ surgical findings.

Ventral laparotomy

The ventral laparotomy has been described for correction of umbilical problems [10,20–25], ruptured bladder [26,27], and left displaced abomasum [7]. The calf is positioned in dorsal recumbency with the legs extended. A V table may be helpful to keep the animal stable. Breathing rate and patterns always should be monitored in field conditions and in the operating room, even if the calf was alert before an elective surgery. Calves with a distended abdomen should be monitored closely for adequate breathing, color of mucosa, and regurgitation while in dorsal recumbency. Pulse oximetry may be used during procedures providing continuous heart rate and oxygen saturation to the surgeon [28,29]. Position of the head relative to the rest of the body is important. If epidural anesthesia has been performed on the animal, the head should be kept elevated. If access and visualization of the caudal abdomen are needed, the gastrointestinal tract should be moved cranially; to achieve this, the head is tilted downward for a short time.

Depending on the diagnosis, a ventral midline laparotomy incision starts cranial to the umbilicus (abomasal surgery) or by an elliptical or fusiform incision around the umbilicus (umbilical infection). Either incision can be extended cranially or caudally during the procedure if needed. Skin incision is followed by a blunt dissection of the subcutaneous tissues until the fibrous ring around the umbilical structures is observed. If umbilical surgery is performed, entrance into the abdomen is by the lateral aspect of the umbilical mass to avoid any infected remnants. Peritoneum is incised, and digital abdominal exploration can be done. The rest of the opening can be performed with Mayo scissors with a good visualization of the underlying structures. Then umbilical structures can be removed en bloc by the same incision [23]. It allows good visualization of the abomasum, forestomachs (variable according to calf's age) greater omentum, a portion of the small intestine, right lobe of the liver, gallbladder, bladder, and kidneys in some calves.

After completion of the surgery, the surgical wound is closed with an interrupted cruciate pattern using a large diameter (USP 1 or 2) absorbable suture material. Tension can be high on the edges of the body wall, making suture difficult. Clamping with another needle driver the first throw of a knot is a solution commonly used to maintain the tension, but also can damage the suture material [30]. Subcutaneous tissue is closed to limit the dead space in the wound with USP 2-0 absorbable suture material in a simple continuous pattern. The skin is closed with a USP 0 nonabsorbable suture material with an interrupted cruciate pattern.

Paralumbar fossa laparotomy

Left paralumbar fossa laparotomy allows the exposure of the rumen in calves older than 2 months. This approach commonly is used only for rumenal tympany to perform ruminotomy or to create a chronic fistula of the rumen. The left kidney moves gradually until it lies to the right of the midline at the same time as the development of the rumen. Left paralumbar fossa laparotomy can be used for left kidney resection [31]. Right paralumbar fossa laparotomy is the main approach in abdominal surgery in calves [5,12,14,16,32–36]. The calf is sedated and positioned in left lateral recumbency. Surgeons may have recourse to general anesthesia depending on the condition [7,10,21,22,25,35,37].

A 15-cm-long dorsoventral skin incision is made in the middle of the paralumbar fossa. Careful attention should be paid when incising the muscles and peritoneum, especially if the abdomen is distended. Flank incision should be opened layer by layer dissecting along muscular fibers. Peritoneum is incised carefully with Metzenbaum scissors to avoid perforation of distended organs. Before manually exploring the abdomen, it is important to identify distended organs protruding from incisions and evaluate the presence of abnormal abdominal fluids. The fluids can be submitted to the laboratory for further analysis (bacteriology and cytology). Manipulation and exteriorization of the organs is done with particular care in calves. The viscera are kept moisturized during long prcoedures with warmed 0.9% saline. The amount of fluid and proteins that can be lost during abdominal surgery in calves must be kept in mind.

After completion of the surgery, the abdominal wall is closed routinely with two muscular layers in a simple continuous pattern using a USP 0 synthetic absorbable suture material: first, the abdominalis transversus muscle, including the peritoneum, and second, the two oblique muscles. If the abdominalis transversus muscle has a tendency to tear during suturing, the internal oblique muscle is included in the first layer. The skin is sutured with a USP 0 nonabsorbable suture material in a continuous interlocking pattern.

Peritonitis is a common complication of abdominal surgery. Two major origins exist: The first is iatrogenic by manipulating the viscera and irritating the serosa, and the second is sepsis that can occur during surgery by the loss of sterility during an enterotomy or before the surgery by a perforated organ (eg, abomasal ulcer) or by the excessive dilation of bowels and translocation of bacteria through the intestinal wall [38]. This bacterial translocation can predispose the calf to septicemia and further secondary complications unrelated to the surgery, such as pneumonia or septic arthritis.

In horses and ewes, 1% sodium carboxymethylcellulose is used to prevent adherences after surgery owing to its lubricative and hydroflotative properties [39,40], without affecting the intestinal healing [41,42] and intra-abdominal defenses [41]. Although there is no case report in cattle, 1% sodium carboxymethylcellulose can be used in calves at a volume of 4 to 6 mL/kg [40] at the end of the surgery before complete closure of the abdominal wall [39].

Surgery of the digestive tract

Numerous gastrointestinal diseases can occur during the first months of life, predisposing the gastrointestinal tract to be one of the most common reasons for abdominal surgery in calves. Based on the authors' hospital population, however, it seems that umbilical problems have a greater incidence. The diagnosis depends on the age of the animal, its nutrition, and its gastrointestinal tract maturity. Weaning is crucial, and if not done properly, it may cause different gastrointestinal problems, such as bloating, abomasal dilation, and abomasal ulcer [1,2]. The surgery itself may not be the definitive treatment in calf gastrointestinal surgery. Feeding regimen changes, pneumonia, or diarrhea treatments should be done at the same time. Postoperative care is extremely important and should not be neglected.

Rumenotomy and rumenostomy

Rumenostomy is performed on calves that are chronically bloated. Tympanism may have several origins, and the origin sometimes is difficult to find. Trichobezoars, rumenitis, fibrous distention of the rumen, chronic rumen acidosis, and rumen putrefaction are the most common diagnoses [1,43]. Failure in closing the esophageal groove or backflow from the abomasum results in milk putrefaction in the rumen by proteolytic bacteria and secondary recurrent bloat in veal calves [1]. Severe pneumonia [44] and a juvenile form of lymphosarcoma [45] have been determined as miscellaneous origins of bloat in calves resulting from the enlarged mediastinal lymph nodes at proximity of the vagal nerve. Chronic rumenal fistula or rumenostomy is the only option to return to a normal abdominal profile and to relieve the abdominal discomfort in case of free gas accumulation without any obstruction.

Rumenostomy is performed under sedation and is the only abdominal surgery in calves that can be done in standing position. Lidocaine infiltration of the planned site or an inverted L infiltration is sufficient to block the surgical site. A 2-cm diameter circular incision is performed in the proximal quarter of the left flank, 7 cm caudally to the last rib. Muscles are bluntly dissected along their fiber orientation up to the peritoneum. The rumen is grasped with an Allis forceps and exteriorized through the wound. Different techniques have been described to anastomose the rumen to the skin, including a two-layer or three-layer technique [46,47]. The three-layer technique adds a suture of the peritoneum and the transversus abdominalis muscle to the dermis on both sides of the wound to protect the abdominal wall with a size 0 absorbable material. Then the rumen is sutured with eight simple interrupted sutures to the skin with a size 0 nonabsorbable material. After incising the rumen, the edges are sutured to the skin in a simple continuous pattern with a size 0 nonabsorbable material. In the authors' opinion, it is preferable to wait 24 to 48 hours before opening the rumen, allowing fibrin deposition in the wound, making the stoma site watertight. The additional suture compared with the two-layer technique increases the surgical time but is a good security if retarded rumenal opening cannot be done.

A syringe case is inserted into the incision and sutured to the skin to prevent premature closure of the fistula if needed [46]. The fistula heals by second intention as soon as the syringe is removed, but healing can take several months, and wound leakage is present until the healing process is completed. Complications related to this procedure include leakage of rumenal juice in the abdominal cavity and severe inflammation of the surgical site. Peritonitis resulting from the leakage is rare and usually localized to the surrounding area of the incision. A large stoma may compromise complete healing of the fistula and leave the animal with permanent leakage of rumen juice. The size of the fistula should be small, just large enough to let free gas out. As long as there is an abnormal positive pressure inside the rumen, the fistula should not close. It may take 4 to 6 months for complete healing of a chronic rumen fistula. For this reason, some surgeons prefer to use a rumen cannula fixed temporarily to the skin. Persistent leakage does not seem detrimental to the animal from a gastrointestinal point of view. The wound has to be cleaned regularly, however.

Circular incision healing is different from any other wound. There is a limit in its healing potential leaving a gap, which explains why large-diameter fistulae never heal even if rumen function returns to normal [47]. Revision of a chronic fistula can be challenging. If the fistula is small, scarification of the inside of the fistula and its closure may be enough. Most often, a complete three-layer revision should be performed, in which the rumen, the muscles, and the skin are sutured separately.

Acute rumenal acidosis in weaned calves induces rumenitis accompanied by an acute bloating [43]. Presence of rumenal trichobezoars, resulting from exclusive milk or roughage-poor diets, has been associated with obstruction of either the cardia or the reticulo-omasal orifice [1]. Rumenotomy is the treatment of choice for those conditions.

The surgical approach is the same as described in adult cows, but the calf is sedated and restrained in right lateral recumbency. Local anesthesia techniques are sufficient for the completion of the surgery. After a left paralumbar laparotomy, the rumen is exteriorized and sutured to the body wall with a simple nonperforating continuous suture pattern using a USP 0 nonabsorbable suture material. It is the authors' opinion that this technique is safer in calves compared with the use of a Weingarth's ring for the removal of rumenal content or foreign bodies [48]. Suture of the rumen is done with a two-layer inverted nonperforating continuous suture pattern using a USP 0 or 1 absorbable suture material before freeing the rumen. Closure of the abdominal wall is routine.

Abomasal surgeries

Abomasal dislocations, although not as frequent as in adult cattle, can be diagnosed easily with physical examination. Diagnosis of abomasal ulceration and abomasitis is more challenging. Even more difficult is the decision whether or not to open the calf. These animals are seriously ill, and elective surgery can be detrimental and fatal.

Abomasal ulcers

Abomasal ulcers have been described thoroughly in adult cattle and classified in four types [49]. Type I is an erosion of the mucosa that does not involve the mucosal basement membrane. It results in minimal blood loss and can heal without any scar. Type II is a nonperforating ulcer with severe intraluminal hemorrhage owing to the penetration of the abomasal wall resulting in melena. Types III and IV are perforating abomasal ulcers. They differ by their location and the amount of peritonitis that they induce—localized for type III and severe diffuse for type IV. Type III occurs most of the time in the area covered by the greater omentum. The etiology of abomasal ulcers in calves is not understood. Four main factors seem to increase risk: trace mineral deficiencies [50,51]; bacterial agents, principally *Clostridium perfringens* [43,51,52]; stress; and abrasive agents, such as hairballs [6].

Signs of abdominal pain are variable and often subtle. Motility of the abomasum is reduced, and a ventral abdominal distention is present. Abdominal palpation may be tense and painful. Sudden death can occur in the case of the involvement of a major blood vessel in the ulcer or acute generalized peritonitis. Definitive diagnosis of an ulcer is challenging. None of the medical imaging techniques available offer good visualization of ulcers. Abdominal ultrasound permits evaluation of the size of the abomasum and surrounding peritonitis, however, which can be compatible with ulcers. Abdominocentesis is a valuable ancillary test to assess the presence of an inflammatory or septic process in the abdomen, especially if ultrasound is not available [13].

Successful surgical treatment of abomasal ulcers has been reported [53]; however, the decision to perform surgery is always difficult and often depends on the size of the abomasums, the presence of fibrin or free fluid in the abdomen, and the clinical course of the calf. The surgery can be performed with sedation and local anesthesia or general anesthesia. The calf is positioned in left lateral recumbency, and a right paralumbar fossa exploratory laparotomy is performed. If the peritonitis is localized and the gastric ulcer is easily exteriorized, an elliptical incision is performed around the ulcer to débride the necrotic tissues, and a double inverting continuous suture is performed with a synthetic absorbable suture material. Abdominal lavage is performed, and the body wall is closed in routine fashion. The prognosis for these ulcers is guarded to poor. Ranitidine or cimetidine can be administered to increase temporarily the pH of the abomasum during the healing process [54]. Type IV abomasal ulcers generally are not treated when discovered at surgery because of the poor prognosis of the diffuse peritonitis they induce (Fig. 1).

Gastric ulcers have been associated with abomasal displacement or abomasal incarceration in umbilical hernia, creating a chronic fistula of the abomasum [7,55–57]. The outcome depends on the location of the ulcers and the extension of the peritonitis. In the authors' experience, the prognosis for such cases is poor, and surgical repair is usually not an option in regard to the severe peritonitis.

Abomasal dislocations

Left and right displacements of the abomasum and abomasal volvulus have been described in calves [7,9,55–59]. The onset of the condition depends on the side of displacement. Right dilation and abomasal volvulus are associated with more severe electrolyte imbalances and acidotic status. Pain is more significant in calves with right displacement of the abomasum than in calves with left displacement of the abomasum. The etiology is uncertain; many hypotheses have been proposed: Dietary changes and ulcers can be predisposing factors. A prospective study of 30 calves indicated an incidence of abomasal displacement in 70% of calves with perforated gastric ulcer [57].

Clinical signs are usually nonspecific with a bilateral distention of the abdomen. Tympanitic or fluid splashing sounds can be heard during percussion or ballottement on the side of displacement. Passing an oral tube into the rumen can help to differentiate rumenal tympany from left abomasal displacement [9], although this can be frustrating. Abdominal

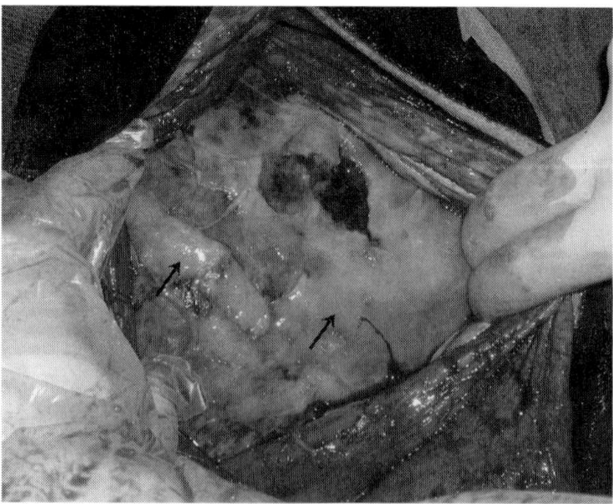

Fig. 1. Surgical view of an extensive diffuse peritonitis in a calf with a perforated abomasal ulcer. Organized fibrin (*arrows*) is present in the entire abdominal cavity. This condition is fatal.

ultrasound with a sectorial 3.5-MHz probe provides good visualization of internal organs. Abomasal mucosa is typically recognizable at ultrasound examination (Fig. 2). If the abomasal content is primarily gas, mucosal ridges are not seen. To verify adequate positioning of the abomasum, the pylorus can be localized. If its position is to the left of the ventral midline, it can be compatible with a left displaced abomasum.

If umbilical infection is associated with left displacement of the abomasum, the ventral midline surgical approach permits the surgeon to remove umbilical remnants and to reduce the displaced abomasum. Procedures can be performed through two distinctive incisions or extending one or the other. An abomasum should not be fixed at the umbilical surgery site because of poor anatomic approximation. If left displacement of the abomasum is the only pathologic finding, a right paralumbar fossa laparotomy approach can be used to perform a better abdominal exploration and reduce displacement.

Right paralumbar fossa laparotomy is the approach of choice for right abomasal disorders [60–62]. A 15-cm linear incision is performed 5 cm caudally to the costal arch. The abdominal wall is thin. This approach allows good visualization of the abomasums and allows a complete abdominal exploration. After reduction of the displacement, the abomasum is fixed by either omentopexy or transfixated abomasopexy [63]. The abdominal wall is sutured as previously described. To the authors' knowledge, there are no reports about the occurrence of further adhesions and related problems when the calves become adults.

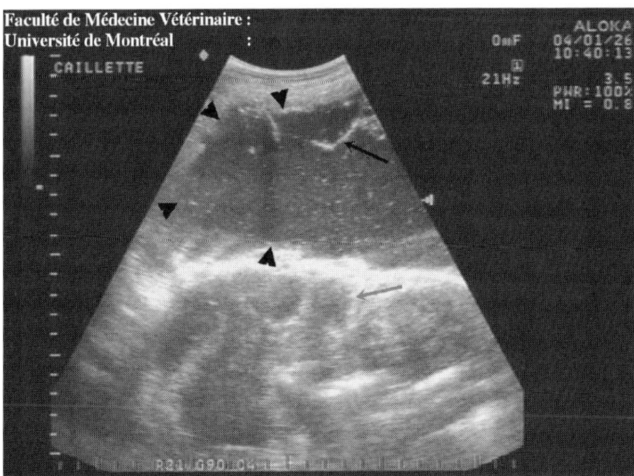

Fig. 2. Normal abdominal ultrasound with a sectorial 3.5-MHz probe in a calf. The abomasum is located ventrally (*arrowheads*). Abomasal mucosal folds appear as hyperechoic filaments inside the lumen (*black arrow*). Small bowels (*gray arrow*) are visible in the greater omentum (hyperechoic line between abomasum and intestine).

Small intestines

The small intestines frequently are involved in distended abdomen in calves [58]. The particularity of the onset of the condition and the side of dilation of the abdomen are helpful to identify the origin of the disease. In adults, per rectum transabominal palpation of the gastrointestinal tract helps the clinician to diagnose a specific gastrointestinal problem. This palpation is not possible in calves. As in any small intestine distention problems, it is often difficult to determine if conservative treatment should be started first or if surgery should be done promptly. Ultrasound is the diagnostic tool of choice. Pertinent ultrasound observations are the diameter of the small bowels, presence of fluid into the intestines or extraluminal fluids, and empty or enlarged portion of small intestines. If ultrasound examination is not possible, exploratory laparotomy is the best option. Sending calves with medical lesions for an exploratory laparotomy does not adversely influence prognosis [59].

Obstruction

Volvulus. Intestinal volvulus in calves is a rotation of a part of the small intestine as in other species, but according to some authors, torsion at the root of the mesentery is more frequent [14,33]. The condition is characterized by a rapid onset. Animals with intestinal volvulus usually show signs of severe colic unresponsive to painkillers [13,14,58]. The abdomen is distended on the both sides. Biochemistry profile shows a metabolic alkalosis in the early stage of the condition followed by a significant acidosis resulting from the ischemic damage in the mesentery and the intestine. Low venous blood pH (7.27 ± 0.2) has been associated significantly with a poor prognosis in cattle with small intestinal volvulus [14]. Predisposition of calves to present with intestinal volvulus is controversial. Anderson et al [14] reported no age-related predisposition (25/190 <2 months old and 17/190 2–6 months old) for the volvulus of the root of the mesentery.

Right paralumbar laparotomy is the approach of choice [14,33]. A surgical decision has to be made quickly to increase the prognosis after the reduction of the volvulus because of the increased vessel injuries and bowel necrosis with time [33,62]. General anesthesia is preferable but not essential. General anesthesia allows more maneuvers to exteriorize the gastrointestinal tract, however. After opening the abdominal cavity, the twisted root of the mesentery can be palpated at its dorsal attachment within the omental bursa for a volvulus of the entire intestine. The volvulus can be limited to the jejunoileal flange. The entire bulk of the involved intestine is rotated in the opposite direction of the torsion by gentle manipulation. Exteriorizing most of the intestinal mass allowed easy reduction of the volvulus [33].

Viability of the intestine is evaluated after the reduction. Parts that stay purple or dark without any arterial flow have to be resected as described for the intussusception. It is not a viable option for the animal to remove the entire length of the intestine.

Incarceration. The umbilical remnants and particularly the umbilical vein are potentially hazardous intra-abdominal structures around which viscus such the abomasum and small bowels can be trapped. Usually the remnants are in close contact with the peritoneum. A rent in their attachment to the peritoneum may leave enough space for a viscus to be trapped or wound up around it [58,64]. Incarceration also can happen around the vas deferens in older steers or in inguinal or umbilical hernia [10,65]. Incarceration results in a partial or complete obstruction of the lumen and ischemic lesions on the digestive tract to different degree. Clinical signs are typical of obstruction with severe abdominal pain. Peritonitis is present depending on the duration of the condition and the state of necrosis of intestine. Ultrasound can be helpful to identify the involved gastrointestinal portion and fetal remnant.

In the case of a small fibrous appearance of the remnant, the correction can be performed with a right paralumbar fossa laparotomy in left recumbency. This approach allows better access to small bowels. The fibrous remnant is cut first proximally. Before cutting it, the surgeon should follow the fibrous chord to its point of origin—most likely the liver (cranial) or vas deferens (caudal direction on steers). It is not always possible to see it and to exteriorize it for ligation. Blind section should be done carefully. The portion of the gastrointestinal tract incarcerated is exteriorized to evaluate any area of necrosis. The surgical correction of the incarceration is more challenging for the surgeon in the case of an infected umbilical remnant. A ventral midline approach combined with an en bloc resection of the umbilical structures is performed to correct the incarceration. Local peritonitis may complicate the surgery by creating multiple adhesions and abscesses. Careful dissection is essential, but impossible to do in field conditions if the lesions are extensive. Ischemic damages are assessed after correction of the incarceration, and enterectomy is performed if needed [66].

Intussusception. Constable et al [32] reported based on a study of 336 cases that there is a significant effect of age, with calves younger than 2 months having increased risk of intussusception compared with older animals associated with a breed predisposition of Brown Swiss. However, The authors' clinical experience is different, however, with intussusception occurring in more Brown Swiss but rarely in calves. *Intussusceptum* defines the segment of bowel invaginated into the other part, and *intussuscipiens* defines the distal part of bowel into which the intussusceptum is invaginated. Colic in calves with intestinal intussusception is less violent than in calves with volvulus, but animals often showed signs of discomfort [5]. Sudden death can occur if surgical treatment is delayed [67]. Calves pass scant feces with blood and fibrin in it.

Two locations are described in the small intestine: the jejunum [32,25], the most common part involved, and the ileocecal junction [32,36,67]. Four types of cecal intussusception are described: cecocecal, cecocolic, ileocolic, and ileocecocolic [36]. The cecocolic form represents half of the cases in a study based on 51 calves [36]. Origin of the intussusception varies. A transitory modification of the motility (eg, diarrhea) or a focal intestinal pathology can be at the origin of the self-invagination of the bowel (Fig. 3) [36].

Ultrasound can be a useful tool to evaluate whether an abdomen is surgical or not. Intussusception and other types of intestinal obstructions are good examples. Visualization of distended small intestine with an absence of gut motility and the concomitant presence of empty small intestine is an indication of a surgical abdomen. Presence of free fluid in the abdomen also can be assessed in more chronically affected calves. Intussusception site can be visualized depending on the location (Fig. 4), and a definitive diagnosis can be made with the appearance of two concentric circles of echogenic tissue looking like a target [68].

Surgery has to be done as soon as possible to decrease the vascular damage and the localized peritonitis that occur around the intussusception. Right paralumbar fossa laparotomy is the approach of choice. The intussusceptum is exteriorized, and Doyen forceps are positioned on both sides. Visualization of mesenteric vessels is easy because of the fat-free mesentery. Hemostasis is performed by ligating the vessels with absorbable suture material. Then the intussusceptum can be resected, and an end-to-end anastomosis is done. Anastomosis is begun by placing mesenteric and antimesenteric suture and continuing with a two-layer semicircular continuous suture pattern or with a simple discontinuous suture pattern with a 3-0 absorbable suture material.

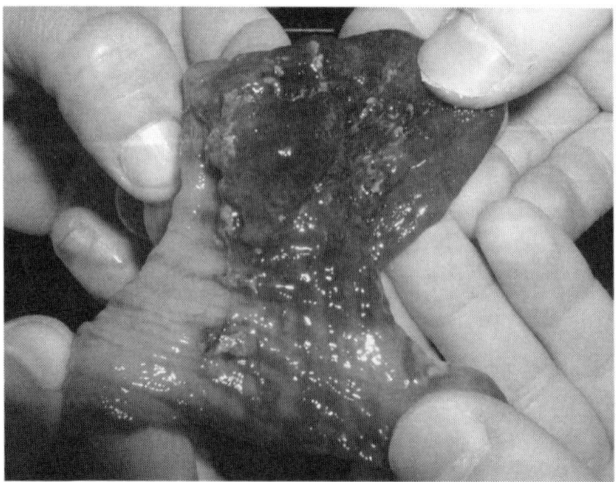

Fig. 3. Anatomic specimen of a necrotic hemorrhagic colitis at the proximal extremity of the intussuscipiens obtained after the resection of an intussusception.

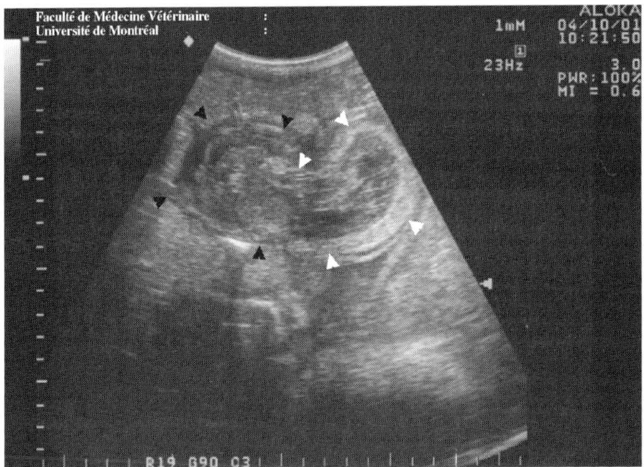

Fig. 4. Abnormal abdominal ultrasound with a sectorial 3.5-MHz probe illustrating an intussusception in a calf with the beginning of intussuscipiens (*black arrowheads*) and intussusceptum (*white arrowheads*).

For cecal intussusceptions, reduction of the intussusceptum can be tried. Cecal amputation is often necessary. Resection of the ileum and the proximal loop of the ascending colon can be added to the cecal amputation depending on the type of cecal intussusception. According to a study on cecal intussusception in calves, 24% of calves that were recovered from anesthesia survived [36].

Atresia. Atresia of the small intestine (ileum and jejunum) is less frequent than atresia of other parts of the gastrointestinal tract [69,70]. The etiology of this condition is not well established, but early pregnancy diagnosis and mild heritability can be involved. Clinical signs are the same as those of atresia of the colon and are discussed further subsequently [20,59,69,70]. Treatment consists of an anastomosis between the blind end of the jejunum and the ileum or the body of the cecum. It is easier first to perform emptying of the blind end by performing an enterotomy before doing the side-to-side anastomosis. A resection of a part of the blind end may be needed to allow a better fit between both ends at the stoma site.

Hairball. Hairballs frequently are associated with gastric ulcers. They have been reported by Abutarbush and Radostits [12] to produce a complete jejunal obstruction in two young beef calves. The removal of the hairballs via an enterotomy through a right paralumbar fossa laparotomy was sufficient to achieve the complete recovery of the calves in both cases.

Dilation of the cecum

Dilation of the cecum can occur in calves and in adult cattle, but torsion around the long axis is less frequent [5,13,58]. The condition is diagnosed by auscultating a "ping" area in the right dorsal abdomen with a distended abdomen on the right side. Electrolytic imbalances are the same as those seen in adults. Dilation of the cecum can be associated with abomasum displacements. Medical treatment can be tried first. Surgical correction of the dilation has to be done, however, if no improvement occurs in the following 24 hours because the impossibility to perform a rectal examination means the diagnosis of torsion is based only on the clinical response. Partial or total cecal amputation can be performed if the cecal wall appears to be nonviable because of an excessive dilation or the presence of necrosis foci. It is performed via a right paralumbar laparotomy. The cecum is exteriorized, and an enterotomy is performed at its apex. If an amputation is needed, a Doyen forceps is positioned preserving the ileocecal valve, ligatures on the vessels in the ileocecal mesentery are positioned, and a typhlectomy is performed. The use of staples to perform typhlectomy has been described in adults [71]; staples can be helpful, but are expensive compared with two inverting suture layers with an absorbable suture material.

Large intestine

Intussusception

Although the jejunum is the main site of intussusception, it also can occur in the spiral colon of calves [32,35,72]. The etiology is the same as for intussusception of the small bowel. Treatment of this condition is resection of the injured colon combined with a side-to-side anastomosis.

Atresia

The origin of atresia coli is not well understood and mostly like is multifactorial. Autosomal recessive inheritance has been proved as a propagation factor in a dairy herd in Illinois [73,74]. Early pregnancy diagnosis at 42 days by palpation of the amniotic vesicle has been suggested as a cofactor in the etiology [73,75]. Breed predisposition seems to exist with an increased risk of atresia coli in Holstein calves [74]. Four types have been described in humans, and the same classification can be used in calves [34]. Type I is a simple mucosal membrane occluding the lumen, type II is a fibrous cord left between intestines with an intact mesentery, type III is a complete separation of the intestine with a V-shaped mesenteric rent, and type IV is a combination of multiple sites of atresia [34]. A modified type III (no mesenteric defect) is reported to be overrepresented in calves with atresia coli [16,34,76]. In accordance with previous studies, in the authors' experience, type III (modified or not) is the most frequently occurring type of atresia coli.

Clinical presentation is typical: The calf appears healthy after birth and usually drinks well its colostrum during the first 24 hours without passing feces but looking alert. Then, 48 to 72 hours after birth, the calf becomes progressively depressed, drifting downward rapidly after 96 hours as the abdomen becomes more distended [5,16,34]. Animals pass no feces, and digital rectal examination reveals mucus with or without blood [5,16,69,76]. No catheter or tubing of any kind should be passed into the rectum to verify its patency. The rectum and the descending colon are thin and fragile, and lacerations are highly possible, especially at the most proximal aspect of the descending colon as it changes to become the transverse colon. The history and physical examination are diagnostic.

Presurgical assessment is crucial. The age at presentation has never been associated with survival rate [34], even with the increased degree of peritonitis in such calves. The surgery should be performed as soon as possible, but it is not a question of minutes. If needed, fluids, plasma, and antibiotics should be administered before going in surgery.

Calves affected with atresia coli drink well for the first 48 hours. Although the calf drinks the expected amount of colostrum, this does not mean that the colostrum was adequately absorbed. Intestinal abnormalities, abnormal intraluminal distention, and ongoing peritonitis affect plasmatic protein concentration and consequently immunity.

If surgery is elected, two options are possible depending on the animal's producing future: (1) bypass of the atresic segment and anastomosis to the descending colon or (2) typhlostomy/cecostomy into the right flank. Typhlostomy is a salvage procedure that allows the animal to grow until market weight is achieved [75,77].

Bypass of the atresic segment is a delicate operation, and in the authors' opinion, it should be performed under general anesthesia. Right paralumbar fossa laparotomy is the approach of choice to expose intestines [5,16,34,69,76,77]. After entrance into the abdomen, the dilated cecum and blind end of the colon are exteriorized (Fig. 5), and a typhlotomy is performed to empty the bowels of meconium [62]. A double-layer suture inverting suture of the Cushing type with USP 3-0 absorbable suture material permits closure of the enterotomy sites. Side-to-side and end-to-side anastomosis are described between the blind end of the ascending colon and the descending colon [34]. This anastomosis can be added to a partial resection of the blind end of the colon to permit a more "anatomic" apposition of the bowels before performing the anastomosis. It seems to increase the survival rate and to reduce the incidence of functional obstruction [16,34]. At this point, a soft stallion urethral catheter can be introduced carefully through the rectum into the descending colon to help the surgeon to localize it. Otherwise, the descending colon is so thin that it is difficult to palpate and manipulate. Lubrication of the catheter by injection of ointment is important to decrease the inflammation during the introduction. Introduction of a catheter without a surgical control can perforate the descending colon.

Use of a staple device (GI-55 stapling instrument) for creating the anastomosis has been described [34,62]. The success rate of the use of such

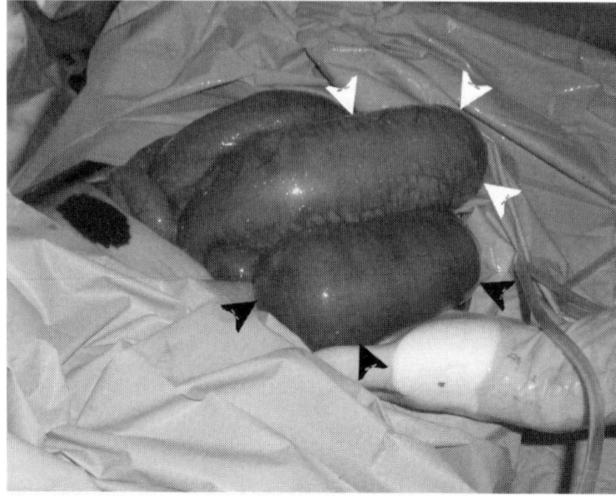

Fig. 5. Surgical view of distended intestine associated with atresia coli after a right paralumbar laparotomy. The cecum (*white arrowheads*) and blind end of the spiral colon (*black arrowheads*) are distended with gas and meconium.

a device compared with hand-sewn colocolostomy is not established. In the authors' opinion, hand-sewn anastomoses are preferable for economical reasons, despite the increased surgical time. It is preferable to create an anastomosis 5 to 7 cm long to ensure that no stricture occurs during healing of the mucosa.

An abdominal lavage with warm isotonic saline is done only if contamination occurred during enterotomy procedures. Closure of the abdominal wall is routine as previously described. The success rate of colocolic anastomosis is approximately 40%, with no difference between end-to-side and side-to-side anastomosis technique [16,34,75].

Typhlostomy, similar to colostomy, can be performed under sedation and an inverted L local anesthesia as a salvage procedure [69,78]. A standard right paralumbar fossa laparotomy is performed. After exploration of the abdominal viscera and decompression of the cecum and the blind end of the colon, the most naturally exposed organs between the blind end of the colon and the cecum are sutured to the body wall at a level distal to the surgical wound, and the proximal part of the wound is sutured with a normal pattern. A three-layer technique of fixation, as described for the rumenostomy, enables the fixation to be safer and more watertight. A resection of the colon may be necessary when a typhlostomy is performed to limit the impaction of the blind end. The successful performance of this procedure allows the calf to grow to approximately 150 kg. This procedure is more useful in beef production [75].

Clinical results

Medical records of calves admitted for colic-related diseases from 1992–2002 at the Centre Hospitalier Universitaire Vétérinaire of the Université de

Montréal were reviewed. Of 1500 calves admitted during this period, 132 fit the search criteria. In examining and managing 87 cases of surgical gastrointestinal abdomen in the hospital, 8 cases involved the rumen (7 bloat and 1 acidosis); 27 involved the abomasum (1 abomasal fistula, 5 left displacement of the abomasum, 8 right displacement of the abomasum, 4 volvulus, 1 incarceration, and 8 ulcers, of which one was nonperforated); and 52 involved the intestines (8 dilation of the cecum, 3 torsions of the mesenteric root, 4 incarcerations around umbilical remnants, 2 intussusceptions, 30 atresia coli, 1 atresia ilei, 3 idiopathic ileus, and 1 diaphragmatic herniated small intestine).

The prognosis highly depended on the diagnosis. None of the calves with perforated abomasal ulcer survived. Twelve calves with an atresia did survive, which represents a success rate of 39%, as reported previously [16,34]. Thirteen (76%) calves with abomasal displacement survived. The overall success rate was 51% [79].

Umbilical surgeries

The external umbilical cord is composed of two veins, two arteries, and one urachus. As it crosses the umbilical ring of the ventral abdominal wall, the umbilical veins become one vessel. The umbilical vein joins the left branch of the portal vein and carries oxygenated blood during fetal life. The two umbilical arteries originate from the internal iliac arteries, travel on each side of the bladder, and follow the urachus to the umbilical cord. They return the oxygen-deprived blood to the placenta. Finally, the urachus is the link between the bladder and the allantoid envelope of the placenta [80].

During normal calving, the umbilical cord breaks by elongation, and left outside is a stalk of 6 to 10 cm. A calf delivered by cesarean section has a short umbilical cord, however, which is a potential problem. Blood vessels contract. The two arteries are retracted inside the abdomen and rapidly decrease in diameter and length during the first week eventually to become the lateral ligament of the bladder. The vein fills up with a thrombus, but remains in the umbilicus [81]. The lumen of the umbilicus is occluded gradually with connective tissues and decreases in size for the next 3 weeks to become the round ligament of the liver. The urachal canal slightly retracts after birth at the level of the internal umbilical ring and rapidly decreases in size over the next week. The umbilical stalk should dry off in a week.

Umbilical hernia and infection are common surgical diseases. There are two causes of umbilical hernia: hereditary or secondary to infection. Umbilical hernia is the most common congenital disease in cattle. The incidence of umbilical hernia was reported to be 0.65% to 1.04% [82,83]. It is more common in female Holsteins. Infection retards the healing process of the umbilical ring. The omentum is the structure most commonly herniated, followed by abomasum, rumen, and small intestine.

More than one umbilical structure can be infected at the same time with or without the presence of hernia. With a meticulous palpation of the tumefaction, an experienced clinician can make an accurate diagnosis without using ultrasound. Palpating the mass with the animal in dorsal recumbency helps to determine if there is an infected internal umbilical structure, provided that the animal is small and docile [22]. To facilitate deep palpation, the animal has to be off feed for 24 hours. Ultrasound is a sensitive examination that can add crucial information before surgery regarding the true size of the structure and its relationship to the rest of the abdominal organs (eg, adhesion of the greater omentum or intestines or presence of free fluid, which can be a sign of peritonitis) [84,85].

Umbilical hernia or infections rarely are associated with colic, unless an organ is adhered in an abnormal position compromising transit or incarcerated into the hernia ring (Figs. 6 and 7). Chronic cystitis is associated with incomplete emptying of the bladder in calves with an infected urachus. Formation of urinary calculi is possible and is observed as small concretions at the ventral commissural aspect of the vulva (see Fig. 7). A young bull with an infected urachus may have urethral obstruction by a calculus secondary to cystitis. Usually the complete blood count indicates a neutrophilia with a high level of serum protein and fibrinogen near the normal values.

Anesthetic considerations

The right ventral laparotomy is the only approach, with the exception of laparoscopic removal of the normal umbilical remnants [86], that permits the en bloc resection of these structures.

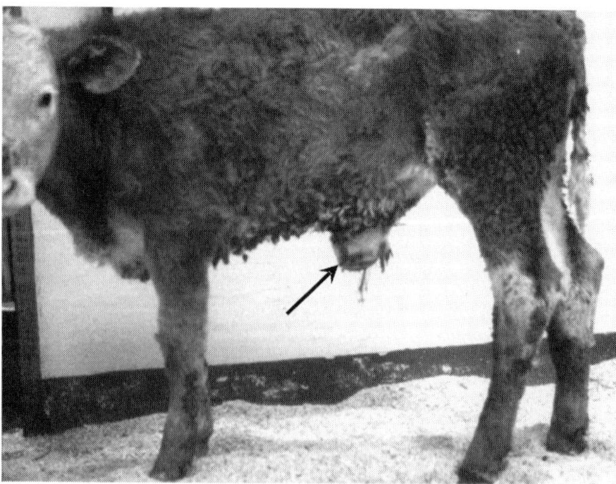

Fig. 6. External conformation of a calf presented with an enlarged painful umbilicus (*arrow*) and complaint of growth loss. Physical examination revealed an umbilical hernia with an incarcerated abomasum.

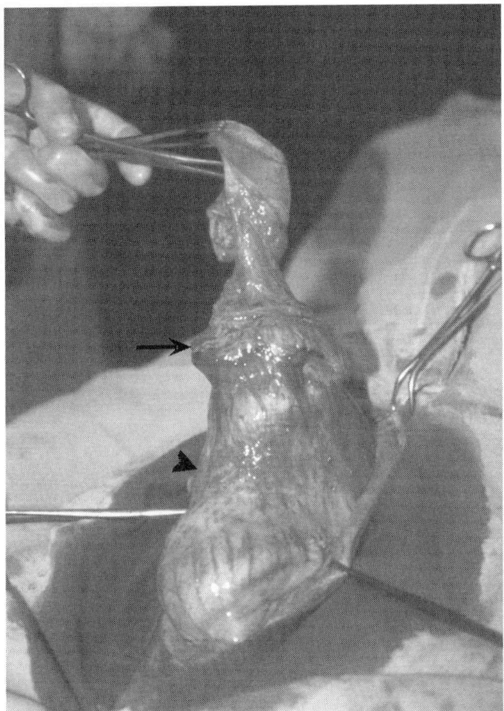

Fig. 7. Surgical view of an umbilical hernia with an incarcerated abomasum in a calf. Tight adherences (*arrowhead*) are present between the abomasal wall and the underlying inflamed tissues. The fibrous annular ring (*arrow*) has been incised close to the median plane to limit the abdominal wall default.

Local anesthesia

Ventral abdomen anesthesia can be obtained by the combination of sedation and lumbosacral epidural administration of lidocaine and xylazine [87]. The duration of the operation was 1 hour, and calves were able to stand within 90 minutes after the reversal effect of xylazine with tolazoline. An additional local anesthesia in a V-shape infiltration might be necessary for the cranial part of the umbilicus. In the authors' institution, a modified protocol with diazepam sedation (0.1 mg/kg intravenously) followed by a lumbosacral epidural containing lidocaine 2% (0.15 mL/kg) and xylazine (0.05 mg/kg) is used for uncomplicated umbilical surgeries. An additional advantage is that pelvic limbs are paralyzed during the surgery, conferring better safety for the surgeon. Prolonged recumbency that follows the surgery until the calf is able to stand up is considered a disadvantage by some surgeons.

General anesthesia

General anesthesia may be required for large umbilical abscess or vein infection. The calf does not move, and the muscle relaxation is as deep as possible, offering the surgeon the space necessary to manipulate the infected organ. Endotracheal or nasotracheal intubation with gas anesthesia is safer.

Infection of the umbilical vein

The umbilical vein extends cranially and to the right from the umbilicus to the liver. After birth, the communication between the umbilical vein and the portal vein closes. When infection of the vein occurs, this separation is the only wall between the abscess and the blood flow, predisposing calves to septicemia and bacteremia (Fig. 8).

Complete resection of the infected umbilical vein depends on the length of the infected part. If a fibrous cord is present at the entry into the liver, an en bloc resection can be done, but if the abscess penetrates the liver, the vein has to be marsupialized to the body wall. This decision is often made in surgery, and appropriate preoperative skin preparation should have been done. The skin is incised in an elliptical fashion around the infected umbilicus followed by a blunt dissection toward the fibrous ring. Special attention is given to hemostasis in this area, which most of the time is well vascularized. The body wall is incised 1 cm laterally to the fibrous ring on the left side until the peritoneum, and a small incision is performed with Metzenbaum scissors to avoid any damage to the underlying organs. Abdominal exploration is performed by digital palpation to confirm the

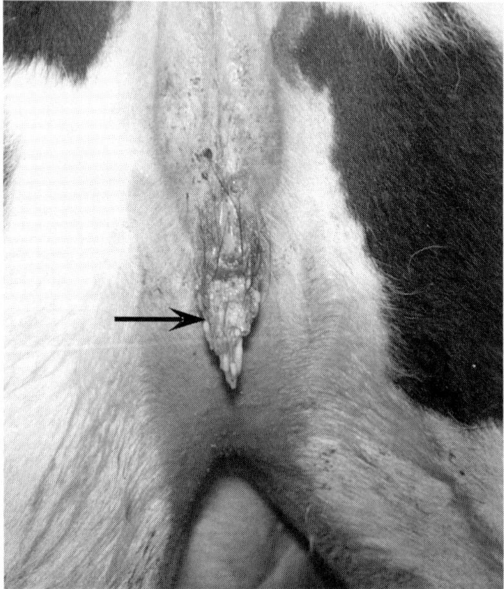

Fig. 8. Heifer with an infected urachus canal. Cranial traction on the apex of the bladder limits bladder emptying and predisposes to the accumulation of calculus at the distal extremity of the vulva. Urination is often painful.

diagnosis. The rest of the body wall opening is done with Mayo scissors in an elliptical fashion. The skin and abdominal wall incision often need to be increased cranially to obtain better visualization of the infected vein. Intraoperative ultrasound with a 10-MHz linear probe inserted in a sterile rectal palpation glove allows better visualization of the proximal extremity of the infected vein and its eventual extension into the liver.

En bloc resection of the vein can be performed if the fibrous occlusion of the vein is distal to the liver. If the infected vein is deeply enlarged or involves the liver parenchyma, marsupialization is necessary. Marsupialization of the umbilical vein has been described in the extended cranial aspect of the midline surgical wound [25] or laterally to the midline surgical wound [22,23,81]. When the vein is dissected out from the surrounding tissue, a circular skin incision is performed on the right side, paracostally, to exteriorize most of the infected vein at the marsupialization site (Fig. 9). The muscles are bluntly dissected. The external part of the umbilicus and the vein is covered by a sterile glove or sutures to prevent any leakage during manipulations to pass the vein through the planned marsupialization site. The vein is sutured to the skin with a nonabsorbable suture material with six interrupted horizontal mattress sutures, and the vein is kept close. Then the body wall is sutured in three separate layers: an interrupted cruciate pattern with monofilament absorbable suture material for the abdominal wall, a single continuous suture pattern with a multifilament absorbable suture material for the subcutaneous layer, and an interrupted cruciate pattern with multifilament nonabsorbable suture material for the skin.

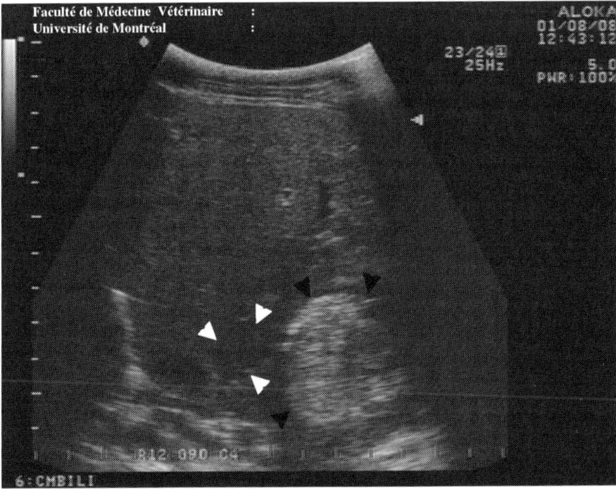

Fig. 9. Abdominal ultrasonography of the liver in a heifer. The infected vein (*black arrowheads*) can be located on the right side of the abdomen from the umbilicus to the liver. It appears as a tubular enlarged structure close to the portal circulation (*white arrowheads*).

Aftercare

The vein is opened transversally at 0.5 cm from the body wall 2 days after surgery to allow fibrin deposition, and drainage of the pus is performed by gentle flushing of the cavity. The part of the vein that is out of the abdomen tends to increase in size and needs to be cut multiple times during the healing process (Fig. 10). Complete drainage of the pus from the vein at the level of the liver has to be reevaluated by ultrasound.

The most common complication is herniation at the marsupialized site. The lack of strength into the abdominal wall created by the marsupialized vein can be the origin of secondary hernia. The percentage of secondary herniation when marsupialization was included in the midline closure was 60% [25]. No herniations have been reported with a lateral marsupialization [22]. The authors currently perform lateral marsupialization of the umbilical vein. The authors have seen herniation with this technique, too (Fig. 11). The hernia is revised 2 months after the surgery with the animal in left lateral recumbency under sedation and local anesthesia. It is a minor procedure, and only a fibrous chord attached to the inside of the herniation is left from the infected umbilical vein (Fig. 12).

Infection of the umbilical arteries

The surgery is performed under epidural anesthesia in dorsal recumbency with sedation. Depending on the deep localization of the extremity of the infected artery, however, general anesthesia may be necessary for some

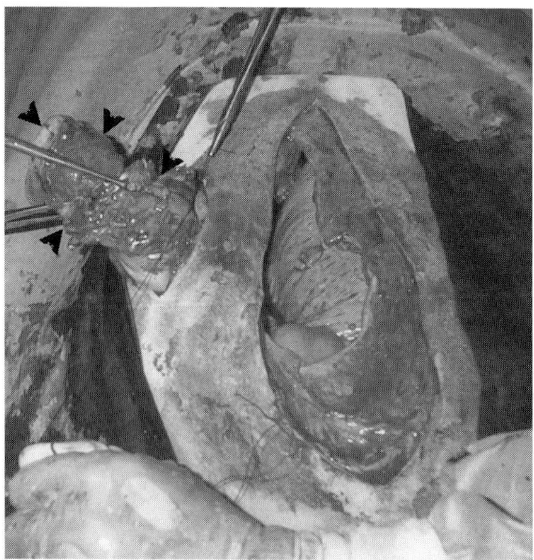

Fig. 10. Umbilical vein marsupialization. The vein (*arrowheads*) is passed through the body wall laterally from the surgical wound. It is sutured to the body wall with a simple interrupted suture. The marsupialization site depends on the ability to mobilize the vein.

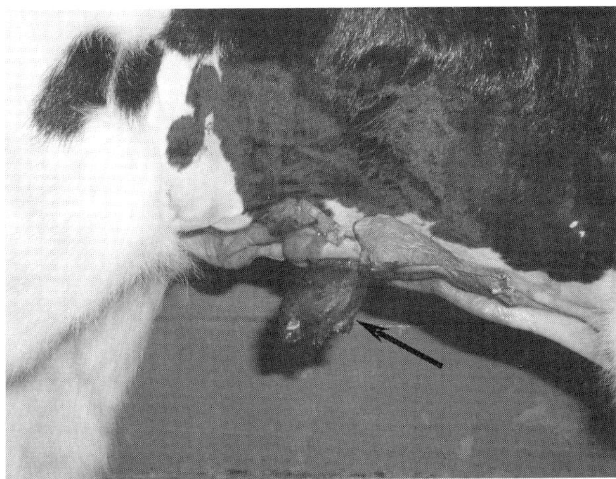

Fig. 11. Lateral view of a marsupialized infected umbilical vein 1 day after surgery. The umbilical vein (*arrow*) is localized on the right side of the abdomen. The exteriorized part of the vein appears swallowed with a red-black color secondary to ischemia of this distal extremity. Repeated resections of the distal end may be necessary to permit complete abscess drainage.

cases. En bloc resection is the treatment of choice for such conditions [23,88]. The approach is similar to the approach for an infected vein, but the perforation of the abdominal wall is performed more cranially. The skin and abdominal wall incisions are continued caudally for a better exposure of the remaining urachus canal and the affected artery (Fig. 13).

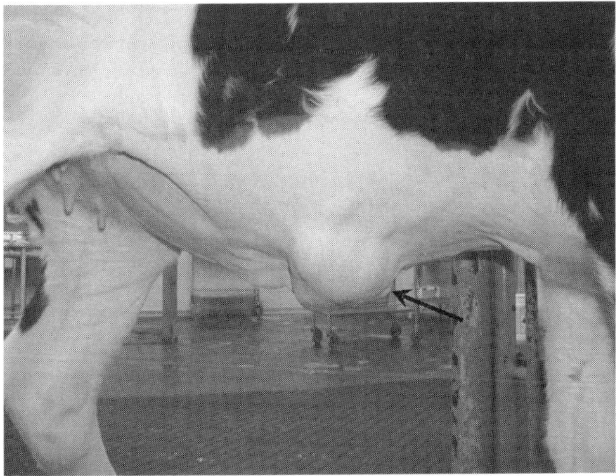

Fig. 12. Abdominal hernia 2 months after umbilical vein marsupialization with the lateral technique. The vein has healed completely, and no drainage is present. A second operation is needed to correct the abdominal wall default.

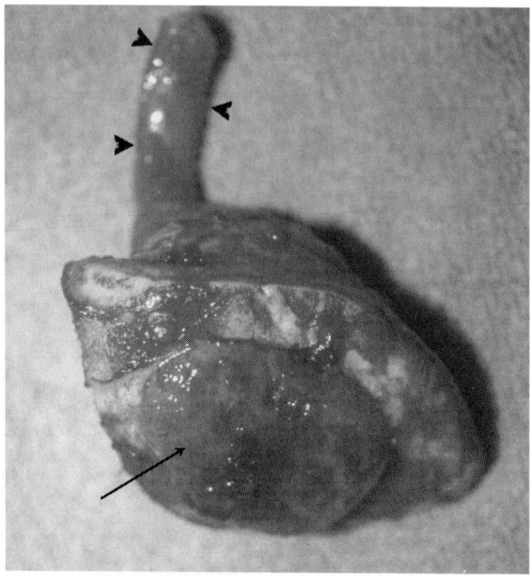

Fig. 13. Anatomic specimen of an umbilical vein after secondary herniorrhaphy. The proximal part (*arrowheads*) is fibrous and can be ligated and sectioned. The external part (*arrow*) looks like granulation tissue.

After isolation of the umbilical remnants by separating the greater omentum, the calf can be positioned with the head tilted downward to increase visualization of the arteries. The arteries have to be ligatured as deep as possible. The use of the three-forceps technique provides maximum safety. The use of an absorbable suture material is preferred, but monofilament or multifilament can be used. Careful traction should be performed on the arteries to avoid any tearing of the internal iliac artery. The urachus canal is removed by partial apical cystectomy. The body wall is closed as mentioned previously for the infected umbilical vein.

Visualization of the arteries can be difficult, and an inexperienced surgeon may try to pull too forcefully on the structure, creating a rent in the aorta and a major hemorrhage. Because it is difficult to ligature the umbilical arteries at their basis, it is the authors' opinion that the ligatures have to be placed at least 1 cm proximally to the extremity of the infection, instead of exercising an excessive traction on the arteries. Marsupialization of the umbilical artery, 6 cm cranial to the forequarter and 5 cm lateral to the midline, has been described by Lopez and Markel [21].

Infection of the urachus canal

The urachus canal infection is the most common infection of an umbilical remnant [23]. The surgical approach is the same as described for infection of the arteries. Adhesion of the greater omentum to the urachal abscess can be tight, and dissection can be challenging to separate both structures (Fig. 14)

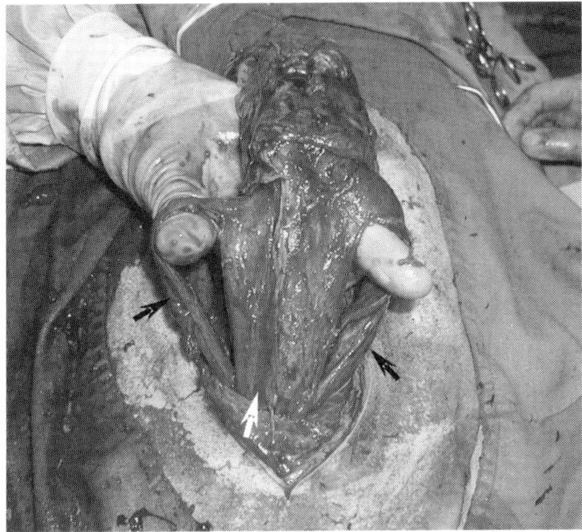

Fig. 14. Caudal umbilical structures in calves. The ventral approach allows visualization of the umbilical arteries (*black arrows*) and the enlarged urachus canal (*white arrow*).

[23,88]. Care is taken not to tear the urachus canal. If omentum is attached firmly, a sharp resection can be done, followed by a suture with a USP 2-0 absorbable suture material in a simple continuous pattern on the greater omentum. After separation and ligature of both umbilical arteries as deep as possible, careful traction is applied to exteriorize the apex of the bladder. Increasing the surgical incision caudally allows better access to the bladder without excessive tension. A linear enterectomy forceps is positioned at 1 cm caudally to the apex of the bladder, and a second one is positioned at the junction between the urachus canal and the bladder. The section of the bladder is performed following the most cranial forceps with a scalpel blade to penetrate the bladder. The suture of the bladder is performed in two inverted layers in a continuous pattern with USP 2-0 absorbable suture material on a swagged on taper needle. Care should be taken to avoid suture penetration of the bladder mucosa [88,89]. Suture of the body wall is routine as previously described.

Surgery of the urinary tract

Ruptured bladder

Ruptured bladder is an uncommon cause of acute painful abdomen [59]. In horses, ruptured bladder is associated with dystocia. In cattle, urethral obstruction seems to be the primary cause of rupture in most cases, but ruptured bladder has been reported in heifers [26,90]. The uroperitoneum brings severe blood chemistry changes, such as increased uremia, hyponatremia, and hypochloremia. Ruminants, including calves, do not develop hyperkalemia, however [91,92]. Diagnosis is made based on the history, ventral abdominal wall distention, and absence of urine flow. Ultrasound shows free abdominal fluid. The diagnosis is confirmed by a high creatinine concentration in the abdominal fluid.

Correcting electrolyte imbalances with appropriate fluids is a prerequisite to surgical correction of the default. Because this condition occurs in young calves, en bloc resection of the umbilical remnants is performed during the surgery. A classic umbilical approach is performed as described earlier, and the incision is extended caudally for a better exposure of the bladder. After localization of the rupture, the bladder is closed in two layers as described for the partial apical cystectomy procedure. Abdominal lavage with sterile warm saline dilutes inflammatory mediators, fibrins, and microorganisms.

Nephrectomy

Pyelonephritis [37], ectopic ureter [93], and polycystic kidneys are rare diseases of the renal system in calves [79]. Unilateral nephrectomy may be required to treat these pathologies if the contralateral kidney is functional as determined by blood chemistry and ultrasound. The right kidney is removed extraperitoneally via a right paralumbar approach close to the last rib [92,94]. The left kidney, because of its dorsal midline position and long renal pedicle, is removed transperitoneally via a right paralumbar fossa laparotomy or via a left paralumbar fossa laparotomy in young calves [31,92]. In one case, an ectopic intra-abdominal infected left kidney concurrent with an infected urachal canal was removed by ventral midline celiotomy [37]. In contrast to adult cattle, the surgery is performed with the calf in lateral recumbency under sedation with a paravertebral anesthesia. After a blind dissection around the kidney, ligatures around the artery, vein, and ureter are done blindly with a USP 1 or 2 absorbable suture material. The abdominal wall is sutured as routinely done for centered paralumbar fossa laparotomy. In the case of a paracostal approach for right kidney removal, the proximal part of the subperitoneal space is left open if it communicates with the abdomen cavity; the closure of the body is routine.

References

[1] Dirksen GU, Garry FB. Diseases of the forestomachs in calves: I. Comp Cont Educ 1987;9: F140–7.

[2] Dirksen GU, Garry FB. Diseases of the forestomachs in calves: II. Comp Cont Educ 1987;9: F173–80.

[3] Von Keindorf HJ. Abomasitis of calf. Monatsh Veterinaermed 1967;20:606–7.

[4] Mass J, Parish SM, Hodgson DR, Valberg SJ. Nutritional myodegeration. In: Smith BP, editor. Large animal internal medicine. 3rd edition. St Louis: Mosby; 2002. p. 1279–82.

[5] Fubini SL. Intestinal obstruction in calves. In: Proceedings of the fourteenth world congress on diseases of cattle. Dublin, 1986. p. 14–7.

[6] Katchuik R. Abomasal disease in young beef calves: surgical findings and management factors. Can Vet J 1992;33:459–61.

[7] Hawkins CD, Fraser DM, Bolton JR, Wyburn RS, McGill CA, Pearse BHG. Left abomasal displacement and ulceration in an eight-week-old calf. Aust Vet J 1986;63:53–5.
[8] Troutt HF, Fessler JF, Page EH, Amstutz HE. Diaphragmatic defects in cattle. J Am Vet Med Assoc 1967;151:1421–9.
[9] Kümper H. A new treatment for abomasal bloat in calves. Bov Pract 1995;29:80–2.
[10] Iselin U, Steiner A. End-to-end anastomosis of the jejunum by use of a biofragmentable anastomosis ring in a calf. J Am Vet Med Assoc 1993;202:1123–5.
[11] Hammond PB, Dziuk HE, Usenik EA, Stevens CE. Experimental intestinal obstruction in calves. J Comp Pathol 1964;74:210–21.
[12] Abutarbush SM, Radostits OM. Obstruction of the small intestine caused by a hairball in 2 young beef calves. Can Vet J 2004;45:324–5.
[13] Fubini SL. Surgical management of gastrointestinal obstruction in calves. Comp Cont Educ 1990;12:591–8.
[14] Anderson DE, Constable PD, St-Jean G, Hull BL. Small-intestinal volvulus in cattle: 35 cases (1967–1992). J Am Vet Med Assoc 1993;203:1178–83.
[15] Iselin U, Lischer CJ, Stocker H, Steiner AL. Kolik beim Kalb, eine retrospektive Studie über 40 Fälle. Wien Tierärztl Mschr 1997;84:20–5.
[16] Smith DF, Ducharme NG, Fubini SL, Donawick WJ, Erb HN. Clinical management and surgical repair of atresia coli in calves: 66 cases (1977–1988). J Am Vet Med Assoc 1991; 199:1185–90.
[17] Barrington GM, Parish SM. Failure of passive transfer. In: Smith BP, editor. Large animal internal medicine. 3rd edition. St Louis: Mosby; 2002. p. 1600–2.
[18] Fecteau G, Palmer M. L'utilisation du plasma en néonatalogie bovine. Med Vet Québec 1996;26:73–6.
[19] Desrochers A, St-Jean G, Anderson DE, Rogers DP, Chengappa MM. Comparative evaluation of two surgical scrub preparation in cattle. Vet Surg 1996;25:336–41.
[20] Hendrickson DA, Rakestraw PC, Ducharme NG. Surgical repair of atresia jejuni in two calves. J Am Vet Med Assoc 1992;201:594–6.
[21] Lopez MJ, Markel MD. Umbilical artery marsupialization in a calf. Can Vet J 1996;37: 170–1.
[22] Edwards RB, Fubini SL. A one-stage marsupialization procedure for management of infected umbilical vein remnants in calves and foals. Vet Surg 1995;24:32–5.
[23] Trent AM, Smith DF. Surgical management of umbilical masses with associated umbilical cord remnant infections in calves. J Am Vet Med Assoc 1984;185:1531–4.
[24] Trent AM. Surgical management of umbilical masses in calves. Bov Pract 1987;22:170–3.
[25] Steiner A, Lischer CJ, Oertle C. Marsupialization of umbilical vein abscesses with involvement of the liver in 13 calves. Vet Surg 1993;22:184–9.
[26] Roussel AJ, Ward DS. Ruptured urinary bladder in a heifer. J Am Vet Med Assoc 1985;186: 1310–1.
[27] Buchoo BA, Sudhan NA. Successful repair of ruptured urinary bladder in male calves—case report. Indian Vet J 1994;71:593–5.
[28] Haskins SC. Monitoring the anesthetized patient. In: Thurmon JC, Tranquilli WJ, Benson GJ, editors. Lumb and Jones' veterinary anesthesia. 3rd edition. Baltimore: Lea & Febiger; 1996. p. 409–24.
[29] Uytepruyst CH, Coche J, Bureau F, Lekeux P. Evaluation of accuracy of pulse oximetry in newborn calves. Vet J 2000;159:71–6.
[30] Stamp CV, McGergor W, Rodeheaver GT, Thacker JG, Towler MA, Edlich RF. Surgical needle holder damage to suture. Am Surg 1988;54:300–6.
[31] Leicht ID. Unilateral pyelonephritis and nephrectomy in a bull calf. Vet Rec 1969;85:686–7.
[32] Constable PD, St Jean G, Hull BL, Rings DM, Morin DE, Nelson DR. Intussusception in cattle: 336 cases (1964–1993). J Am Vet Med Assoc 1997;210:531–6.
[33] Tulleners EP. Surgical correction of volvulus of the root of the mesentery in calves. J Am Vet Med Assoc 1981;179:998–9.

[34] Ducharme NG, Arighi M, Horney FD, et al. Colonic atresia in cattle: a prospective study of 43 cases. Can Vet J 1988;29:918–24.
[35] Horne MM. Colonic intussusception in a Holstein calf. Can Vet J 1991;32:493–5.
[36] Doll K, Klee W, Dirksen G. Blinddarminvaginationen beim Kalb. Tierärtzl Prax Ausg G Grosstiere Nutztiere 1998;26:247–53.
[37] Mueller PO, Hay WP, Allen D, Collatos C, Watson E. Removal of an ectopic left kidney through a ventral midline celiotomy in a calf. J Am Vet Med Assoc 1999;214:532–4.
[38] Akcay MN, Capan MY, Gundogdu C, Polat M, Oren D. Bacterial translocation in experimental intestinal obstruction. J Intern Med Res 1996;24:17–26.
[39] Moll HD, Wolfe DF, Schumacher J, Wright JC. Evaluation of sodium carboxymethylcellulose for prevention of adhesions after uterine trauma in ewes. Am J Vet Res 1992;53: 1454–6.
[40] Hay WP, Mueller POE, Harmon B, Amoroso L. One percent sodium carboxymethylcellulose prevents experimentally induced abdominal adhesions in horses. Vet Surg 2001;30: 223–7.
[41] Murphy DJ, Peck LS, Detrisac CJ, Widenhouse CW, Goldberg EP. Use of a high-molecular-weight carboxymethylcellulose in a tissue protective solution for prevention of post operative abdominal adhesions in ponies. Am J Vet Res 2002;63:1448–54.
[42] Eggleston RB, Mueller POE, Parviainen AK, Groover ES. Effect of carboxymethylcellulose and hyaluronate solutions on jejunal healing in horses. Am J Vet Res 2004;65:637–43.
[43] Navarre CB, Belknap EB, Rowe SE. Differentiation of gastrointestinal diseases of calves. Vet Clin North Am Food Anim Pract 2000;16:37–57.
[44] Dirksen GU. Tympany, displacement and torsion of the abomasum in calves: pathogenesis, diagnosis and treatment. Bov Pract 1994;28:120–6.
[45] Thurmond MC. Bovine lymphosarcoma. In: Smith BP, editor. Large animal internal medicine. 3rd edition. St Louis: Mosby; 2002. p. 1067–71.
[46] Ducharme NG, Fubini SL. Ruminal distension in calves. In: Ducharme NG, Fubini SL, editors. Farm animal surgery. Philadelphia: WB Saunders; 2004. p. 466–8.
[47] Sattler N. La ruminostomie chez les bovines. Point Vétérinaire 2000;31:725.
[48] Dehghani SN, Ghadrdani AM. Bovine rumenotomy: comparison of four surgical techniques. Can Vet J 1995;36:693–7.
[49] Smith DL, Muson L, Erb HN. Abomasal ulcer in adult dairy cattle. Cornell Vet 1983;73: 213–24.
[50] Lebreton P, Mathevet P. Ulcères de la caillette: la piste des oligo-éléments. Point Vétérinaire 2003;34:44–6.
[51] Mills WM, Johnson JL, Jensen RL, Woodard LF, Doster AR. Laboratory findings associated with abomasal ulcers/tympany in range calves. J Vet Diagn Invest 1990;2:208–12.
[52] Roeder BL, Chengappa MM, Nagaraja TG, Avery TB, Kennedy GA. Isolation of *Clostridium perfringens* from neonatal calves with ruminal and abomasal tympany, abomasitis, and abomasal ulceration. J Am Vet Med Assoc 1987;190:1550–5.
[53] Tulleners EP, Hamilton GF. Surgical resection of perforated abomasal ulcers in calves. Can Vet J 1980;21:261–4.
[54] Ahmed AF, Constable PD, Misk NA. Effect of orally administered cimetidine and ranitidine on abomasal luminal pH in clinically normal milk-fed calves. Am J Vet Res 2001;62:1531–8.
[55] Albert TF, Ramey DB. Abomasal torsion and ulceration in two calves. J Am Vet Med Assoc 1967;150:408–11.
[56] Mueller K, Merrall M, Sargison ND. Left abomasal displacement and ulceration with perforation of abdominal musculature in two calves. Vet J 1999;157:95–7.
[57] Lorch VA, Rademacher G. Pathologish-anatomische Befunde bei Kälbern mit perforierendem Labmagengeschwür. Tierärtl Umschau 2001;56:572–81.
[58] Wendel H, Rademacher G, Klee W. Differentiadiagnostik der Kolik bei Kalb und Jungrind. Teil 1: Prüfung des diagnostischen Wertes von Schweregrad der Kolik und Krankheitsdauer. Tierärzt Prax 1999;27(G):199–206.

[59] Naylor JM, Bailey JV. A retrospective study of 51 cases of abdominal problems in the calf: etiology, diagnosis and prognosis. Can Vet J 1987;28:657–62.

[60] Navetat H, Rizet C. Chirurgie des troubles de la caillette chez le veau. Point Vétérinaire 2000; 31(numéro spécial):742–5.

[61] Navetat H, Schelcher F, Rizet C, Cabanie P, Espinasse J. Differential diagnosis between abomasum torsion, mesenteric torsion and caecum dilatation/volvulus in calves. Bov Pract 1998;32:53–4.

[62] Bristol DG, Fubini SL. Surgery of the neonatal bovine digestive tract. Vet Clin North Am Food Anim Pract 1990;6:473–93.

[63] Saint-Jean GD, Hull BL, Hoffsis GF, Rings MD. Comparison of the different surgical techniques for correction of abomasal problems. Comp Cont Educ 1987;9:F377–82.

[64] Hylton WE, Rousseaux CG. Intestinal strangulation associated with omphaloarteritis in a calf. J Am Vet Med Assoc 1985;186:1099.

[65] Wolfe DF, Mysinger PW, Robert LC, Powers RD, Rice DN. Incarceration of a section of small intestine by remnants of the ductus deferens in steers. J Am Vet Med Assoc 1987;191: 1597–8.

[66] Smith DF. Surgery of the bovine small intestine. Vet Clin North Am Food Anim Pract 1990; 6:449–60.

[67] Julian RJ, Hawke TW. Cecalcolic intussusception in a calf. Can Vet J 1963;4:54–5.

[68] Braun U, Marmier O, Pusterla N. Ultrasonographic examination of the small intestine of cows with ileus of the duodenum, jejunum or ileum. Vet Rec 1995;137:209–15.

[69] Martens A, Gasthuys F, Steenhaut M, De Moor A. Surgical aspect of intestinal atresia in 58 calves. Vet Rec 1995;136:141–4.

[70] Steenhaut M, De Moor A, Vershooten F, Desmet P. Intestinal malformations in calves and their surgical correction. Vet Rec 1976;98:131–3.

[71] Steiner A, Braun U, Waldvogel A. Comparison of staple and suture techniques for partial typhlectomy in the cow: A clinical prospective study of 40 cases. J Am Vet Med Assoc 1992; 39:26–37.

[72] Hamilton GF, Tulleners EP. Intussusception involving the spiral colon in a calf. Can Vet J 1980;21:32.

[73] Syed M, Shanks RD. Incidence of atresia coli and relationships among the affected calves in one herd of Holstein cattle. J Dairy Sci 1992;75:1357–64.

[74] Syed M, Shanks RD. Atresia coli inherited in Holstein cattle. J Dairy Sci 1992;75: 1105–11.

[75] Constable PD, Huhn JC, Morin DE, Nelson DR. Atresia coli in calves: etiopathogenesis and surgical management. Bov Pract 1999;33:70–3.

[76] Kiliç N, Sarierler M. Congenital atresia in calves: 61 cases (1999–2003). Rev Med Vet (Toulouse) 2004;155:381–4.

[77] Dreyfuss DJ, Tulleners EP. Intestinal atresia in calves: 22 cases (1978–1988). J Am Vet Med Assoc 1989;195:508–13.

[78] Bouisset S, Daviaud L, Ruckebusch Y. Atrésie du colon terminal chez un veau. Point Vétérinaire 1985;17:485–7.

[79] Mulon PY, Desrochers A, Babkine M, Couture Y, Fecteau G, Francoz D. Surgical abdomen in calves: 132 cases (1992–2002). Méd Vétérinaire Québec 2004;34:157.

[80] Barone R. Topographie abdominale du veau. In: Barone R, editor. Anatomie comparée des mammifères domestiques. Tome4 Splanchnologie II. 3rd edition. Paris: Edition Vigot; 2001. p. 769–79.

[81] Baxter GM. Umbilical masses in calves: diagnosis, treatment, and complications. Comp Cont Educ 1989;11:505–13.

[82] Priester WA, Glass AG, Waggoner NS. Congenital defects in domesticated animals: general considerations. Am J Vet Res 1970;31:1871–9.

[83] Hayes HM. Congenital umbilical and inguinal hernias in cattle, horses, swine, dogs and cats: risk by breed and sex among hospital patients. Am J Vet Res 1974;35:839–42.

[84] Buczinski SMC. Étude clinique de cas de pathologie ombilicale chez le veau—comparaison de la palpation et de l'examen échographique. Thèse de doctorat vétérinaire. Ecole Nationale Vétérinaire d'Alfort; 2002.

[85] Staller GS, Tulleners EP, Reef VB, Spencer PA. Concordance of ultrasonographic and physical findings in cattle with an umbilical mass or suspected to have infection of the umbilical cord remnants: 32 cases (1987–1989). J Am Vet Med Assoc 1995;206:77–82.

[86] Bouré L, Foster RA, Palmer M, Hathway A. Use of an endoscopic suturing device for laparoscopic resection of the apex of the bladder and umbilical structure in normal neonatal calves. Vet Surg 2001;30:319–26.

[87] Lewis CA, Constable PD, Huhn JC, Morin DE. Sedation with xylazine and lubosacral epidural administration of lidocaine and xylazine for umbilical suregry in calves. J Am Vet Med Assoc 1999;214:89–95.

[88] Rings DM. Umbilical hernias, umbilical abscesses, and urachal fistulas—surgical considerations. Vet Clin North Am Food Anim Pract 1995;11:137–48.

[89] Hooper RN, Taylor TS. Urinary surgery. Vet Clin North Am Food Anim Pract 1995;11: 95–121.

[90] Bertone AL, Smith DF. Ruptured bladder in a yearling heifer. J Am Vet Med Assoc 1984; 184:981–2.

[91] Wilson DW, MacWilliams PS. An evaluation of the clinical pathologic findings in experimentally induced urinary bladder rupture in pre-ruminant calves. Can J Vet Res 1998; 62:140–3.

[92] Sockett DC, et al. Metabolic changes due to experimentally induced rupture of the bovine urinary bladder. Cornell Vet 1986;76:198–212.

[93] Hammer EJ. Nephrectomy for treatment of ectopic ureter in a Holstein calf. Bov Pract 2000; 34:101–3.

[94] Baird AN. Surgery of the kidney. In: Wolfe DF, Moll HD, editors. Large animal urogenital surgery. 2nd edition. Baltimore: Williams & Wilkins; 1998. p. 367.

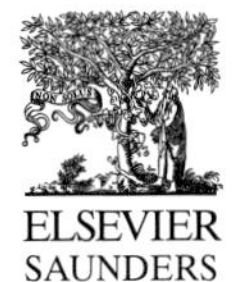

ELSEVIER
SAUNDERS

Vet Clin Food Anim 21 (2005) 133–154

VETERINARY
CLINICS
Food Animal Practice

Intestinal Surgery of Adult Cattle

David E. Anderson, DVM, MS[a,*],
Jennifer M. Ivany Ewoldt, DVM, MS[b]

[a]*Department of Veterinary Clinical Sciences, College of Veterinary Medicine, The Ohio State University, 601 Tharp Street, Columbus, OH 43210, USA*
[b]*Scott County Animal Hospital, Eldridge, IA 52748, USA*

Principles of bovine intestinal surgery

Three factors influence bovine intestinal surgery: anatomy, surgical approach, and anesthesia/analgesia. In cattle, the forestomachs occupy most of the abdominal compartment. In late pregnant cows, the uterus occupies much of the remainder of abdominal space. The remainder of the gastrointestinal tract is limited by space and influenced by abnormalities of the forestomachs and uterus. The cranial part of the descending duodenum courses cranially from the pylorus to the ansa sigmoidea duodenalis medial to the liver. The descending duodenum courses caudally, wraps around the omental curtain, and turns cranially as the ascending duodenum. This portion of the duodenum courses cranial to the root of the mesentery medial to the omentum and joins the jejunum. The entire duodenum is contained by two mesenteries: mesoduodenum and omentum. The jejunum is restricted by a short mesentery except for the distal third of the jejunum and proximal segment of the ileum, which are suspended by a long mesenteric segment often referred to as the "jejunoileal flange." This segment can be exteriorized from the abdomen easily, but the remainder of the jejunum and ileum are poorly exteriorized because of the short mesentery.

Although the demeanor of cattle allows for standing paralumbar fossa laparotomy, excessive tension on the mesentery is likely to stimulate the patient to lie down and interfere with surgical procedures. The authors prefer to perform intestinal surgery with the patient standing after proximal paravertebral anesthesia with or without epidural analgesia when possible, but perform many intestinal resections with the cow recumbent with or without general anesthesia. Right paralumbar fossa laparotomy is preferred

* Corresponding author.
E-mail address: Anderson.670@osu.edu (D.E. Anderson).

0749-0720/05/$ - see front matter
doi:10.1016/j.cvfa.2004.12.010

for access to most of the gastrointestinal tract (duodenum, kidneys, liver, small intestine, large intestine, and cecum). Left paralumbar fossa laparotomy provides limited access and is used most commonly for surgery of the rumen and uterus. Ventral midline laparotomy provides limited access to the intestinal tract in cattle older than 30 days. This approach is used most commonly for surgery of the umbilicus, bladder, and abomasum.

Duodenal obstruction

Duodenal outflow problems occur as a result of obstruction or dysfunction. Duodenal dysfunction occurs as a result of peracute duodenitis, duodenal ulcers with or without perforation, clostridial duodenitis, and electrolyte abnormalities [1–4]. Duodenal obstruction occurs as a result of trichobezoars (discussed later), foreign bodies (eg, gravel), duodenal stricture after an ulcer, obstruction by displacement of viscera (eg, gallbladder, uterus), iatrogenic duodenal obstruction after omentopexy or pyloropexy, and extraluminal compression caused by liver abscess, omental abscess, or lymphosarcoma [3–8].

Clinical signs

Animals affected with duodenal obstruction may be observed to have severe bloat caused by fluid distention of all forestomachs, acute collapse and dehydration, decreased appetite, weight loss, decreased fecal production, lethargy, and apparent depression (Fig. 1) [3]. Affected animals initially show clinical signs of abdominal pain (restlessness, kicking at the abdomen,

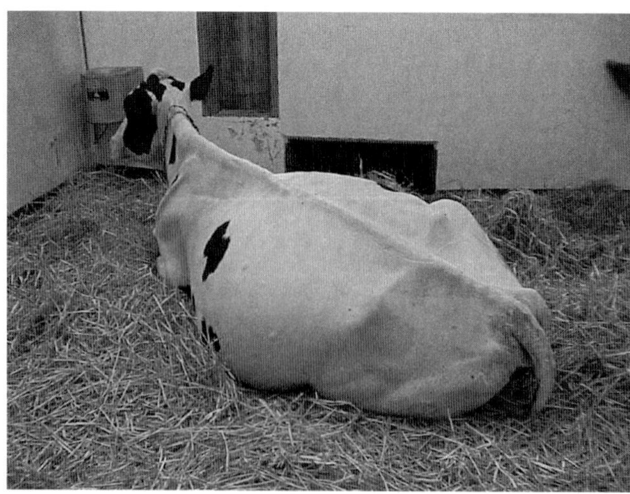

Fig. 1. Holstein cow, recumbent, with severe forestomach distention caused by proximal intestinal outflow obstruction.

lying down and getting up frequently, arching the back, stretching out of the legs while standing) and progress to severe rumen distention, recumbency, and apparent depression. Death ensues because of dehydration and severe electrolyte disturbances.

Clinical pathology

Serum biochemistry analysis reveals profound hypokalemic, hypochloremic metabolic alkalosis, the severity of which depends on the duration of the lesion [3]. These changes are most severe with proximal intestinal obstruction and become more severe with increasing duration. Cows with duodenal disease were reported to have severe hyperglycemia (range 263–990 mg/dL) [10]. If ischemic necrosis of the intestinal wall has occurred, an inflammatory leukogram with increased numbers of immature neutrophils may be seen. As peritonitis develops, and organic acids are released into the bloodstream, the serum biochemistry changes to a metabolic acidosis with relative hyperkalemia. These changes are consistent with a poor prognosis, but death may occur before these changes occur. Perforation of the duodenum with contamination of the abdomen with ingesta carries a poor to grave prognosis.

Diagnosis

In affected cattle, serum biochemistry changes are consistent with intestinal obstruction. Rumen chloride concentration may be elevated (rumen chloride >30 mEq/L). Although not routinely done, rumen fluid bile acid concentration is helpful in differentiating duodenal and proximal jejunum obstructions from abomasal outflow obstruction. Bile acid concentrations in cattle with proximal duodenal or jejunum obstruction had significantly higher rumen bile acid concentration compared with cattle affected with reticuloperitonitis, abomasal displacement, or cecal dilation. The cause of intraluminal obstruction is rarely palpable per rectum, but small intestinal distention may be palpable. Ultrasound examination of the abdomen may be useful [9]. The intestinal tract appears normal, but severe distention of the duodenum and forestomachs is noted. Edema may be observed in the mesoduodenum. Duodenal obstruction should be suspected in cattle with severe rumen tympanites with marked increase in rumen chloride and classic electrolyte changes, especially if there is a history of recent surgery to correct abomasal displacement. Differential diagnoses include trichobezoars, intussusception, vagus indigestion syndrome, intestinal lymphosarcoma, fat necrosis, intestinal entrapment around anomalous fibrovascular bands, and volvulus of the jejunoileal flange.

Treatment

When obstruction of the duodenum is suspected, a right paralumbar fossa celiotomy and exploration of the abdomen should be performed. The obstruction is found by careful palpation and inspection of the duodenum, paying special attention to the ansa sigmoidea. If an intraluminal mass is found, this segment of intestine is exteriorized from the abdomen and isolated using moistened surgical towels, and an enterotomy is performed. After removal of the foreign body, the enterotomy is closed with absorbable suture material (eg, No. 2-0 polydioxanone, polyglactin 910) using two lines of an inverting suture pattern. The enterotomy may be closed transversely to maximize the lumen of the affected segment of intestine and to minimize the tension endured by the suture line during contraction of the intestinal wall. When the perceived economic value of the affected cattle is high, surgery may be performed with the patient under general anesthesia; this minimizes the risk of ingesta contamination of the abdomen during surgery. If a duodenal stricture is found, a duodenoduodenostomy or jejunoduodenostomy may be performed. This procedure may be accomplished by hand-sewn anastomosis or by staple techniques. In the authors' experience, staplers designed for use in human intestine are prone to dehiscence when used in bovine intestine. Staplers designed for use in horse intestine have a sufficient staple arm length for clinical use in bovine bowel, but these instruments are cost prohibitive in most cases. Surgical correction is best performed by side-to-side anastomosis of the cranial part of the descending duodenum to the descending duodenum. The side-to-side anastomosis should maximize the dimension of the stoma created. The most accessible segment of duodenum is placed alongside the cranial part of the descending duodenum, and seromuscular stay sutures are placed to maintain positioning without tension of the anastomotic site. A 5- to 10-cm-long enterotomy is performed, and a side-to-side anastomosis is performed.

Intravenous fluid therapy is based on the clinical estimate of dehydration, severity of intestinal lesion identified at surgery, and severity of serum biochemistry changes. In general, cattle should receive 20 to 60 L of isotonic saline intravenously over 12 hours. The authors routinely add calcium (1 mL of 23% calcium gluconate/kg body weight) and dextrose (to create a 1.25% solution) to the intravenous fluids. Nonsteroidal anti-inflammatory drugs (eg, flunixin meglumine, 1 mg/kg body weight intravenously every 12 hours × 3 days) and antibiotics (for 3–5 days) also are administered.

Prognosis

The prognosis for return to productive use is based on the animal's body condition, severity of changes in serum biochemistry variables [11], presence of visceral perforation or peritonitis, and ability to perform surgical removal of the foreign body without contaminating the abdomen. Cattle that are less than 10% dehydrated and have mild-to-moderate hypochloremia (eg, chloride >80 mEq/L) and metabolic alkalosis (eg, bicarbonate >32 mEq/L) have a fair-to-good prognosis for recovery. Cattle that are more than 10% dehydrated, have severe hypochloremia (eg, chloride <80 mEq/L) and metabolic acidosis (eg, bicarbonate <20 mEq/L), or have visceral perforation have a poor prognosis for survival. Immediate surgical intervention is required for alleviation of clinical signs caused by intraluminal foreign bodies. In one study, 23 cows with duodenal ileus were reported [3]. Of these cows, 10 were slaughtered after diagnosis, and 13 cows had phytobezoars, of which 11 survived.

Prevention

Duodenal obstruction occurs infrequently in cattle. The sporadic nature of the problem limits recommendations for prevention. Adequate dietary roughage should be made available to cattle at all times.

Intussusception

Intussusception refers to the invagination of one segment of intestine into an adjacent segment of intestine. The invaginated portion of intestine is termed the *intussusceptum,* and the outer, or receiving, segment of intestine is termed the *intussuscipiens* (Fig. 2). Intussusception occurs sporadically in cattle of all ages, breeds, and gender and may be seen anytime during the year [12,13]. In a case-control epidemiologic study of 336 cattle, intussusception occurred most commonly in calves less than 2 months old, Brown Swiss cattle seemed to be overrepresented, and Hereford cattle seemed to be underrepresented compared with Holstein cattle [12]. Although the inciting cause is rarely identified, intussusception may occur secondary to enteritis, intestinal parasitism, sudden changes in diet, mural granuloma or abscess, intestinal neoplasia (especially adenocarcinoma), mural hematoma, and administration of drugs that affect intestinal motility. Any focal disturbance of intestinal motility may facilitate the invagination of an orad segment into an aborad segment of intestine. Intussusception occurs most commonly in

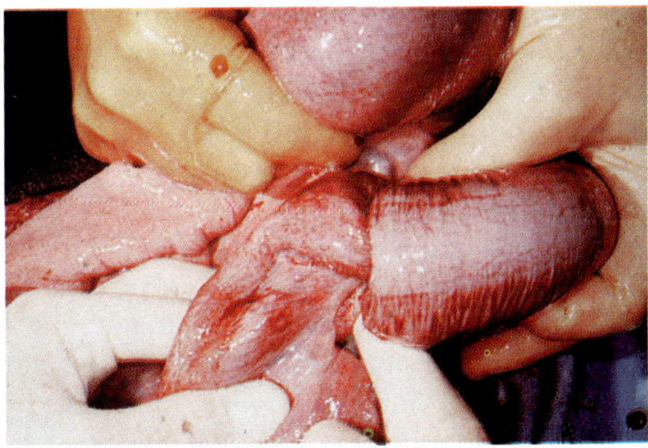

Fig. 2. Intussusception in an adult Holstein cow.

the distal portion of the jejunum, but intussusception has been found affecting the proximal jejunum, ileum, cecum, and spiral colon [12–18]. In a review of 336 intussusceptions in cattle, 281 affected the small intestine; 7 were ileocolic, 12 were cecocolic, and 36 were colocolic [12].

Clinical signs

Cattle affected with intussusception show clinical signs of abdominal pain (restlessness, kicking at the abdomen, lying down and getting up frequently, assuming abnormal posture) for 24 hours after the onset of disease. Cattle frequently are anorectic, lethargic, and reluctant to walk. After the initial signs of abdominal pain subside, affected cattle become progressively lethargic, are recumbent, and show apparent depression. Abdominal distention becomes apparent after 24 to 48 hours. Abdominal distention is caused by gas and fluid distention of the forestomach and intestines, and sequestration of ingesta within the gastrointestinal tract results in progressive dehydration and electrolyte depletion. Heart rate increases proportionally to abdominal pain, intestinal necrosis, and dehydration. Fecal production may be normal for 12 hours after the occurrence of the intussusception, but minimal fecal production is noted after 24 hours. Passage of blood and mucus from the rectum is common at this time.

Clinical pathology

Hemoconcentration is usually present (increased packed cell volume and total protein), and an inflammatory leukogram may be seen if ischemic necrosis of the intussusceptum has occurred. Often, changes in the white blood cell count and differential are minimal, and changes in peritoneal fluid constituents are not seen because the intussusceptum is isolated by the intussuscipiens. Hypochloremic metabolic alkalosis is found with serum biochemistry analysis. Hyponatremia, hypokalemia, hypocalcemia, azotemia, and hyperglycemia also may be found. The magnitude of these changes depends on the location and duration of the lesion. Proximal jejunal intussusception causes rapid and severe dehydration, electrolyte sequestration, and metabolic alkalosis. Most lesions occur in the distal jejunum and may require more than 48 hours to develop these changes. Elevation of rumen chloride concentration ($>$30 mEq/L) may be found if fluid distention of the rumen is present.

Diagnosis

Diagnosis of intussusception usually is made during exploratory laparotomy. Occasionally the intussusception can be felt during rectal palpation, but distention of multiple loops of small intestine is most commonly identified. In the authors' experience, an intussusception may be present for 48 hours or more in adult cattle without being able to find

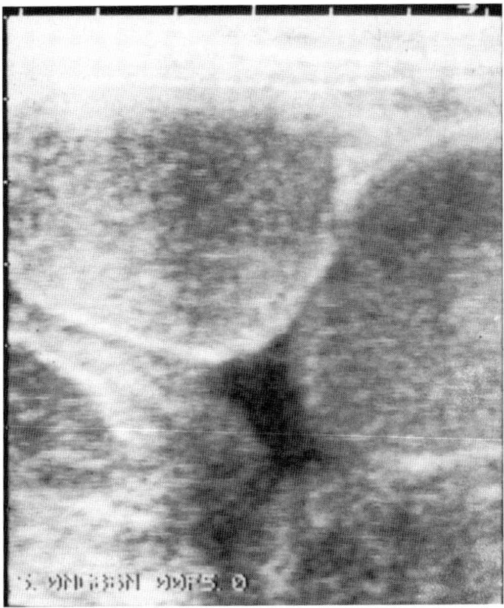

Fig. 3. Ultrasound of the abdomen shows fluid-distended intestinal loops with increased peritoneal fluid.

intestinal distention during rectal palpation. In calves and small ruminants, percutaneous palpation and ultrasound examination of the abdomen may be used to identify intestinal distention and, possibly, the intussusception (Figs. 3 and 4). It should be suspected in cattle with a history of abdominal pain and distention, scant feces consisting of blood and mucus, and palpable distention of the intestine. Differential diagnoses include primary indigestion, functional ileus, trichobezoar, foreign bodies, intestinal incarceration or strangulation, vagal syndrome, intestinal neoplasia, fat necrosis, and jejunoileal flange volvulus.

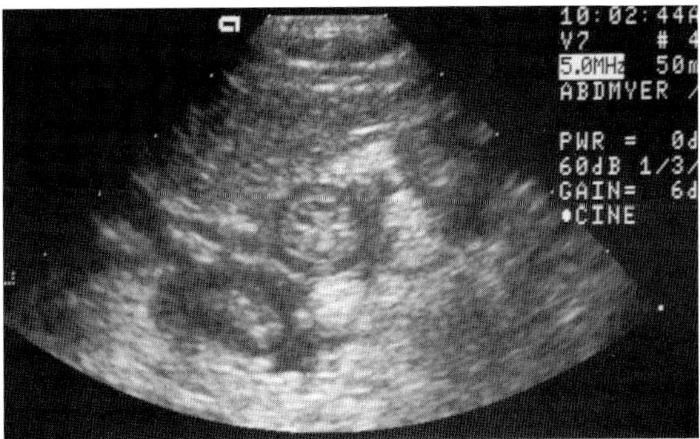

Fig. 4. Ultrasound of abdomen shows "target" lesion suggesting intussusception.

Treatment

Affected cattle must be stabilized before surgical intervention is performed. Fluid therapy should be administered to replace fluid and electrolyte deficits. Surgical correction may proceed after the patient has been assessed as a suitable candidate. Right paralumbar fossa exploratory laparotomy is the surgical approach of choice for treatment of intussusception. Most of the small intestine of cattle has a short mesentery, preventing adequate exteriorization of the intussusception through a ventral midline incision. Also, the attachments of the greater omentum limit exposure with this approach. The presence of the rumen in the left hemiabdomen prevents adequate exteriorization of the intussusception through a left paralumbar incision. Most often, diagnostic exploratory laparotomy is performed with the cow standing after regional anesthesia. Tension on the mesentery of the small intestine results in pain, and cattle may attempt to lie down during the procedure. Of 35 cattle having standing right paralumbar fossa laparotomy for resection of intussusception, 14% became recumbent and 26% attempted to become recumbent during the surgery [12]. Preoperative planning should include anticipation of this possibility. When intussusception is suspected and the animal is of high perceived economic value, right paralumbar fossa celiotomy may be performed with the patient under general anesthesia and in left lateral recumbency. The intussusception may be more difficult to elevate through the incision in recumbent cattle because the fluid-filled bowel gravitates away from the surgical site, but isolation and resection of the intussusception can be done without risk of the animal lying down during the procedure and with minimal risk of contamination of the abdomen.

Surgical removal by resection and anastomosis is the treatment of choice for intussusception. The intussusception is exteriorized from the abdomen and isolated using a barrier drape and moistened towels. Manual reduction of the intussusception is not recommended because of the risk for rupture of the intestine during manipulation, probable ischemic necrosis of the intestine after surgery, possible reoccurrence of the intussusception, and prolonged ileus caused by motility disturbance and swelling in the affected segment of bowel. The margins for excision are selected in healthy-appearing intestine. In general, the distal margin may be 10 cm aborad to the lesion, but the proximal margin should be a minimum of 30 cm orad to the lesion. The larger proximal segment is chosen because chronic distention, inflammation, microvascular thrombosis, relative ischemia, and noxious ingesta accumulated in this segment may cause severe and prolonged postoperative ileus. Cattle have a short mesentery; traction on it is painful, and the animal may go down at this moment. This short mesentery precludes adequate exteriorization of some segment of the small bowel. Only the portion to be resected should be exteriorized to avoid excessive traction and contamination during the resection and anastomosis.

Infiltration of lidocaine 2% into the mesentery where it is planned to be resected may decrease the pain of traction.

The mesenteric vessels (arteries and veins) are ligated using "mass ligation" with absorbable suture material (No. 3 chromic gut, No. 1 polyglactin 910), making sure not to compromise the blood supply to the intestine to be preserved. Mass ligation is required because cattle do not have an arcuate vascular anatomy as do horses, and the fatty mesentery renders vessel identification difficult and time-consuming. The sutures are placed in an overlapping pattern such that double ligation of the vessels is accomplished. This technique may be performed rapidly and efficiently. In the authors' experience, stapling instrumentation is highly unreliable for occlusion of mesenteric vessels because of the large amount of fat normally found in the intestinal mesentery of cattle. When the authors used stapling instruments, extensive manual ligation was required to control hemorrhage. After completion of mesentery ligation and transection, Doyen intestinal forceps are used to occlude the lumen of the normal and abnormal bowel (Fig. 5). Then the intussusception and associated bowel are resected and discarded. The proximal segment of bowel is exteriorized carefully to its maximal length, and the Doyen forceps is removed. Ingesta within the intestine orad to the lesion is "milked" out through the enterectomy site, being careful not to contaminate the incision or abdomen with ingesta. This procedure lessens the severity of postoperative ileus and shortens convalescence.

The two segments of intestine are reunited by end-to-end or side-to-side anastomosis with an absorbable suture material (No. 2-0 polydioxanone or polyglactin 910) using a simple continuous suture pattern. The anastomosis is performed in three overlapping suture lines, each placed in one third of the circumference, or in four overlapping suture lines, each placed in one fourth of the circumference so that a purse-string effect is not created. The

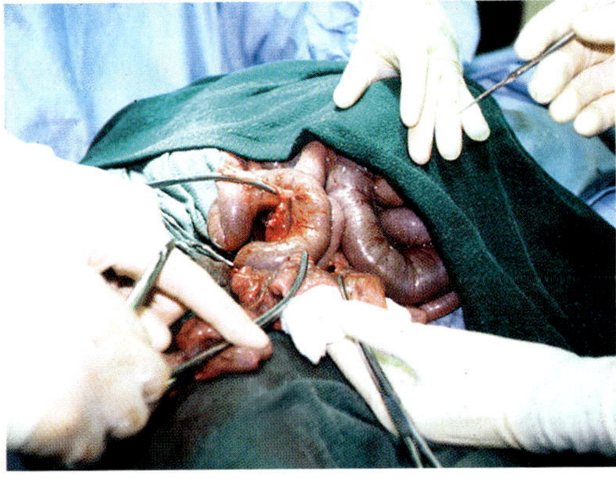

Fig. 5. Doyen intestinal clamps used to isolate segment of intestine during resection to minimize risks of contamination of surgical field or abdomen with ingesta.

initial suture line should be placed at the mesenteric attachment because this is the most likely site for leakage to occur. A second row of sutures is placed to prevent leakage using interrupted segments of inverting suture patterns (eg, Cushing or Lembert). The affected intestine is washed thoroughly with sterile isotonic fluids, checked for the presence of leakage, and replaced into the abdomen. The authors place a solution of antibiotic (5 million U of potassium penicillin G or 1 g of ceftiofur sodium), heparin (20 U/kg body weight), and saline (1000 mL) into the abdomen before closing the abdominal wall in routine fashion.

Postoperative management should be directed to prevent dehydration, maintain optimal blood electrolyte concentration, control for infection and inflammation, and stimulate appetite. Intravenous fluids are beneficial during the first 24 hours after surgery. The authors routinely perform rumen transfaunation 12 to 24 hours after surgery to stimulate forestomach motility and appetite. Withholding food after surgery should not be done. Administration of butorphanol tartrate (0.02–0.04 mg/kg intravenously) may help with pain induced ileus by providing mild visceral analgesia without direct adverse effects on intestinal motility.

Prognosis

The prognosis for return to productivity after surgical correction of intussusception varies and depends on the duration of the lesion. In the authors' experience, cattle respond favorably to surgery if operated within 48 hours of the onset of the disease. Cattle presenting with severe dehydration (>12%), tachycardia (heart rate >120 beats/min), severe decrease in serum chloride concentration (chloride <80 mEq/L), and severe abdominal distention are considered to have a poor prognosis for survival. In the authors' experience, calves respond more favorably to surgery than adult cattle. If viscera rupture is present at the time of surgery, the prognosis is grave. Of cattle in which surgical correction was attempted, 85 of 143 cattle with small intestinal intussusception, 0 of 4 with ileocolic, 10 of 11 with cecocolic, and 10 of 20 with colocolic were discharged from the hospital [12].

Prevention

Recommendations for prevention of intussusception are difficult because the cause is seldom identified, and a seasonal predilection has not been shown. Changes in dietary management should be made gradually, and good hygiene and control strategies should be practiced to minimize transmission of enteric diseases or internal parasites.

Intestinal volvulus

Volvulus refers to the rotation of viscera about its mesenteric attachment. Torsion refers to the rotation of viscera about its own (or long) axis.

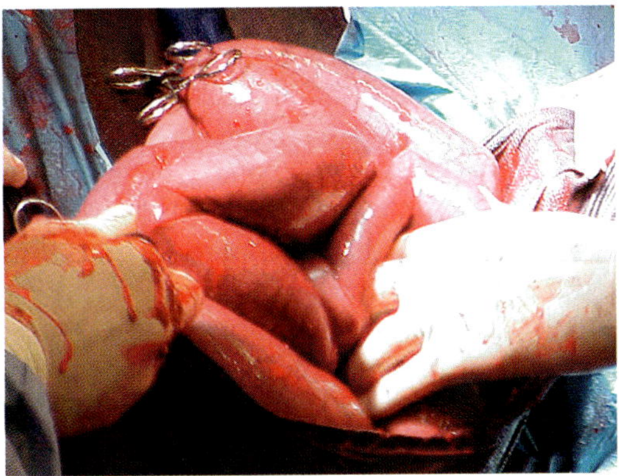

Fig. 6. Volvulus of root of the mesentery results in extreme dilation of bowel and severely limits exteriorization during surgery.

Although torsion of the abomasum and uterus are found in cattle, torsion of the small intestine is rare. Small intestinal volvulus may occur in different forms [11,19,20]. The most severe form of intestinal volvulus originates from the root of the mesentery and involves the entirety of the small intestine and mesenteries (Fig. 6). Volvulus of the root of the mesentery causes obstruction of venous outflow and arterial blood supply to the intestines. Ischemic necrosis of the intestine occurs rapidly, which causes metabolic acidosis, shock, and death. Volvulus of the jejunoileal flange refers to volvulus of the mid to distal jejunum and proximal ileum where the mesentery is long (Fig. 7). This long mesentery and associated bowel has been termed the *flange* and may rotate about its mesentery without involving the remaining small intestine. Often, arterial occlusion is not found with volvulus of the jejunoileal flange, possibly because extensive fat

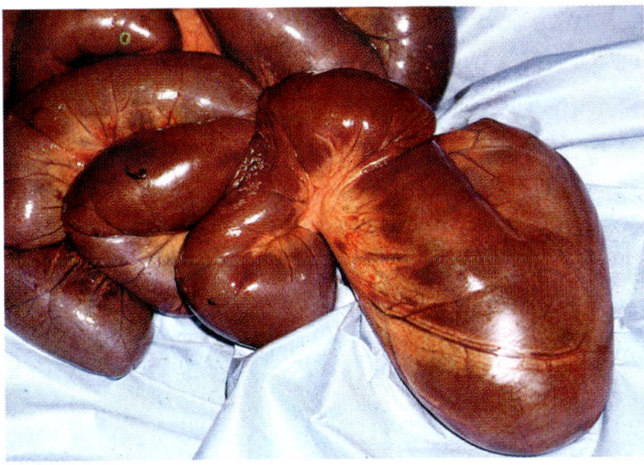

Fig. 7. Volvulus of the jejunoileal flange, possibly associated with a jejunal diverticulum in an adult Brown Swiss cow.

deposits within the mesentery may prevent compression of the muscular wall of the arteries until the volvulus becomes severe. Obstruction of outflow of venous blood may be equally detrimental, however, because of mural edema, shunting of blood away from the mucosa, and progressive ischemia.

Cattle of any breed, age, or sex may be affected by intestinal volvulus at any time during the year. In a review of 190 cattle having intestinal volvulus, dairy breeds were at a higher risk of developing volvulus compared with beef breeds [11]. This difference was thought to be associated with differences in management. Neither lactation nor gestation was identified as a risk factor, and calves were not found to be at an increased risk compared with adult cattle. In a separate study of 100 cattle having intestinal volvulus, 86 were calves between 1 week and 6 months old [21].

Clinical signs

Cattle having volvulus of the root of the mesentery may be found dead with severe abdominal distention. Early in the course of the disease, affected cattle show acute, severe abdominal pain (kicking at the abdomen, rolling, lying down and getting up frequently, grunting) and have marked elevation in heart rate (>120 beats/min) and respiratory rate (>80 breaths/min). The rapid progression of the disease precludes development of significant dehydration, but cardiovascular shock is usually present.

Cattle having volvulus of the jejunoileal flange may present similarly to cattle having volvulus at the root of the mesentery. These cattle often show clinical signs consistent with acute intestinal obstruction, however, rather than cardiovascular shock. Cattle show signs of abdominal pain, are tachycardic (80–120 beats/min), and pass minimal feces. Cattle may be dehydrated at the time of examination.

Clinical pathology

Because of the rapid onset and progress, cattle having intestinal volvulus may not show changes in serum biochemistry or hematology data. The changes expected with intestinal volvulus are consistent with intestinal obstruction, stress, and dehydration and include azotemia, hypocalcemia, hyperglycemia, and a leukocytosis with a mild left shift [11]. In the early stages of the disease, cattle develop alkalemia with normal serum potassium concentration. As cardiovascular compromise and intestinal ischemia proceed, cattle develop metabolic acidosis and hyperkalemia. Cattle having the shift to acidosis and hyperkalemia have a poor prognosis for survival [11].

Diagnosis

Diagnosis of intestinal volvulus is by exploratory laparotomy. Rectal palpation reveals multiple loops of distended intestine filling the caudal abdomen and excessive tension on the intestinal mesentery. Simultaneous auscultation and percussion of the abdomen yields multifocal pings of variable pitch and location. Findings of scant feces, abdominal pain, sudden onset of abdominal distention, and multiple loops of distended intestine on rectal palpation in cattle are highly suggestive of intestinal volvulus. Differential diagnoses include intussusception, cecal volvulus, abomasal volvulus, intraluminal obstruction, and severe indigestion.

Treatment

Immediate surgical correction is the treatment of choice. Intravenous fluids should be administered to treat cardiovascular shock, but preparation for surgery should not be delayed. The volvulus must be corrected before irreversible ischemic injury or thrombosis of the mesenteric arteries has occurred. A right paralumbar fossa laparotomy with the cow standing is the approach of choice. Restoration of normal anatomic position of the intestines is done more easily with the patient standing. Cattle that are believed to be at great risk of becoming recumbent during surgery should be placed under general anesthesia, in left lateral recumbency, and the laparotomy should be performed through the right paralumbar fossa. The presence of the volvulus and the direction of the twist are assessed by palpating the root of the mesentery and, in the case of jejunoileal flange volvulus, following this ventrally to the location of the twist. The intestinal mass is derotated gently, being careful not to cause rupture of the viscera. This procedure may require exteriorization of various portions of the intestinal mass. After correction of the volvulus, the intestinal tract should be examined for evidence of nonviable bowel. If the intestine is compromised (arterial thrombosis, blackened serosa, friable wall of the affected segment, mural edema), intestinal resection and anastomosis is indicated (see section on intussusception). Also, exploration of the abdomen should be done to rule out the presence of a second lesion (eg, abomasal displacement, fecalith, intussusception, anomalous fibrovascular bands, peritonitis).

Postoperative management is directed toward maintaining optimal hydration, electrolyte, and acid-base status. Antibiotics and anti-inflammatory drugs are indicated. Ileus may be seen during the first 48 hours after surgery, but the use of prokinetic drugs should be weighed against the risk of leakage at the site of the anastomosis if intestinal resection was performed. Passage of large volumes of diarrhea within 24 hours after surgery is considered to be a favorable prognostic indicator.

Prognosis

Prognosis varies with the severity and duration of the lesion. Prognosis for survival for cattle having volvulus of the root of the mesentery (44%) is less than for volvulus of the jejunoileal flange (86%) [11]. Overall, dairy cattle had a better prognosis for survival (63%) than beef cattle (22%). This difference was presumed to be due to the fact that dairy cattle are observed more frequently, and treatment is sought earlier in the progression of the disease. Of 92 cattle in which surgical correction of intestinal volvulus was attempted, 13 were killed during surgery, 25 died within 24 hours after surgery, 13 died between 2 and 7 days, and 41 (45%) survived [21].

Prevention

Specific recommendations for strategies to prevent intestinal volvulus are not possible because no risk factor has been identified. Some authors have suggested that turning out to graze lush pastures is a risk factor for intestinal volvulus [22]; this has not been the authors' experience. Feeding of concentrates, frequent dietary changes, confinement housing, and selection for high productivity may place dairy cattle at higher risk compared with beef cattle. These management techniques also are used in feedlot operations, but these cattle may not be presented for treatment to teaching hospitals because of their lower perceived economic value. Recommendations should be aimed to optimize cattle health by gradual changes in diet and environment.

Trichobezoars

Intraluminal obstruction of the intestinal tract of cattle, sheep, and goats most commonly is caused by a trichobezoar, phytobezoar, or enterolith [23,24]. These foreign bodies form in the rumen or abomasum and may pass into the intestinal tract, where they become lodged within the small intestine or spiral colon. Hairballs (trichobezoar) are caused by frequent ingestion of hair; this is seen most commonly in cattle infested with lice or mange or during the spring when shedding of the winter hair coat occurs. Phytobezoars and enteroliths form around undigested materials (eg, nylon fibers, cotton fabric). In a necropsy survey of 166 dead calves less than 90 days old in Western Canada, 56 calves died because of perforation of an abomasal ulcer [25]. Calves having an abomasal ulcer were 2.74 times more likely to have an abomasal hairball. Calves less than 31 days old and having an abomasal ulcer were 3.81 times more likely to have an abomasal hairball. The authors of the study were unable, however, to establish a causative relationship between the presence of abomasal hairballs and a perforating ulcer. During a study of confined cattle being fed a roughage-limited diet, cows began biting hair from each others' hair coat and developed multiple ruminal hair balls (range 2–10 hair balls weighing 0.2–3.8 kg each) [26]. The investigators speculated that the cows began "grazing" hair because of the lack of roughage in the diet, boredom, and high stocking density. One report described clinical findings in 2 sheep having 107 individual hairballs [27]. The authors of the report speculated that pruritus or some unknown dietary deficiency was the cause of excessive ingestion of the wool.

Clinical signs

Animals affected with ruminal or abomasal bezoars may be observed to have decreased appetite, weight loss, decreased fecal production, lethargy, and apparent depression. Multiple bezoars present in the rumen or abomasum of calves, sheep, and goats may be found during transabdominal palpation or on abdominal radiographs. When an obstruction of the small intestine or spiral colon occurs, affected animals initially show clinical signs of abdominal pain (restlessness, kicking at the abdomen, lying down and getting up frequently, arching the back, stretching out the legs while standing) and progress to recumbency and apparent depression. Progressive bloat or abdominal distention and lack of fecal production are noted.

Clinical pathology

Serum biochemistry analysis reveals hypokalemic, hypochloremic metabolic alkalosis, the severity of which depends on the duration and location of the lesion. These changes are most severe with proximal intestinal obstruction and become more severe with increasing duration. If ischemic necrosis of the intestinal wall has occurred, an inflammatory leukogram with increased numbers of immature neutrophils may be seen. As peritonitis develops and organic acids are released into the bloodstream, the serum biochemistry changes to a metabolic acidosis with relative hyperkalemia. These changes are consistent with a poor prognosis. Perforation of an abomasal ulcer or rupture of the intestine and contamination of the abdomen with ingesta carries a poor-to-grave prognosis.

Diagnosis

In affected cattle, serum biochemistry changes are consistent with intestinal obstruction. Rumen chloride concentration may be elevated (rumen chloride >30 mEq/L). The cause of intraluminal obstruction is rarely palpable per rectum, but small intestinal distention may be palpable. Ultrasound examination of the abdomen may be useful in calves and small ruminants. Intraluminal intestinal obstruction should be suspected in cattle with recurrent rumen tympanites, which is transiently responsive to decompression and is associated with minimal fecal production. Differential diagnoses include intussusception, vagus indigestion syndrome, intestinal lymphosarcoma, fat necrosis, intestinal entrapment around anomalous fibrovascular bands, and volvulus of the jejunoileal flange.

Treatment

Trichobezoars, phytobezoars, or enteroliths located within the rumen are unlikely to cause clinical signs, unless the number and magnitude of the foreign bodies are severe (eg, two sheep in which hairballs accounted for >10% of the animals' body weight [27]). A cow had esophageal obstruction after suspected attempted regurgitation of a rumen trichobezoar [28]. Ruminal foreign bodies are removed via a left paralumbar fossa celiotomy and rumenotomy (see section on traumatic reticuloperitonitis). The authors prefer to close the rumen with absorbable monofilament suture material (eg, No. 1 polydioxanone) using two layers of an inverting suture pattern (eg, Cushing or Lembert patterns). Abomasal hairballs may cause pyloric obstruction, which leads to rapid onset of abdominal distention. The authors prefer to perform a right paramedian or ventral paracostal laparotomy to exteriorize the abomasum. An abomasotomy is performed along the greater curvature of the abomasum, the foreign bodies are removed, and the abomasum is closed with absorbable monofilament suture material (eg, No. 0 polydioxanone) using two layers of an inverting suture pattern. When obstruction of the duodenum, jejunum, or spiral colon is suspected, a right paralumbar fossa celiotomy and exploration of the abdomen should be performed. The foreign body is found by exteriorizing a segment of normal or distended intestine and tracing this segment orad or aborad until the obstruction is found. This segment of intestine is exteriorized from the abdomen and isolated using moistened surgical towels, and an enterotomy is performed. After removal of the foreign body, the enterotomy is closed with absorbable suture material (eg, No. 2-0 polydioxanone, polyglactin 910) using two layers of an inverting suture pattern. The enterotomy may be closed transversely to maximize the lumen of the affected segment of intestine and to minimize the tension endured by the suture line during contraction of the intestinal wall. When the perceived economic value of the affected cow is high, surgery may be performed with the patient under general anesthesia; this minimizes the risk of ingesta contamination of the abdomen during surgery.

Intravenous fluid therapy is based on the clinical estimate of dehydration, severity of intestinal lesions identified at surgery, and severity of serum biochemistry changes. In general, cattle should receive 20 to 60 L of isotonic saline intravenously over 12 hours. The authors routinely add calcium (1 mL of 23% calcium gluconate/kg body weight) and dextrose (to create a 1.25% solution) to the intravenous fluids. Nonsteroidal anti-inflammatory drugs (eg, flunixin meglumine, 1 mg/kg body weight intravenously every 12 hours × 3 days) and antibiotics (for 3–5 days) also are administered.

Prognosis

The prognosis for return to productive use is based on the animal's body condition, severity of changes in serum biochemistry variables [11], presence of visceral perforation or peritonitis, and ability to perform surgical removal of the foreign body without contaminating the abdomen. Cattle that are less than 10% dehydrated and have mild-to-moderate hypochloremia (eg, chloride >80 mEq/L) and metabolic alkalosis (eg, bicarbonate >32 mEq/L) have a fair-to-good prognosis for recovery. Cattle that are more than 10% dehydrated, have severe hypochloremia (eg, chloride <80 mEq/L) and metabolic acidosis (eg, bicarbonate <20 mEq/L), or have visceral perforation have a poor prognosis for survival. Immediate surgical intervention is required for alleviation of clinical signs caused by intraluminal foreign bodies.

Prevention

Intraluminal obstruction of the intestinal occurs infrequently in cattle. The sporadic nature of the problem limits recommendations for prevention. Adequate dietary roughage should be made available to cattle at all times. Lice control strategies, particularly during the winter months, prevent pruritus-associated ingestion of hair.

Intestinal hematoma syndrome (hemorrhagic bowel syndrome, intraluminal-intramural hematoma)

A syndrome has been recognized in adult dairy cows involving intraluminal and intramural intestinal hemorrhage and necrosis with subsequent clot formation and intestinal obstruction (Fig. 8). This syndrome has been called *jejunal hemorrhage syndrome (JHS), hemorrhagic bowel syndrome, intraluminal-intramural hematoma, bloody gut,* and *hemorrhagic enteritis*. Clinical signs of this peracute disease include recumbency, dehydration, shock, abdominal distention, anorexia, abdominal pain, and lack of feces or the production of tarry feces with blood clots [29–37]. In many cases, the cow is found dead. Affected cows are usually in early lactation, producing large quantities of milk, and are fed silage or total mixed ration [33–36]. The case-mortality rate for this syndrome is 77%

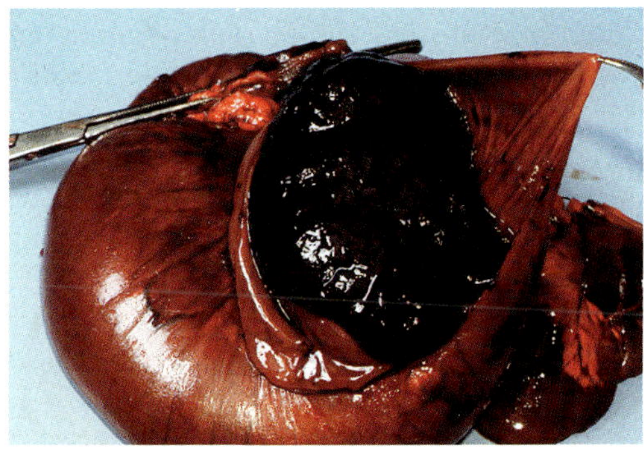

Fig. 8. Intestinal obstruction caused by intraluminal blood clot in an adult Brown Swiss cow diagnosed as hemorrhagic bowel syndrome.

[38,39]. In the search for the cause of this disease, much speculation has fallen on *Clostridium perfringens* type A. *C. perfringens* type A was suspected as a cause or contributing factor in this disease because this organism has been cultured from the intestinal contents or feces of many cows affected with JHS [34,38,39]. Evidence regarding pathogenicity of these isolates has not been produced, however, to link *C. perfringens* type A to development of JHS. Similar hemorrhagic enteritis syndromes have been reported in other species, some of which have been related to *C. perfringens* [40–52]. *C. perfringens* type A has been linked to abomasal ulcers and abomasitis in calves [51–59]. *C. perfringens* type A also is found in the gastrointestinal tract of cattle, however, without causing clinically apparent disease [51,52,60]. *C. perfringens* type E also has been described to cause hemorrhagic enteritis of calves [62].

Clinical signs

The most common clinical signs reported for cows affected with JHS were apparent depression, decreased milk production, tachycardia, ruminal stasis, abdominal distention, and dark clotted blood in feces [38].

Diagnosis

Definitive diagnosis of JHS is made during exploratory laparotomy or necropsy. Clinical diagnosis can be made based on clinical signs, presence of scant volume feces composed of blood clots, evidence of intestinal stasis or obstruction on rectal palpation, ultrasound examination, and serum biochemistry. These clinical signs are common among several intestinal diseases (eg, *Salmonella,* intussusception, coccidiosis), and diagnosis is presumptive unless confirmed by ruling out other disease or by exploratory laparotomy or necropsy.

Treatment

Exploratory laparotomy is done via the right paralumbar fossa approach after proximal paravertebral anesthesia. On entering the abdomen, dilated small intestine is found immediately. The dilated intestine is examined throughout its length until the obstruction is found. The obstruction is spongy and smooth in texture, friable on compression, and movable within the lumen if the hematoma is not transmural. The obstruction can be loosened by massage of the hematoma into small fragments and replaced in the abdominal compartment, the obstruction can be removed via an enterotomy, or the affected segment of intestine can be resected and an end-to-end anastomosis performed. The authors initially treated these cases with intestinal resection and anastomosis, but the survival rate after such treatment was approximately 25%. More recently, the authors have used medical therapy consisting of intravenous fluids, antibiotics (eg, procaine penicillin G at 22,000–44,000 U/kg body weight daily), and deep analgesic therapy. Multimodal analgesic therapy is advised, such as a combination of flunixin meglumine (1 mg/kg intravenously every 12 hours), butorphanol tartrate (0.05 mg/kg body weight subcutaneously every 6 to 8 hours), and lidocaine (50 mL of 2% lidocaine HCl administered in 20 L of intravenous fluids over 8 hours). These cows are walked (light exercise for 20 minutes two or three times daily) as their condition permits to stimulate the enteric nervous system. Surgical diagnosis, massage of the hematoma, and medical therapy in combination has improved success rates to greater than 50%. In one study of 22 cattle with JHS, 7 of 8 cows treated medically died, and 9 of 13 cows treated surgically died [38].

Prevention

At present, it is thought that JHS is a multifactorial disease [30,34–36, 38–39]. Proposed risk factors include feeding of silage or total mixed ration, feeding finely ground corn in the ration, early stage of lactation, high level of production, and free-choice feeding. These factors may create an environment in which stress, excess gastrointestinal starch, and subclinical rumen acidosis allow overgrowth of *C. perfringens* type A bacteria in the gastrointestinal tract. Studies in calves, lambs, and chickens had induced clinical disease by direct inoculation of the rumen, duodenum, and ligated intestinal loops with pure cultures of *C. perfringens* type A or C [45,51–53,58,61–63]. The diseases produced included hemorrhagic enteritis, enterotoxemia, abomasal ulceration, and abomasitis. Spontaneous cases of hemorrhagic enteritis caused by *Clostridium* species also have been reported in dogs [44,47], foals [40,41,43,46,50,51], lambs [49,50], goats [48], and calves [55–57,59]. Inoculation of live calves or ligated intestinal loops with *C. perfringens* type A produced no clinical signs of enterotoxemia or enteritis, however [62]. Jelinski et al [56] found no difference in the prevalence of *C. perfringens* type A in calves with and without abomasal ulcer/abomasitis syndrome.

Prevalence of *C. perfringens* type A in the intestine of normal cattle has been reported to be 36.8% to 78.6% [53,56,64,65]. Most studies have used samples obtained at necropsy. The high prevalence of *Clostridium* may be an overestimation associated with rapid postmortem overgrowth. *C. perfringens* type A grows rapidly in the intestine after death, so the prevalence in live animals may be lower than reported [51]. Amtsberg et al [53] reported *C. perfringens* in only 33.9% of live calf feces. *C. perfringens* type A produce α-toxin, and some may produce a β_2-toxin. Excess grain or starch in the small intestine is more likely to lead to sudden bacterial overgrowth. This passage of grain particles into the small intestine may be a factor in the pathogenesis of JHS in dairy cows fed high-grain total mixed ration. Excess mixing of total mixed ration causing finely powdered corn was suspected to be related to an outbreak of clinical cases of JHS on one farm [34].

References

[1] Pfeiffer CJ. A review of spontaneous ulcer disease in domestic animals: chickens, cattle, horses, and swine. Acta Physiol Hung 1992;80:149–58.
[2] van der Velden MA. Functional stenosis of the sigmoid curve of the duodenum in cattle. Vet Rec 1983;112:452–3.
[3] Braun U, Steiner A, Gotz M. Clinical signs, diagnosis, and treatment of duodenal ileus in cattle. Schweiz Arch Tierheilkd 1993;135:345–55.
[4] Braun U, Hausammann K, Forrer R. Reflux of bile acids from the duodenum into the rumen of cows with a reduced intestinal passage. Vet Rec 1989;124:373–6.
[5] Cebra CK, Cebra ML, Garry FB. Gravel obstruction of the abomasums or duodenum of two cows. J Am Vet Med Assoc 1996;209:1294–6.
[6] Koller U, Lischer C, Geyer H, et al. Strangulation of the duodenum by the uterus during late pregnancy in two cows. Vet J 2001;162:33–7.
[7] Boerboom D, Mulon PY, Desrochers A. Duodenal obstruction caused by malposition of the gallbladder in a heifer. J Am Vet Med Assoc 2003;223:1475–7.
[8] Steiner A, Muller L, Pabst B. An unusual complication after the partial resection of the ascending duodenum of a cow. Tierarztl Prax 1989;17:17–20.
[9] Braun U, Marmier O, Pusteria N. Ultrasonographic examination of the small intestine of cows with ileus of the duodenum, jejunum, or ileum. Vet Rec 1995;137:209–15.
[10] Garry F, Hull BL, Ringd DM, et al. Comparison of naturally occurring proximal duodenal obstruction and abomasal volvulus in dairy cattle. Vet Surg 1988;17:226–33.
[11] Anderson DE, Constable PD, St-Jean G, et al. Small-intestinal volvulus in cattle: 35 cases (1967–1992). J Am Vet Med Assoc 1993;203:1178–83.
[12] Constable PD, St-Jean G, Hull BL, et al. Intussusception in cattle: 336 cases (1964–1993). J Am Vet Med Assoc 1997;210:531–6.
[13] Pearson H. Intussusception in cattle. Vet Rec 1971;89:426–37.
[14] Smart ME, Fretz PB, Gudmundson J, et al. Intussusception in a Charolais bull. Can Vet J 1977;18:244–6.
[15] Archer RM, Cooley AJ, Hinchcliff KW, et al. Jejunojejunal intussusception associated with a transmural adenocarcinoma in an aged cow. J Am Vet Med Assoc 1988;192:209–11.
[16] Horne MM. Colonic intussusception in a Holstein calf. Can Vet J 1991;32:493–5.
[17] Hamilton GF, Tulleners EP. Intussusception involving the spiral colon in a calf. Can Vet J 1980;21:32.
[18] Strand E, Welker B, Modransky P. Spiral colon intussusception in a three-year-old bull. J Am Vet Med Assoc 1993;202:971–2.
[19] Fubini SL, Smith DF, Tithof PK, et al. Volvulus of the distal part of the jejunoileum in four cows. Vet Surg 1986;15:150–2.
[20] Tulleners EP. Surgical correction of volvulus of the root of the mesentery in calves. J Am Vet Med Assoc 1981;179:998–9.
[21] Rademacher G. Diagnosis, therapy, and prognosis of the intestinal mesenteric torsion in cattle. Proceedings, XVII World Buiatrics Congress and XXV American Association of Bovine Practitioners Conference, St Paul. 1992. Vol 1:137–42.
[22] Willet MDJ. Intestinal torsion in cattle. N Z Vet J 1970;18:42–3.
[23] Pearson H, Pinsent PJN. Intestinal obstruction in cattle. Vet Rec 1977;101:162–6.
[24] Pearson H. The treatment of surgical disorders of the bovine abdomen. Vet Rec 1973;92: 245–54.
[25] Jelinski MD, Ribble CS, Campbell JR, et al. Investigating the relationship between abomasal hairballs and perforating abomasal ulcers in unweaned beef calves. Can Vet J 1996;37:23–6.
[26] Cockrill JM, Beasley JN, Selph RA. Trichobezoars in four Angus cows. Vet Med Sm Anim Clin 1978;73:1441–2.
[27] Ramadan RO. Massive formation of trichobezoars in sheep. Agric Practice 1995;16:26–8.

[28] Patel JH, Brace DM. Esophageal obstruction due to a trichobezoar in a cow. Can Vet J 1995; 36:774–5.
[29] Anderson BC. 'Point source' haemorrhages in cows. Vet Rec 1991;128:619–20.
[30] Godden S, Frank R, Ames T. Survey of Minnesota dairy veterinarians on the occurrence and potential risk factors for jejunal hemorrhage syndrome in adult dairy cows. Bov Pract 2001; 35:97–103.
[31] Hattel A, Maddox C, Drake T, et al. Type A *Clostridium perfringens* associated with hemorrhagic and necrotizing enteropathy in adult dairy cattle. 50th Annual American Congress of Veterinary Pathologists Meeting, Chicago. November 1999.
[32] Hermann JA. Thoughts on bowel treatment in cattle. J Am Vet Med Assoc 2002;221:1250.
[33] Kirkpatrick MA, Timms L, Kersting KW, Kinyon J. Jejunal hemorrhage syndrome of dairy cattle [abstract]. Bov Pract 2001;35:135–6.
[34] Kirkpatrick MA, Timms LL, Kersting KW, et al. Case report: jejunal hemorrhage syndrome of dairy cattle. Bov Pract 2001;35:104–16.
[35] Maddox CW, Hattel AL, Drake TR, et al. Beta2 toxin positive *Clostridium perfringens* type A and fatal hemorrhagic enteritis of adult dairy cows. Winter-Spring Conference, Pennsylvania Vet Lab, Pennsylvania Anim Diag Lab System. March 1999.
[36] Maddox C, Hattel A, Drake T, et al. *Clostridium perfringens* type A strains recovered from acute hemorrhagic enteritis of adult dairy cattle. Am Assoc Vet Lab Diagnosticians, 42nd Annual Meeting, AAVLD Abstracts. October 1999.
[37] St Jean G, Anderson DE. Intraluminal-intramural hemorrhage of the small intestine in cattle. In: Howard JE, Smith RA, editors. Current veterinary therapy: food animal practice. 4th edition. Philadelphia: WB Saunders; 1999. p. 539.
[38] Dennison AC, VanMetre DC, Callan RJ, et al. Hemorrhagic bowel syndrome in dairy cattle: 22 cases (1997–2000). J Am Vet Med Assoc 2002;221:686–9.
[39] Dennison AC, VanMetre DC, Callan R, et al. Hemorrhagic bowel syndrome in dairy cattle. Proceedings 19th Am Coll Vet Intern Med, Denver, CO. 2001. p. 354–5.
[40] Bueschel D, Walker R, Woods L, et al. Enterotoxigenic *Clostridium perfringens* type A necrotic enteritis in a foal. J Am Vet Med Assoc 1998;213:1305–7.
[41] East LM, Savage CJ, Traub-Dargatz JL, et al. Enterocolitis associated with *Clostridium perfringens* infection in neonatal foals: 54 cases (1988–1997). J Am Vet Med Assoc 1998:212;1751–6.
[42] Estrada Correa AE, Taylor DJ. Porcine *Clostridium perfringens* type A spores, enterotoxin and antibody to enterotoxin. Vet Rec 1989;124:606–10.
[43] Jones RL, Adney WS, Alexander AF, et al. Hemorrhagic necrotizing enterocolitis associated with *Clostridium difficile* infection in four foals. J Am Vet Med Assoc 1988;193:76–9.
[44] Kruth SA, Prescott JF, Welch MK, et al. Nosocomial diarrhea associated with enterotoxigenic *Clostridium perfringens* infection in dogs. J Am Vet Med Assoc 1989;195: 331–4.
[45] Niilo L. Experimental production of hemorrhagic enterotoxemia by *Clostridium perfringens* Type C in maturing lambs. Can J Vet Res 1986;50:32–5.
[46] Pearson EG, Hedstrom OR, Sonn R, et al. Hemorrhagic enteritis caused by *Clostridium perfringens* type C in a foal. J Am Vet Med Assoc 1986;188:1309–10.
[47] Prescott JF, Johnson JA, Patterson JM, et al. Haemorrhagic gastroenteritis in the dog associated with *Clostridium welchii*. Vet Rec 1978;103:116–7.
[48] Russell WC. Type A enterotoxemia in captive wild goats. J Am Vet Med Assoc 1970;157: 643–6.
[49] Shaw WB. Intestinal haemorrhage syndrome in artificially reared lambs [letter]. Vet Rec 1971;88:700.
[50] Sims LD, Tzipori S, Hazard GH, et al. Haemorrhagic necrotising enteritis in foals associated with *Clostridium perfringens*. Aust Vet J 1985;62:194–6.
[51] Songer JG. Clostridial enteric diseases of domestic animals. Clin Microbiol Rev 1996;9: 216–34.

[52] Songer JG. *Clostridium perfringens* Type A infection in cattle. Bov Pract 1999;32:40–4.
[53] Amtsberg G, Bisping W, Matthiesen I, et al. Zum Vorkommen und zur pathogenen Bedeutung von *Clostridium perfringens* beim Kalb 2. Mitteilung: Infektionsversuche, Ligaturtest und Prüfung auf Enterotoxinbildung zur Klärung der pathogenen Bedeutung von *Clostridium perfringens* Type A. Zbl Vet Med B 1977;24:183–97.
[54] Amtsberg G, Bisping W, Krabisch P, et al. Zum Vorkommen und zur pathogenen Bedeutung von *Clostridium perfringens* beim Kalb 1. Mitteilung: Quantitative bakteriologische Untersuchungen zum *Clostridium perfringens*-Keimgehalt im Kot und Darminhalt von gesunden und erkrankten Kälbern. Zbl Vet Med B 1977;24:104–13.
[55] Hogle RM. Clinical and laboratory diagnosis of enterotoxemia of cattle. Vet Med/SAC 1975;70:983–6.
[56] Jelinski MD, Ribble CS, Chirino-Trejo M, et al. The relationship between the presence of *Helicobacter pylori*, *Clostridium perfringens* type A, *Campylobacter* spp., or fungi and fatal abomasal ulcers in unweaned beef calves. Can Vet J 1995;36:379–82.
[57] Mills KW, Johnson JL, Jensen RL, et al. Laboratory findings associated with abomasal ulcers/tympany in range calves. J Vet Diagn Invest 1990;2:208–12.
[58] Roeder BL, Chengappa MM, Nagaraja TG, et al. Experimental induction of abomasal tympany, abomasitis, and abomasal ulceration by intraruminal inoculation of *Clostridium perfringens* type A in neonatal calves. Am J Vet Res 1988;49:201–7.
[59] Roeder BL, Chengappa MM, Nagaraja TG, et al. Isolation of *Clostridium perfringens* from neonatal calves with ruminal and abomasal tympany, abomasitis, and abomasal ulceration. J Am Vet Med Assoc 1987;190:1550–5.
[60] Mylrea PJ. The bacterial content of the small intestine of young calves. Res Vet Sci 1969;10:394–5.
[61] Al-Sheikhly F, Truscott RB. The pathology of necrotic enteritis of chickens following infusion of broth cultures of *Clostridium perfringens* into the duodenum. Avian Dis 1977;21:230–40.
[62] Billington SJ, Wieckowski EU, Sarker MR, et al. *Clostridium perfringens* Type E animal enteritis isolates with highly conserved silent enterotoxin gene sequences. Infect Immunol 1998;66:4531–6.
[63] Niilo L, Dorward WJ. The effect of enterotoxigenic *Clostridium welchii (perfringens)* Type A on the bovine intestine. Res Vet Sci 1971;12:376–8.
[64] Vance HN. A survey of the alimentary tract of cattle for *Clostridium perfringens*. Can J Comp Med Vet Sci 1967;31:260–4.
[65] Yoo HS, Lee SU, Park KY, et al. Molecular typing and epidemiological survey of prevalence of *Clostridium perfringens* types by multiplex PCR. J Clin Microbiol 1997;35:228–32.

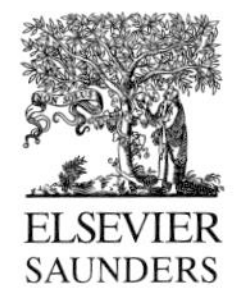

ELSEVIER
SAUNDERS

Vet Clin Food Anim 21 (2005) 155–171

VETERINARY
CLINICS
Food Animal Practice

Management of Peritonitis in Cattle

Gilles Fecteau, DMV

Department of Clinical Sciences, Université de Montréal, CP 5000, St-Hyacinthe, Québec J2S 7C6, Canada

Peritonitis is an inflammatory process that involves the peritoneal cavity and its serosal surface—the peritoneum. Peritonitis is not a true synonym of intra-abdominal infection because the latter is defined as an inflammatory response of the peritoneum to microorganisms and their toxins, which results in purulent exudates in the abdominal cavity. Peritonitis should be considered as the localized equivalent of systemic inflammatory response syndrome, whereas intra-abdominal infection is the localized equivalent of sepsis. An intra-abdominal abscess is an intra-abdominal infection that is confined within the abdominal cavity. Because peritonitis in farm animals is caused most often by bacteria, the two terms often are used synonymously.

A variety of conditions can cause peritonitis of varying severity, including traumatic incidents, surgery, intestinal obstruction, compromised intestinal vascularization, or gastrointestinal ulceration. In farm animals, the terms "acute" or "chronic," "septic" or "chemical," and "localized" or "generalized" are used most often to describe better the suspected pathologic problem. The terms "primary peritonitis," "secondary peritonitis," and "tertiary peritonitis" are used commonly in human medicine. Primary peritonitis is associated with systemic infection, secondary peritonitis occurs as a consequence of a viscus perforation or after surgery, and tertiary peritonitis is a particular case of chronic peritonitis with a small number of bacteria or fungi [1].

Normal anatomy of the peritoneal cavity

Abdominal viscera are located outside of the peritoneal cavity, but inside the abdominal cavity. To illustrate this concept, remember that during a flank laparotomy, the parietal peritoneum is incised first to enter the peritoneal cavity and allow palpation of the different viscera; however, all viscera are covered by the visceral peritoneum (Fig. 1). The parietal and

E-mail address: gilles.fecteau@umontreal.ca

doi:10.1016/j.cvfa.2004.12.007 *vetfood.theclinics.com*

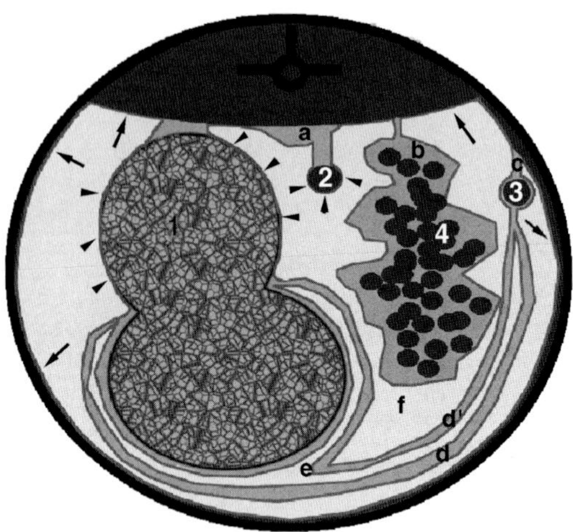

Fig. 1. Anatomic disposition of the parietal and visceral peritoneum. 1, dorsal sac of the rumen; 2, descending colon; 3, descending duodenum; 4, jejunum; black arrows, parietal peritoneum; black arrowheads, visceral peritoneum or serosa; a, mesocolon; b, mesentery; c, mesoduodenum; d, external sheath of the greater omentum; d′, internal sheath of the greater omentum; e, omental bursa; f, supraomental recess. (Courtesy of André Desrochers, DVM, Saint-Hyacinthe, Québec, Canada.)

visceral peritoneum constitutes the major parts of the peritoneum. The minor parts are the omentum, the mesenteries, and ligaments. The dorsal reflected folds of the peritoneum are called the mesenteries. They connect visceral and parietal peritoneum and suspend organs from the dorsal abdominal wall. The ligaments are folds of the peritoneum that enclose sheets or cords of connective tissue (eg, suspensory ligament of the ovary). The omentum is a special fold of the peritoneum that extends from the stomach to the adjacent viscera. The omentum is a unique type of connecting peritoneum that contains adipose tissue, blood vessels, nerves, and lymphatics. The omental bursa is the cavity between the two layers of omentum. Its only access is by way of the epiploic foramen that is situated ventrally to the caudate lobe of the liver. The normal anatomy of the omentum is particular in ruminants. The greater omentum creates an envelope or "sling" in which is contained the major part of the small intestine. This area of the abdomen is named the supraomental recess. Peritonitis outside the supraomental recess generally has fewer consequences compared with a peritonitis that involves the serosa of the small intestine.

Three natural openings of the abdominal cavity are located in the diaphragm: the esophageal, vena cava, and aortic hiatus. At these sites, the pleura and the peritoneum are in close contact which allows infection to spread from one cavity to the other. The umbilicus also is a normal opening that is present in utero but normally closes soon after birth. Infection from the environment and development of peritonitis is possible from this opening. The peritoneal cavity is completely closed in males, whereas in females the ovarian bursa opening creates a communication between the genital tract and the peritoneal cavity. Extension of a severe metritis to the peritoneal cavity and development of peritonitis is possible (Fig. 2) [2].

Histology of the peritoneum

The peritoneal cavity is lined by a serous membrane that is composed of two layers (the peritoneum). The deeper layer (subserosa) is composed of loose connective tissue that contains collagen, fat cells, reticular cells, and macrophages. Covering that layer is a single surface layer of mesothelial squamous cells (serosa). The peritoneal mesothelial cells (PMCs) contain lamellar bodies which produce surfactant that acts as a lubricant. PMCs have the same mesodermal origin as the endothelial cells which indicates that they may be the source of effector mechanism during peritonitis [3]. On the surface of the diaphragm, special lymphatic-collecting vessels are located under the mesothelial basement membrane. Small stomata are found between mesothelial cells. They act as channels for lymphatic drainage from the peritoneal cavity to the thoracic duct. The omentum also has the ability to absorb particles from the peritoneal spaces [3]. The peritoneum is a highly permeable membrane that acts as a bidirectional semipermeable barrier. Diffusion of water and low molecular weight solutes between blood and the peritoneal fluid is possible. Normal peritoneal fluid provides lubrication for the movement of abdominal organs and apposed peritoneal surfaces. It is formed and resorbed constantly. Peritoneal fluid movement is achieved by movement of the viscera and contraction of the diaphragm during respiration. In humans, during peritoneal dialysis, a net flow of 300 mL

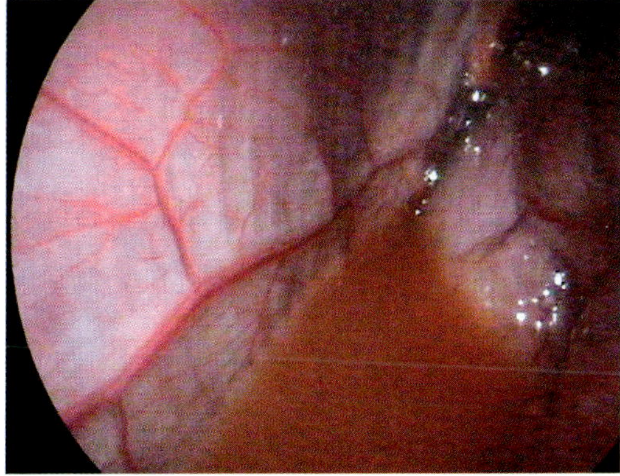

Fig. 2. Abdominal fluid observed by laparoscopic examination on a cow that is suffering from uterine aplasia. Severe dilation of the affected uterine horn causes accumulation of peritoneal fluid. (Courtesy of André Desrochers DVM, Saint-Hyacinthe, Québec, Canada).

to 500 mL of water per hour into the peritoneal space may be induced [4]. Acute severe peritonitis may induce a net flow of many liters of proteinaceous fluid into the peritoneal cavity.

Pathophysiology of peritonitis

Healing of the mesothelium and adhesion formation

The mesothelium of the peritoneum is sensitive; minimal trauma can initiate exfoliation of cells. Regeneration is completed rapidly. Healing can occur by reperitonealization or creation of an adhesion with an adjacent nearby mesothelial surface. This adherent type of healing occurs more frequently if the inflammation is severe, with the presence of bacteria or foreign material. Adhesions are defined as fibrinous or fibrous bands that create an abnormal attachment of two or more surfaces. Formation of adhesions is part of the healing process and should be interpreted as an effort to control an injury. The omentum often is involved in adhesions and acts as a natural sealing device to control the acute phase of inflammation. Prevention of undesired adhesions is achieved best by careful hemostasis. Whole blood potentiates adhesion formation by providing more fibrinogen.

Adhesion may or may not be reversible, depending on the amount of organization that took place during the process. The three major elements that are responsible for dissolution of fibrinous adhesions are: (1) adequate oxygen and nutriment supply of the mesothelium, (2) liberation of plasminogen-activating substance by mesothelial and submesothelial cells, and (3) control of the inflammatory process. Adhesions that are cut or broken reform rapidly in bovines. Attempts to cut an adhesion surgically should be attempted only if the adhesions prevent normal gastrointestinal transit or cause other organ failure.

Host defenses against infection

The first mechanism of defense is physical removal of the bacteria. In normal dogs, for example, it is possible to retrieve bacteria in the blood stream 12 minutes after an experimental peritoneal injection [4]. The second mechanism of defense relates to the response to noxious stimuli. This intense acute inflammatory response includes degranulation of peritoneal mast cells with release of vasoactive substances. The mesothelial cells initiate an inflammatory response that modifies the permeability of the peritoneum and its vascular supply. Several blood constituents are able to move into the peritoneal cavity. Macrophages and polymorphonuclears, humoral opsonins, natural antibodies, serum complement, and a protein-rich fluid are the most important. Thirdly, the omentum contributes to the defense mechanism by adhering to an infected or damaged area to circumscribe a problem. The omentum contains cells that previously were referred to as "milky spots." These aggregates contain mainly macrophages and lymphocytes. The cells are supported by reticular fibers and infiltrated by nonmyelinated nerve fibers. The number of milky spots decreases with age, except during peritonitis when they appear as tiny, cotton-wool–like masses (Fig. 3) [3]. Finally, the rapid movement of neutrophils, and later, macrophages is one of the most important mechanisms of control against infection.

Systemic effect of the inflammatory response

The initial inflammatory response induces several systemic abnormalities that the clinician must recognize and treat adequately. In acute diffuse septic peritonitis, the major adverse effects of peritoneal contamination are: (1) rapid clearance of bacteria that produce **endotoxemia** or **bacteremia**, (2) rapid influx of fluid that is rich in protein toward the peritoneal cavity that leads to **hypovolemia** and **hypoproteinemia**, (3) deposition of fibrin that occludes lymphatic drainage, contributes to the abdominal distension, and enhances the chance of abscess formation, and (4) **ileus**, and (5) **adhesion** formation, which may lead to obstruction (Fig. 4).

Pain response

Painful responses to palpation of the abdomen are due to stimuli that are perceived by the somatic afferent nerve endings in the parietal peritoneum. During surgery, palpation of the different viscera is not painful, except in the presence of severe distension, acute inflammation (breaking of adhesions), or if important traction is made on the root of the mesentery. Stimulation of the parietal peritoneum by a painful sensation also is believed to be responsible for the abdominal wall rigidity that is observed during peritonitis.

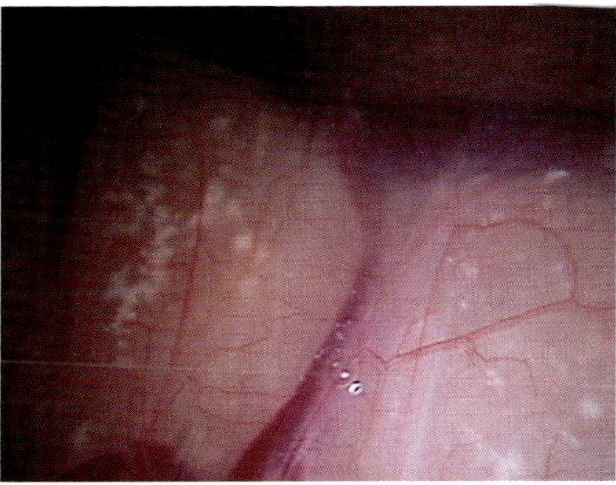

Fig. 3. Presence of "milky spots" observed by laparoscopic examination in an adult cow that is suffering from septic peritonitis. (Courtesy of André Desrochers DVM, Saint-Hyacinthe, Québec, Canada).

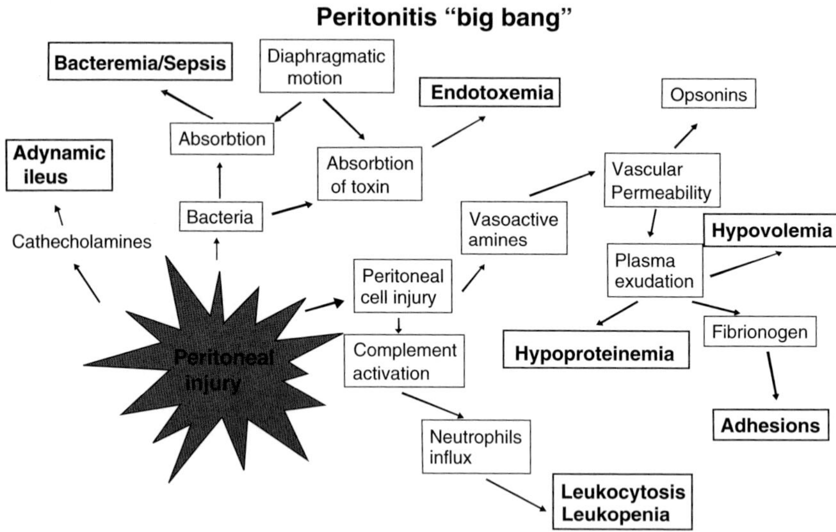

Fig. 4. Pathophysiology of peritonitis. (*From* Smith BP, editor. Large animal internal medicine. St. Louis (MO): Mosby; 2002. p. 751; with permission.)

Clinical signs

A detailed history often leads to high suspicion of peritonitis (eg, recent surgery or dystocia). Acute stages tend to be associated with more characteristic clinical signs. As the disease evolves toward chronicity, clinical signs become nonspecific. The severity of clinical signs ranges from a mild, recurrent discomfort that is caused by a localized abscess, to an acute, severe onset of toxemia and hypovolemia that lead rapidly to death.

Abdominal rigidity and tenderness, abdominal distension, scleral injection, fever, anorexia, and sudden reduction in milk production (in dairy cattle) are classic findings of acute peritonitis. In the acute stage, abdominal pain and the release of catecholamines often lead to a complete gastrointestinal stasis and ileus. The rumen is completely atonic and feces are present in small amounts and often are dry. In chronic cases, feces tend to be diarrheic. Persistent pain, decreased plasma volume, and endotoxemia often result in tachycardia. Anterior abdominal pain, evaluated by the "skootch test" may be identified in some cases. Abdominal discomfort in cattle often is expressed by reluctance to move.

Diagnostic procedures

Peritoneal fluid analysis

Normal bovine peritoneal fluid should be clear, with a specific density of less than 1.016. Protein content should be less than 3 g/dL, although some investigators reported normal values up to 6.3 g/dL (the major part being albumin). According to one investigator, it may contain fibrinogen and clot when exposed to air [5]. Nucleated cells count should be less than 10,000 cells per μL, with a majority of macrophages. Lymphocytes, eosinophils, and desquamated mesothelial cells also may be present. Neutrophils are rare. Periparturient cattle have significantly more peritoneal fluid with a decreased protein concentration. Cytologic examination of the peritoneal fluid is a useful aid in making a definitive diagnosis of peritonitis. A needle, blunt teat canula, or a bitch catheter may be used with success (Fig. 5). Failure to secure fluid is common, and may be explained by the presence of fibrinous peritonitis with fluid loculation (Fig. 6). At least two sites should be evaluated if no fluid is secured from the first site (Figs. 7 and 8). Table 1 summarizes the normal value for bovine peritoneal fluid as reported by several investigators.

Because most cases of peritonitis are secondary in cattle, one may assume that a mixed flora with the presence of obligate anaerobes may be cultured, at least in the acute phase. In humans, most cases of secondary peritonitis eventually are associated with an *Escherichia coli* and *Bacteroides fragilis* infection. The concept of biphasic infection means that after an initial phase of infection in which numerous bacteria are involved, there is a second phase in which only bacteria that are capable of surviving well outside of their regular environment survived [10]. Little is known in bovine medicine about the most common bacteria that are isolated from acute or chronic peritonitis; however, because *Arcanobacter pyogenes* commonly is isolated from abscesses in the bovine, one could assume that it may be of importance in chronic abcedative cases.

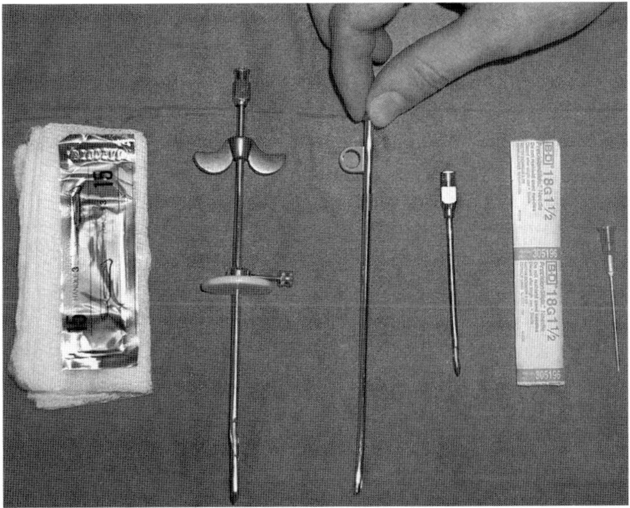

Fig. 5. Materials used to obtain peritoneal fluid.

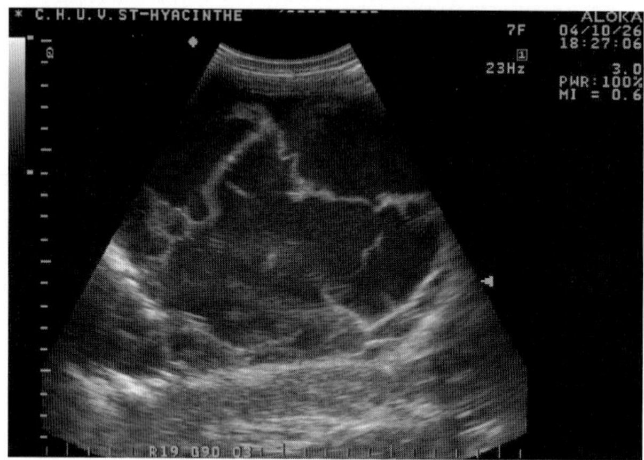

Fig. 6. Accumulation of peritoneal fluid observed during ultrasound examination. Note the multiple pockets and the location appearance.

Abdominal radiographs

Abdominal radiographs that use a high-power unit are extremely useful in cases in which reticuloperitonitis is suspected (Fig. 9). They have limited value in other causes of peritonitis. A review of radiographic interpretation of the bovine cranio-ventral abdomen was published by Partington and Biller [11].

Abdominal echographic examination

Ultrasound examination is useful in the assessment of the presence of abdominal fluids (see the article by Braun elsewhere in this issue). Abscesses

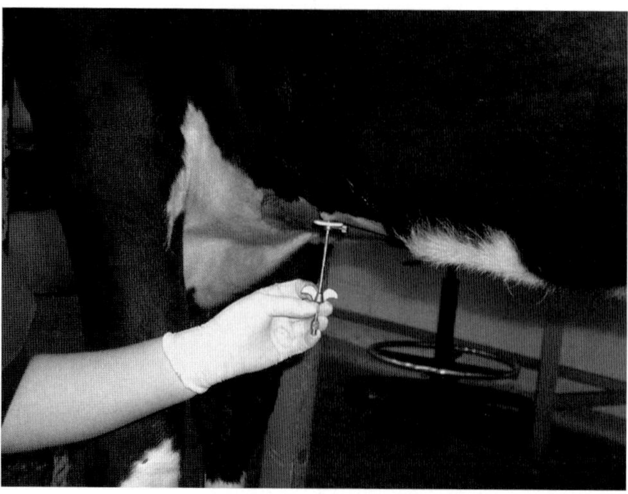

Fig. 7. Cranial site of abdominocentesis.

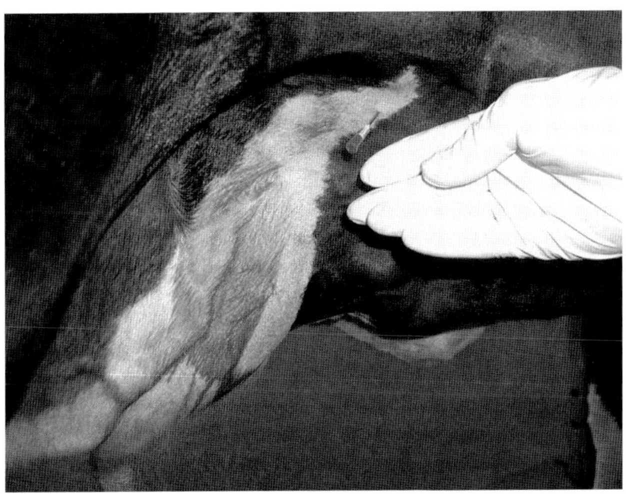

Fig. 8. Caudal site of abdominocentesis.

can be located and fluid aspiration can be performed. Adequate knowledge of the topographic anatomy is important to avoid misinterpretation of images. Abscesses can have mixed echogenicity that vary from anechoic (absence of internal echoes) to echogenic, depending on the relative amounts of fluid, fibrin, and gas (Fig. 10). The fibrous capsule of an abscess may be identified as echogenic bands around the area in question (see Fig. 10). Ultrasound also is useful to guide peritoneal tap. During an exploratory

Table 1
Normal range for the classification of bovine peritoneal fluid

Parameters	Normal values	References
Turbidity	Clear	[6–8]
Total protein (g/dL)	0.1–3.1	[8]
	<3.0	[6]
	2.2–4.0	[9]
	1.2–6.3	[7]
Specific gravity	1.005–1.015	[8]
Total cell count (× 1000/μL)	425–2950	[9]
	300–5300	[8]
	2000–5000	[7]
	<10,000	[6]
Differential	Ratio 1:1 neutrophils to mononuclear	[6,8]
Neutrophils	45–2183	[9]
Lymphocytes	8–168	[9]
Mononuclear	36–960	[9]
Eosinophils	5–545	[9]
Comments	Eosinophils may predominate	[6]
	Serosa cells may predominate	[7]

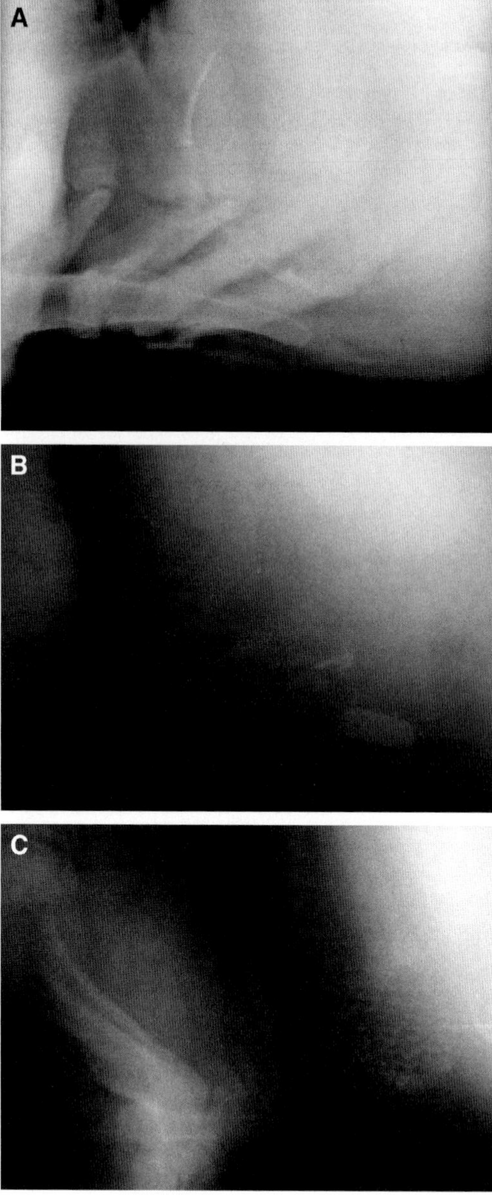

Fig. 9. (*A,B*) (Courtesy of Marie Babkine, DMV, St-Hyacinthe, Québec, Canada). Cranial abdominal radiographs showing the presence of a linear foreign body that is causing peritonitis. (*C*) Normal radiographic appearance of the reticulum. (*D*) Presence of two magnets on rumen pili just in between the reticulum and the atrium of the rumen.

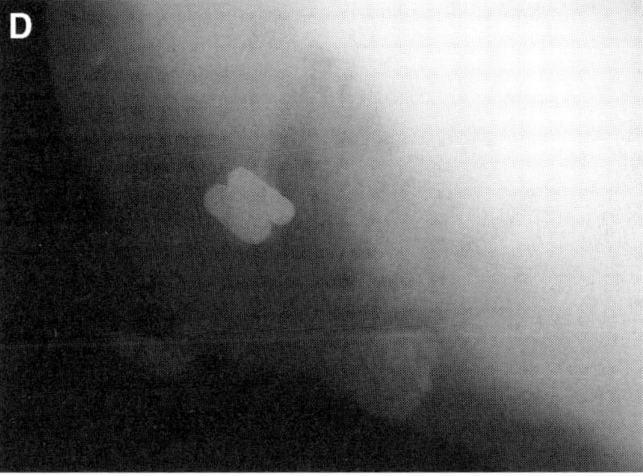

Fig. 9 (*continued*)

surgery, ultrasound can be used to visualize an internal mass or an abnormal viscus. Intraoperative ultrasound is performed by placing the probe in a sterile sleeve that is filled with ultrasound gel. Of particular interest, would be the thickness of the capsule of an abscess and the possibility of establishing drainage outside of the peritoneal cavity without causing severe diffuse peritonitis.

Diagnostic surgery

Surgical exploration is used often to confirm or rule out an intra-abdominal problem. Immediate action to correct the identified problem may be indicated (eg, drainage of an abscess or closure of an ulcer). Cattle are particularly amenable to exploratory surgery because the procedure is

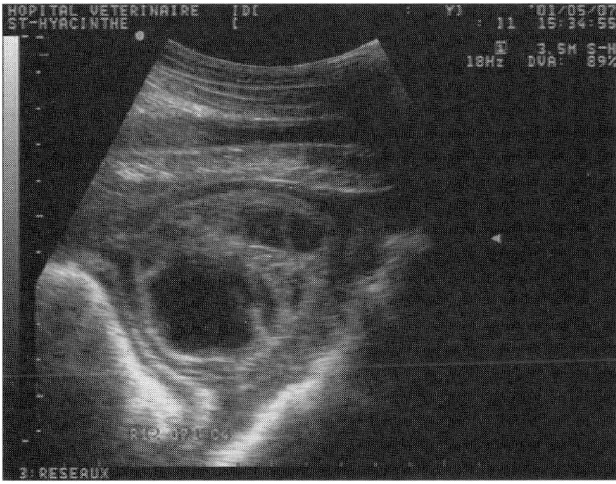

Fig. 10. Ultrasound view of an abdominal abscess. (Courtesy of Marie Babkine, DMV, St-Hyacinthe, Québec, Canada)

performed standing and is associated with few complications. The inexpensive cost of surgery often makes multiple, expensive tests irrelevant in bovines. Important structures to evaluate are presented in Fig. 11.

Recent advances in minimally-invasive surgical techniques in cattle are promising. Laparoscopy can be used to diagnose acute and chronic peritonitis that otherwise is difficult to identify with ultrasound or abdominocentesis. It is easier to evaluate the extent of the lesions with the organs in situ [12].

Ancillary tests

Hematologic findings that are associated with peritonitis range from a completely normal hemogram to severe leukopenia with degenerative left shift and presence of toxic neutrophils, depending on the severity and cause of the peritoneal contamination. A neutrophilic leukocytosis and a hyperfibrinogenemia are observed commonly. Because of the rapid influx of fluid that is rich in proteins toward the peritoneal cavity, packed cell volume tends to increase as protein concentration decreases. In chronic cases, plasma proteins often tend to increase as a result of hyperglobulinemia and hyperfibrinogenemia. Hematology also is a useful tool to monitor response to therapy. Persistence of immature cells in the peripheral blood or

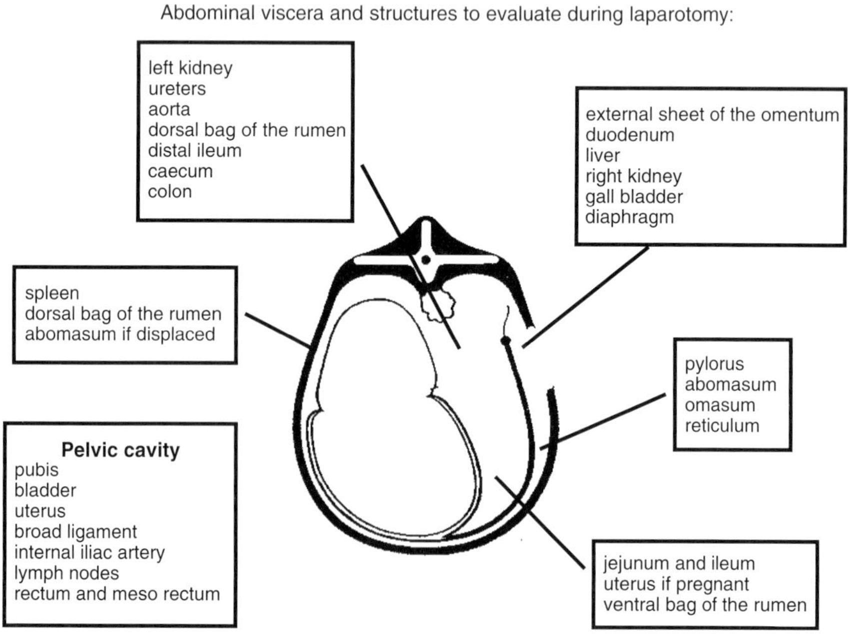

Fig. 11. Checklist of abdominal structures to verify during an exploratory laparotomy.

leukocytosis are indications that the therapy should be continued. Plasma fibrinogen concentration also is used to monitor the response to therapy. Acute phase proteins (APP) contribute to restore homeostasis and limit infection. Their clinical use is not common; however, several studies indicate that some particular APP may be of interest in the diagnosis of infection in cattle. α1-Acid glycoprotein, ceruloplasmin, haptoglobin, protease inhibitors, and transferrin are the most promising because they are specific to infection in bovines [13].

Changes in the serum chemistry profile are nonspecific and often reveal secondary problems. Chronic inflammation may cause an increase in serum globulin concentration. In acute cases, secondary findings may include increased serum urea nitrogen and creatinine, mild elevation of liver enzymes, and reduction in serum protein (albumin and globulins). Ileus and stasis of the upper gastrointestinal system may result in hypochloremia, hypokalemia, and metabolic alkalosis.

Therapeutic management

The basic types of therapy should be supportive therapy, antibiotic therapy, and surgical therapy.

Supportive therapy

Depending on the severity of the process, the patient may present in shock. Large volumes of isotonic intravenous fluids are indicated. Correction of any acid-base deficit is indicated. Electrolyte abnormalities (hypokalemia and hypocalcemia) should be identified and corrected. If the animal is hypoproteinemic, plasma or whole blood transfusions may be beneficial. Nonsteroidal or steroidal anti-inflammatory drugs may be of importance to prevent the synthesis of more inflammatory mediators. Pain control also is important. Transfaunation may be beneficial in cases of prolonged anorexia. In one study, rumen transfaunation reduced ketonuria and increased feed intake and milk yield after surgical correction of left displaced abomasum [14].

Antibiotic therapy

Systemic antibiotic therapy should be instituted as soon as a decision to treat is made. Until results of culture and antimicrobial susceptibility become available, a broad spectrum antibiotic should be used. The choice should take into consideration the cost of treatment, withdrawal period in food animals, spectrum of activity, and treatment regimen (frequency and route). Tetracycline or a B-lactam antibiotic (third-generation cephalosporin or the synthetic penicillin) seem to be good choices. Diffusion into the peritoneal cavity is not a major limiting factor, because the permeability of the peritoneum always is increased in peritonitis. When fibrin becomes organized and form multiple, small pockets of infected peritoneal fluid, diffusion becomes more problematic. In human medicine, single antimicrobial therapy with a broad-spectrum agent is effective in patients who suffer from secondary peritonitis [15,16].

Surgical therapy

Surgical control of peritonitis includes peritoneal debridement, irrigation, and drainage. Using ultrasound guidance, it is possible to establish drainage from the abdominal cavity safely. A thoracic chest trocar can be used temporarily until all fluid has been removed (Fig. 12). Aseptic preparation is important.

The concept of abdominal lavage during surgery was adopted by human surgeons around the turn of the century and has been accepted as a part of treatment of peritonitis since then with fluctuating support [17]. Although the principle of removal of any gross contamination is not under question, the level of aggressiveness with which we should institute abdominal lavage during surgery is open to debate in the human and veterinary literature. There is evidence of a negative effect of lavage on the mesothelial cells and the peritoneal defense mechanism and the risk of spreading the infection [17,18]. The solution that is used to irrigate also is under debate. There is no significant advantage to adding antibiotics to the lavage solution [17,18] and there controversy about the possible advantages of adding an antiseptic [17]. In our experience, drainage of the abdomen with Foley catheters or negative pressure drains has been unsuccessful consistently in bovines. Large amounts of fibrin may be deposited in a short period of time in combination with the omentum; this causes those drains to plug and become ineffective rapidly.

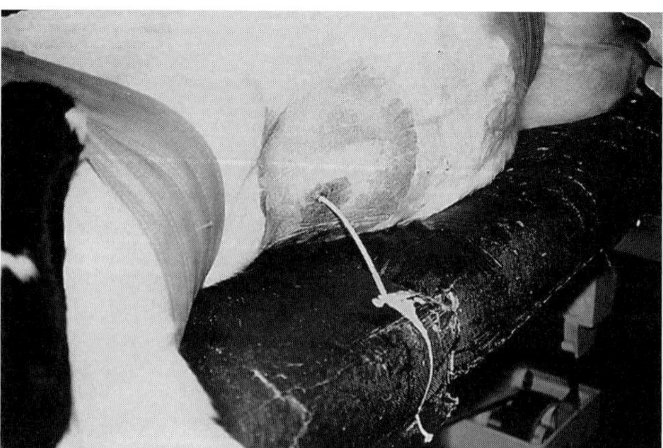

Fig. 12. Chest trocar used to drain an abdominal abscess percutaneously using echographic guidance.

Prognosis

The ultimate outcome of an episode of bacterial peritonitis is determined by many factors, some of which are controlled by the clinician. The early decision to treat (medical and surgical), adequate choice of antimicrobials, and supportive therapy contribute to the success or failure of a therapy. The owner's delay in seeking therapy, the primary cause of peritonitis, and the patient's age are examples of important factors that are beyond the clinician's control. In humans, the development of an objective scoring system has proven to be extremely useful to predict outcome in cases of peritonitis and to allow comparison of patients who are enrolled in clinical trials. The APACHE II (acute physiology and chronic health evaluation) is a severity of disease classification system that uses 12 routine physiologic measurements [19].

In animals, where aggressive therapy is economically possible, survival rates may be good, but long-term sequelae and recurrence could compromise a complete recovery.

Miscellaneous conditions

Ascites

Ascites is a collection of serous fluid in the peritoneal cavity. The primary cause must be identified to treat the patient adequately. Common causes of ascites in ruminants include congestive right-sided heart failure. Young cattle who have mesothelioma accumulate large amounts of ascites. Ascites remains an uncommon condition that needs to be differentiated from septic causes of peritonitis and from urine accumulation with ruptured bladder.

Pneumoperitoneum

Pneumoperitoneum is observed commonly after surgery. Simultaneous percussion and auscultation reveal a low-pitch resonance in the upper flank on both sides of the abdomen. Pneumoperitoneum normally resolves in the week after surgery and no clinical signs seem to be associated, although some clinicians believe that it is associated with abdominal pain. Pneumoperitoneum that is not associated with surgery is indicative of bacterial peritonitis and the presence of gas-producing bacteria.

Retroperitoneal abscess

Retroperitoneal abscess is a particular condition that occurs in cattle following a flank laparotomy. The animal often is presented several days after surgery. They are mildly febrile, not performing adequately, and show clinical signs that are compatible with peritonitis. The skin wound often is unremarkable, but some pain may be elicited while palpating the flank area. A substantial mass could be palpated per rectum, that is localized in the upper quadrant of the side of the previous surgical approach. The mass will be firm, smooth, unmovable, and close to the previous flank incision. Transabdominal or rectal ultrasound examination reveals a large amount of fluid located between the peritoneum and the rectus abdominis or the internal oblique of the abdomen. A needle aspiration allows visual inspection of a thick, opaque, foul-smelling fluid. Treatment is aimed at establishing drainage and systemic antimicrobial therapy. A large volume of purulent and fibrinous material (up to 40 L) can be removed from the abscess. Rapid decompression may provoke hypovolemic shock; intravenous fluids should be administered in prevention. Prognosis is good but the recovery phase is extremely long because of the large cavity that is left after drainage. Early closure of the drain often is observed which necessitates reopening.

References

[1] Borgonovo GAA, Varaldo E, Mattioli FP. Definition and classification of peritonitis. Med Mal Infect 1995;25:7–12.
[2] Kirby BM. Peritoneum and peritoneal cavity. In: Slatter D, editor. Textbook of small animal surgery. New York: WB Saunders; 2003. p. 414–45.
[3] Hall JC, Heel KA, Papadimitriou JM, et al. The pathobiology of peritonitis. Gastroenterology 1998;114:185–96.
[4] Ahrenholz D, Simmons R. Peritonitis and other intra-abdominal infections. In: Simmons R, Howard R, editors. Surgical infectious diseases. New York: Appleton-Century-Crofts; 1982. p. 795–841.
[5] Wilson A, Hirsch V, Osborne A. Abdominocentesis in cattle: technique and criteria for diagnosis of peritonitis. Can Vet J 1985;26:74–80.
[6] Kopcha M, Schultze AE. Peritoneal fluid. Part I. Pathophysiology and classification of nonneoplastic effusions. Compend Contin Educ Pract Vet 1991;13:519–26.
[7] Rosenberger G. Abdomen and abdominal cavity. In: Co WS, editor. Clinical examination of cattle. Philadelphia: WB Saunders; 1979. p. 252–8.
[8] Radostits OM, Guay CC, Blood DC, et al. Veterinary medicine. In: Hinchcliff KW, editor. 9th edition. New York: WB Saunders; 2000. p. 179–81.
[9] Anderson DE, Cornwell D, Anderson LS, et al. Comparative analyses of peritoneal fluid from calves and adult cattle. Am J Vet Res 1995;56:973–6.
[10] Wittmann DH, Schein M, Condon RE. Management of secondary peritonitis. Ann Surg 1996;224:10–7.
[11] Partington BP, Biller DS. Radiography of the bovine cranioventral abdomen. Vet Radiol 1991;32:155–68.
[12] Franz S, Baumgartner W. Laparoscopy in upright position of the animal as a diagnostic tool in bovine medicine. Société Française de Buiatrie 2004;127.
[13] Murata H, Shimada N, Yoshioka M. Current research on acute phase proteins in veterinary diagnosis: an overview. Vet J 2004;168:28–40.
[14] Rager KD, George LW, House JK, et al. Evaluation of rumen transfaunation after surgical correction of left-sided displacement of the abomasum in cows. J Am Vet Med Assoc 2004; 225:915–20.
[15] Hopkins JA, Wilson SE, Bobey DG. Adjunctive antimicrobial therapy for complicated appendicitis: bacterial overkill by combination therapy. World J Surg 1994;18:933–8.
[16] Stone HH, Strom PR, Fabian TC, et al. Third-generation cephalosporins for polymicrobial surgical sepsis. Arch Surg 1983;118:193–200.

[17] Platell C, Papadimitriou JM, Hall JC. The influence of lavage on peritonitis. J Am Coll Surg 2000;191:672–80.
[18] Schein M, Gecelter G, Freinkel W, et al. Peritoneal lavage in abdominal sepsis. A controlled clinical study. Arch Surg 1990;125:1132–5.
[19] Knaus WA, Draper EA, Wagner DP, et al. APACHE II: a severity of disease classification system. Crit Care Med 1985;13:818–29.

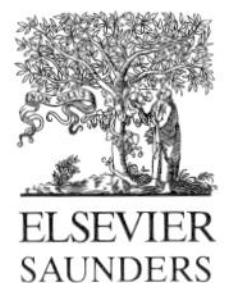

ELSEVIER
SAUNDERS

Vet Clin Food Anim 21 (2005) 173–204

VETERINARY
CLINICS
Food Animal Practice

Procedures and Surgeries of the Teat

Yvon Couture, DVM*, Pierre-Yves Mulon, DMV

Department of Clinical Sciences, Université de Montréal, Faculté de Médecine Vétérinaire, C.P. 5000, St Hyacinthe, Québec, J2S 7C6, Canada

Traumatic injuries to the teat or the mammary gland are frequent in dairy cattle. These lesions, consequences for the most part of accidents, greatly interfere with milk production and, in certain cases, can compromise the production of the quarter or of the whole gland. Because of the genetic and economic value of high-producing animals, producers need expertise from well-trained veterinarians. Teat surgery can be frustrating, and good knowledge of the anatomy, udder development, milk ejection mechanism, and healing process is essential.

Major improvements have been made in the field of teat surgery since the 1980s, such as determination of the ultimate suturing technique; new imaging technologies, such as radiography, ultrasound, and theloscopy, have helped in the diagnosis of the different afflictions of the teat. These diagnostic tools are important to determine the best possible interventions and to obtain better results with therapeutic approaches. Compared with blind intervention, such as the use of the conventional teat knife, theloscopy allows for a lot more precision in fibrous tissue removal.

A completely different approach has been used more recently to manage streak canal fibrosis with rethinking of certain procedures and treatments. Use of dilator rods (Dr Naylor teat dilators, Morris, NY; or Colombus, Jorgen Krusse Marslev, Denmark) and of their components is being questioned. Complete rest (no milking) when the papillary canal is affected, depending on the gland's infection status, is an approach that merits attention. Absence of milking for 3 to 5 days should not be a major inconvenience to a healthy gland. Silicone rods and natural fatty acid rods, both of which favor better healing of the papillary canal lesions, should replace fiber dilator rods.

* Corresponding author.

0749-0720/05/$ - see front matter
doi:10.1016/j.cvfa.2004.12.005

vetfood.theclinics.com

Epidemiology aspects

Annual reports from the Quebec Dairy Livestock Analysis Program from 1998–2002 indicate that approximately 2% of lactating cows were eliminated from the herd because of teat or mammary gland problems, other than those related to mastitis [1]; in Michigan in 1981, 3% of cows were excluded from the herd for similar reasons [2]. These teat lesions are associated with subclinical infections of the gland [3,4] even after healing [5]. A similar distribution of these lesions is observed according to different authors [6,7]. Lesions can be superficial, deep, or penetrating, and they can involve the internal structures of the teat's cisterna. Of 154 observed lesions, 12% involved the superior half of the teat; 29%, the inferior half; 52%, the inferior extremity of the teat; and 7%, the whole teat. Of the 52% located at the distal extremity, 36% affected the papillary canal [6]. These conditions of the papillary canal tend to favor infections and interfere with mechanical milking—hence the importance of proper treatment and speedy recovery while respecting this delicate structure.

Approximately 10% of lesions to the teat cause internal lesions to the teat's cisterna. The posterior quarters are affected more than the anterior quarters by 60% [7]. Of 105 cases referred to the Faculty of Veterinary Medicine of the Université de Montréal from 1990–2003 for deep lesions involving the cisterna's lining (teat), with milk loss at the lesion site, the authors have not observed a difference in frequency: front left, 24; rear left, 27; front right, 28; and rear right, 26.

Integrity of the papillary canal is important to the health of the mammary gland and its conformation. The length of this canal varies between 5 and 13 mm, with an average of approximately 8.5 mm; its diameter in the distal part is 0.45 mm and in the proximal part is 0.94 mm. When comparing infected and noninfected quarters, an increase in diameter of the papillary canal in the infected quarters of 30% is observed [8]. An illustration by Seeh et al, as reported by Frémont et al [9], indicates the types of lesions and their importance (Fig. 1).

Anatomy

The alveolus is the basic unit of a group of cells that drain in a simple epithelium interlobular duct. These milk-gathering ducts join in double-epithelium collecting ducts of increasing lumen size [10]. In the cow, lactiferous ducts include wide parts, separated by narrowings that open in a lactiferous sinus, the gland's cisterna; there can be more in some quarters. The lactiferous sinus has a glandular part and a papillary part, separated by an annular relief (Fig. 2). The large glandular part (cisterna) is egg-shaped and has ramifications that affect the lactiferous ducts. The cisterna's volume varies greatly, from 100 to 2000 mL [11]. Occasionally, these loosely organized structures can be responsible for milking outflow [12]. The

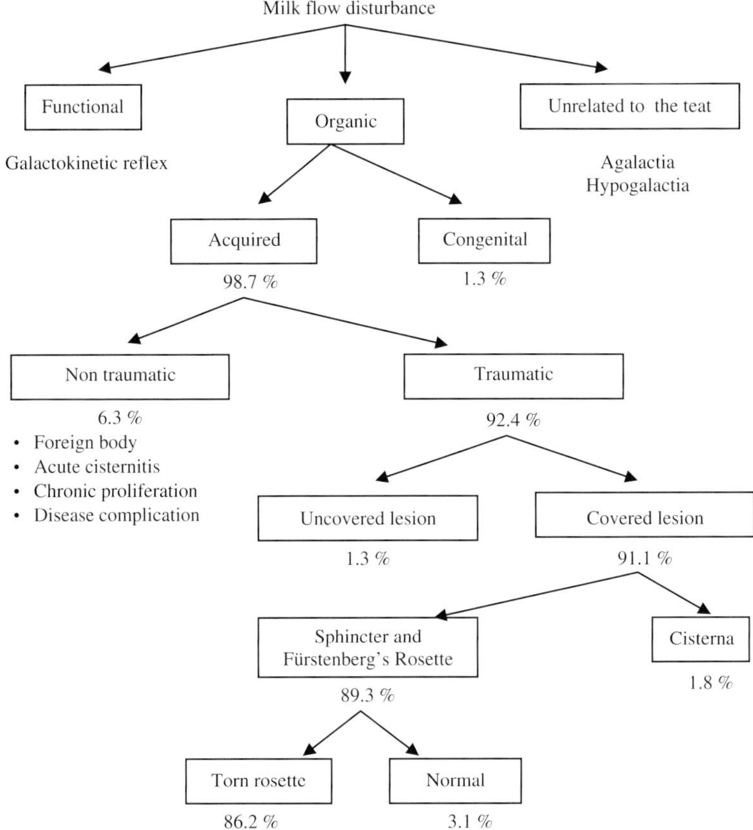

Fig. 1. Relative importance of different teat conditions. A covered lesion involves mucosa, muscularis, or both. Skin can be traumatized but not lacerated. An uncovered lesion involves laceration of the mucosa, muscularis, and skin. (*From* Frémont A, Bergonier D, Berthelot X, et al. Intérêt de l'endoscopie pour le diagnostic et le traitement des sténoses du trayon chez la vache laitière: étude d'un cas clinique. Rev Med Vet 2002;153:40–6; with permission.)

annular relief, or fold, supports a well-developed vascular network, which is important to identify clearly during surgery.

The teat's lining is composed of five different histologic layers. From the inside working out, the mucosa and submucosa; a highly vascularized layer of conjunctive tissue; the muscularis, made up of circular and longitudinal fibers; and finally the skin, covered by a stratified squamous epithelium, can be observed. The cisterna's mucosa, in the papillary part, has limber longitudinal folds that spread easily to allow for dilation. They start at the annular fold and converge toward the teat's distal extremity to form a rosette (Fürstenberg rosette). The role of this structure is believed to be to block the papillary duct between milking. The Fürstenberg rosette also protects against microbial invasion because it holds a large quantity of

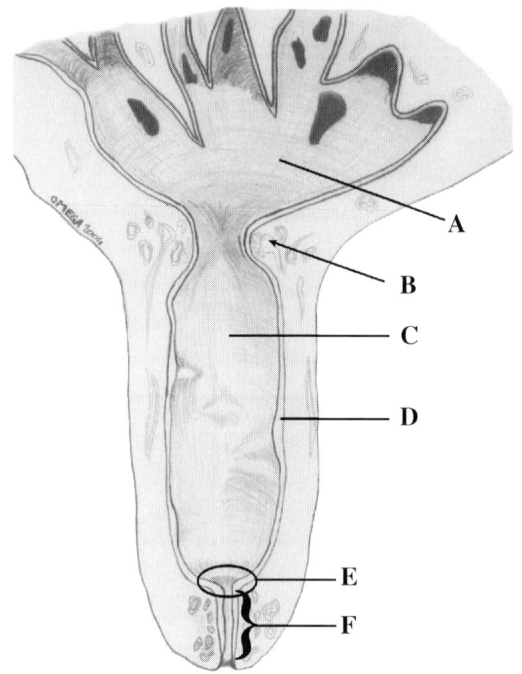

Fig. 2. Teat anatomy. Gross anatomy. (*A*) Glandular cisterna. (*B*) Annular relief. (*C*) Teat cisterna. (*D*) Mucosa. (*E*) Rosette of Fürstenberg. (*F*) Papillary canal.

intraepithelial lymphocytes [11]. This structure often is involved in traumas to the teat's extremity [9]. A slight fibrosis may interfere greatly with milking. According to Phillipron et al, as reported by Gourreau [7], "heritability of clinically known lesions is around 28%."

The papillary duct or teat's canal completes the mammary gland's excretory system. The internal lining of this passage consists of a stratified squamous epithelium and circular nonstriated muscular fibers composing a vaguely defined sphincter. It seems to be a multispiraled, elastic-muscular structure, which would allow the opening or closing of the canal according to the physiologic status of the gland. The presence of Langerhans' cells in the internal epithelium adds to the defense mechanisms by acting as antigen detectors [13]. The internal epithelium, by renewing itself, promotes the keratinization process; keratin (lipids, fatty acids, and proteins) is manufactured, and plaques of this substance are deposited like tiles on a roof to facilitate occlusion of the papillary canal between milking. This substance also is a barrier against bacterial invasions [11]. Repeated interventions involving this canal, with milking cannulas, particularly metallic ones, can destroy this layer of biologic protection. When acutely dilated, it should regain its diameter within 24 to 48 hours, and the keratin should regenerate [7]. Prolonged use of milking cannulas and pipe cleaner–type dilators has a major impact on the incidence of mastitis. Traditionally, quarters are identified by numbers 1 to 4: *1*, the left front quarter; *2*, the left rear; *3*, the right front; and *4*, the right rear.

At its production peak, the mammary gland produces large amounts of milk. The vascular system must be well developed; the blood supply (arteries) and the blood return (the venous and lymphatic systems). In the cow, the mammary arteries stem mostly from divisions of the external pudendal artery and a few branches from the internal pudendal artery; the main artery can reach diameters of 2 cm easily. Generally, the veins that drain the gland, run along with and have the same names as the arteries. The external pudendal vein is the main carrier of blood from the gland. Part of the blood is drained through the cranial epigastric vein (milk vein). At the teat's level, the main artery follows a path parallel to the longitudinal axis—laterally, caudal, or medial, depending on its origin. The venous part of the teat is more complex. The highly muscle-lined veins form a plexus starting with the one surrounding the sphincter and create many anastomoses. This drainage of blood from the teat finishes at the venous ring at the base of the teat. This disposition is believed to favor a better blood return when the animal is lying down [14]. Understanding the teat's vascular system allows clinicians to understand why injuries can lead to significant bleeding and that vertical lacerations heal better than transverse ones.

Diagnosis of traumatic conditions affecting the teat

Diagnosis is easy when there is a full-thickness laceration and milk is leaking out of the teat. If the mucosa is intact or there is a nonpenetrating injury, locating and assessing the type of lesion becomes more difficult. A complete and thorough examination helps assess the situation, plan treatment, and establish a prognosis [15,16]. Fig. 3 [15] shows that a structured step-by-step method leads to a certain precision in dealing with teat problems. A step-by-step examination procedure to teat lacerations is as follows:

- Visual examination and description of the lesion (type and location of the problem)
- Complete palpation of the gland and the teat (extraction of a few squirts of milk from each teat and rolling each teat between fingers helps assess location and importance of the problem)
- Insertion of a graduated rod in the teat, via the papillary canal, to help locate obstruction or assess damage to the canal
- Milk bacterial culture and sensitivity, if necessary, particularly for chronic problems and accessory glands
- Medical imaging, such as ultrasound, contrast radiographs, or thelo-scopy, to refine diagnosis, determine a therapeutic plan, and establish a prognosis

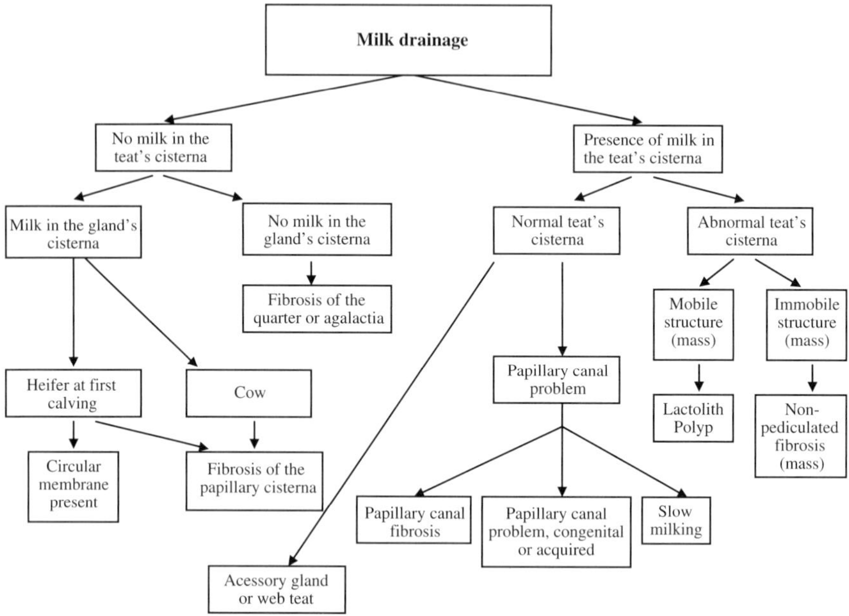

Fig. 3. Diagnostic approach to milk flow problems. (*Adapted from* Modransky P, Welker B. Diagnosing and treating milk flow problems. Vet Med 1993;88:788–804; with permission.)

Lesions can be grossly located in the following regions: papillary duct, Fürstenberg rosette, papillary sinus, or glandular sinus; stenosis can affect many of these sites at the same time. In such cases, clinical examination (palpation) does not allow sufficient precision regarding the nature and location of the lesion; consequently, prognosis is uncertain. The insufficient precision of palpation is particularly true for lesions situated at the lactiferous sinus or papillary or glandular part of the mammary gland.

Papillary canal examination merits particular attention because it is often the site of traumatic lesions. A graduated teat probe is available to measure the length of the papillary canal and to gather information about it (Fig. 4) [17]. Geishauser and Querengässer [17] examined 133 cows presenting with papillary canal dysfunction problems; results indicate that compared with the counter-lateral papillary canal, the affected papillary canal tends to stretch. This is an important observation, and a more accurate diagnosis can be determined with theloscopy.

Imaging techniques, particularly ultrasound and radiology, show an image of the suspected lesions, whereas theloscopy shows the lesion directly. The major advantage with theloscopy is that intervention can occur at the same time. Theloscopic examination can be performed through the papillary duct or the teat lining.

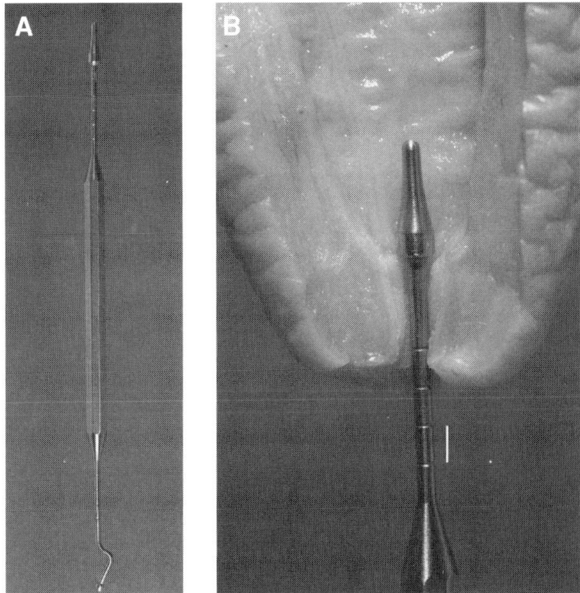

Fig. 4. (*A*, *B*) Teat probe (Dr Fritz GmbH, Tuttlingen, Germany) for teat canal measurement. Length of the landmark is 3 mm.

Ultrasound

Many authors have described teat examination by ultrasound. Teat examination is a procedure that suits neophytes in cattle ultrasound well because a rectal linear ultrasound probe can be used, and results can be compared easily with normal teats of the same animal (Figs. 5 and 6) [18–24].

	Histological plane	Ultrasound images
External	Skin	Hyperechoic
↓	Muscular layers: longitudinal and circular	Medium echogenicity
	Conjunctive tissue layers,	Medium echogenicity
	blood vessels	Hyperechoic
	Sub-mucosa	Medium echogenicity
	Mucosa	Hyperechoic
Internal	Fürstenberg's Rosette	Hyperechoic
	Papillary duct	Hyperechoic

Fig. 5. Normal structures visible by ultrasound.

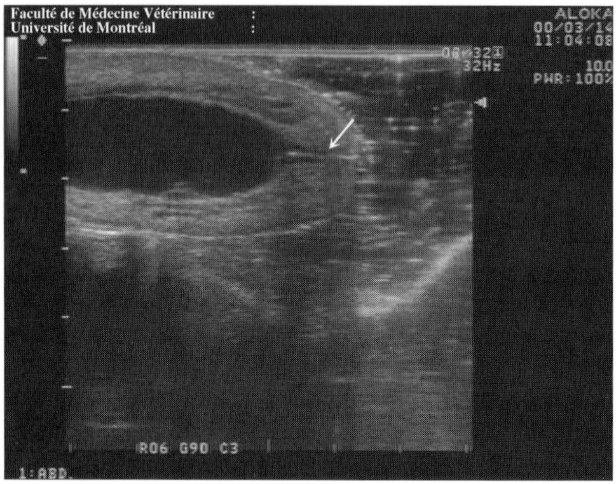

Fig. 6. Ultrasound of a normal teat. The teat cisterna appears hypoechoic, and the papillary canal appears as a narrow hyperechoic line surrounded by two hypoechoic lines (*arrow*).

Probes

Transrectal linear probes of 5 MHz or 7.5 MHz can be used for teat examination. Variable-frequency probes are available but are more expensive (eg, 5 MHz and 7.5 MHz or 5 MHz, 7.5 MHz, and 10 MHz). Teat examination is a relatively simple technique compared with the technique needed for other organs; the structures are easily accessible, tissues are simple, and comparison between healthy structures from a neighboring quarter and the affected teat is easy.

Preparation

Preparation is simple, consisting of a thorough cleansing of the area and shaving of hairs, if necessary, to obtain a good contact between the probe and the skin; addition of gel helps facilitate this contact. Use of an acoustic pad on the probe allows for better image quality with less powerful machines. Water can be used as an interface liquid. The teat is immersed in a small plastic container (acrylic), and the probe, with the gel, is applied to the external surface of the container [23]. This method makes teat examination easy because neither the pressure from the probe nor the examiner's hand modifies the teat's shape.

Procedure

The probe is applied sagittally, starting at the distal part; following this, it is directed toward the lactiferous sinus of the gland. This procedure is repeated on the four aspects of the teat. Second, the probe is applied transversely, at a 90° angle with the teat, allowing for observation of transverse sections of the teat. This procedure helps in localizing lesions or anomalies on the circumference of the teat or of the papillary sinus mucosa. The sagittal position is more appropriate for the papillary canal, whereas the transverse position of the probe is more appropriate for examination of the gland's cisterna. The reference regarding tissue echogenicity is the contents of the papillary sinus—milk. Colostrum and mastatic milk have a different echogenicity than regular milk. When interpretation is difficult, a quarter is milked out, and saline or sterile water is infused into the teat. As mentioned before, reference to another teat for comparison is always easy.

Lesions commonly identified with ultrasound include the following:

- Fibrosis or papillary canal lesions
- Fibrosis or trauma to or near Fürstenburg rosette
- Lesions or fibrosis at the teat's sinus
- Lesions or fibrosis at the gland's sinus
- Venous dilation (varicose vein) in the teat of origin of the vascular ring.

Good localization of the lesion on the circumference of the mucosa of the teat's cisterna is essential to choose the appropriate surgical approach.

Radiography

The veterinary literature reports few references on radiography. Researchers have used this method to study certain aspects such as evolution of the papillary canal's diameter during first lactation and to measure its length and importance of this diameter in relation to protection from infection [25–28]. Witzig et al [28] studied this technique in regard to stenosis of the papillary gland and of the teat's cisterna. The radiographic image of a lactiferous sinus contrast study varies greatly depending on whether the gland is in drying or lactating period and time after milking. Particularly in the proximal part of the glandular sinus, the papillary sinus' diameter is greater immediately after milking than 4 or 6 hours later. A double-contrast study can be performed allowing better visualization of the teat's sinus' contours and localization of certain lesions (fibrosis, occlusion, presence of membrane, or damage to Fürstenberg rosette). Fibrosis of the gland's cisterna is observed easily when approximately 30 mL of contrast substance, or less if the fibrosis is important, is infused. In a normal glandular cisterna, contrast liquid appears as a cloud in the distal part of the gland (Fig. 7), whereas in the presence of fibrosis, this liquid traces sinuous lines traveling to the proximal part of the gland.

Technique

Radiographic technique is as follows:

Radiopaque contrast solution, Hypaque (50% diatrizonate sodium solution; Amersham, Oakville, Ontario), is prepared.

Volume infused is 20 to 30 mL or volume possible to infuse; occasionally, lesions limit the quantity possible to infuse.

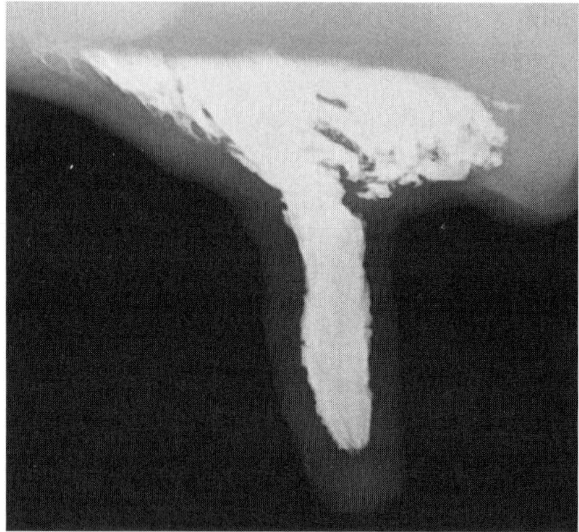

Fig. 7. Contrast radiograph of normal cisterna, teat, and gland parts.

After appropriate cleansing and sterilization, a teat cannula is inserted, and a radiopaque contrast substance is injected slowly, maintaining a constant pressure during injection.

The double-contrast method for papillary sinus examination is as follows:

1. Place a clamp (Doyen or teat clamp), or any other means to obstruct the superior part of the papillary sinus, as close to the gland as possible.
2. Inject radiopaque contrast substance in the teat's cisterna; generally, a 4- to 8-mL volume is sufficient.
3. Take a lateral radiographic view; this step is not always necessary.
4. Milk the excess injected radiopaque contrast solution.
5. Inject a volume of air equivalent to the volume of liquid injected in step 2. The teat should be well distended.
6. A second radiographic view is taken.
7. The clamp is removed, and the injected contrast material is milked out.

Injecting the radiopaque contrast substance with a positive pressure allows it to adhere to all the surfaces of normal or pathologic linings of the teat's sinus mucosa. Removal of the excess liquid followed by injection of air distends the cisterna and allows visualization of the contour of the mucosa or the pathologic formation. Similar to ultrasound, it can be useful to examine another quarter or another teat on the same side as reference. Many factors justify this control; from one animal to another, the shape, length, and even the diameter of the teat's sinus are not always identical.

Position of the cartridge

The cassette is placed in the crease separating the left and right quarters of the mammary gland. It is pushed as far up as possible in this space. This cartridge position gives a lateral view; it also is possible to obtain a front and rear quarter image at the same time but with more difficulty. Contrary to ultrasound, radiologic technique does not allow localization of lesions on the circumference of the mucosa. As reported by Frémont et al [9], Kiossis and Stocker compared the sensitivity of three diagnostic imaging techniques (ultrasound, radiology, and theloscopy) with clinical diagnosis. According to their results, endoscopy is more accurate in identification of lesions in the teat's canal than ultrasound and radiology. For damages to Fürtensberg rosette, imaging techniques are of similar precision but superior than physical examination and palpation. For lesions located at the teat's cisterna, all three imaging techniques and physical examination were of equal precision. For lesions located at the base of the teat, radiology had a 21% sensitivity, whereas sensitivity of the other two imaging techniques and clinical diagnosis was almost 100% [9]. It is the authors' opinion that radiographic study has superior results than described for lesions at the base of the teat when simultaneously analyzing the cisterna's and the gland's image.

Theloscopy

Theloscopy is a new noninvasive surgical technique that offers the visualization of the internal cavity of the teat. It has been described and used since the 1990s and is explained thoroughly in a subsequent article. Theloresectoscopy is a surgical procedure that allows visualization via a theloscope and intervention via a wire snare connected to an electrosurgical unit for monopolar cutting. There are two advantages to this technique. The first is that one port is necessary to visualize and débride the lesions. The second is the use of an electrosurgical wire snare, which decreases bleeding during débridement. It is more cumbersome to use for beginners, and because of all the small parts, cleaning and sterilization could be a potential problem [29].

Restraint, anesthesia, and preparation of the site

Adequate restraint is a crucial, yet often neglected, factor for successful reconstruction of a teat laceration. In contrast to any other bovine surgery under field conditions, tissue handling and suturing techniques should be precise and delicate. Lacerated tissues and normal teat tissues are fragile, and the use of appropriate suture material is extremely important [30].

For a simple procedure, such as opening or resection of the sphincter, the surgery is performed with the animal standing in a chute if available. Light sedation and local anesthesia are used as needed. A technique of intravenous anesthesia is described in a subsequent chapter; 5 mL of local anesthetic solution also can be injected into the teat's cisterna. For a more invasive procedure, such as laceration repair or thelotomy, the animal must be sedated and placed in lateral or dorsal recumbency. The dorsal position is often favored, granting better access to the surgical site and partially preventing milk seepage from the site.

Sedation and anesthesia

Intramuscular or intravenous xylazine can be administered at the recommended dose; occasionally, in an extremely anxious animal, butorphanol (0.05 mg/kg) can be added by the intramuscular route. For xylazine, depending on administration method and dosage, and if the animal is placed on its back, a fasting period of 24 hours is preferable if possible. Acepromazine given intramuscularly 30 minutes before surgery at a dose of 0.1 mg/kg can be a substitute to xylazine. After surgical preparation of the site, lidocaine 2% without epinephrine is used to infiltrate the teat. Three different local anesthesias have been used according to the situation and surgeon preference: (1) a ring block at the base of the teat, (2) an inverted V above the laceration or the planned incision, and (3) intravenous injection in one of the teat's veins after putting a tourniquet at the base of the teat. In the authors' opinion, circular injection at the teat's base is easy to perform, does not interfere with healing, and is a satisfactory method for the repair of lacerations to the teat. A small-gauge needle (eg, 22G to 25G) is used to infiltrate the lidocaine solution. When the papillary mucosa is intact, it is recommended to inject 5 to 10 mL of local anesthetic agent (2% solution) into the teat's cisterna via the papillary canal. Preparation of the surgical site is completed by shaving of the area surrounding the teat and cleansing and sterilization of the site. To these basic anesthetic methods, others can be added, such as paravertebral anesthesia of L3 and L4; for posterior teats, anesthesia of the pudendal nerve's mammary ramus must be added along with epidural anesthesia combining lidocaine and xylazine and finally general anesthesia, particularly for ablation of the mammary gland [31,32].

Suture material

Even if the teat laceration heald well, it does not mean that quarter will be milked out properly. Today, with sophisticated milking systems, teats need to be perfect; otherwise the cow is undermilked or overmilked. With automatic computerized milking machines, the cow may not be milked at all. Surgeons working on teats should aim for perfection and not just healing. One good start is to use the appropriate suture material with the appropriate suture pattern.

Synthetic absorbable sutures should be used on all internal tissues (mucosa and submucosa) because of minor tissue reactions. This material should be easy to manipulate, does not tend to cut tissues, and is sewn with a swaged atraumatic needle. Small-diameter suture decreases the chance of milk leaking around it and fistula creation. The authors use suture sizes of

USP 3-0 to 4-0. For the skin, nonabsorbable multifilament or monofilament material of 2-0 caliber is preferable. Polybutester (Novafil; Tyco, Ville St-Laurent, Québec) with its slightly elastic characteristic is a good choice.

Suture types

Many suture techniques have been described in the literature [33–39]. Ghamsari et al [39] compared four suture patterns on lactating cows; their evaluation criteria were based on clinical observation, radiology, biomechanics, and histopathology. According to their research, a three-layer closing was superior to a two-layer closing: simple continuous suture on the mucosa, simple continuous suture on the stoma (musculosa and connective tissues), and simple interrupted suture on the skin. Polyglactin USP 3-0 was used for internal sutures, and USP 2-0 was used for the skin.

As mentioned before, other types of sutures can be used, such as Cushing for the mucosa, simple interrupted for the muscle layers, and mattress sutures for the skin. Based on research findings and authors' experiences, a three-layer technique with simple continuous sutures gives superior results. Skin sutures should be removed no later than 8 to 10 days after surgery; when left in place for a longer period, suture tract infection or inflammation appears around the stitches. Teat wall swelling and fibrous reaction, which are not desired, may result. A small dressing can be applied on the incision for 24 to 48 hours after surgery.

Mechanical milking

If the swelling of the teat is under control after surgery, mechanical milking should be resumed at the second or third milking. If swelling is too severe, a larger teat cup can be used for the affected teat until improvement. Milking mechanics allow even circumferential pressure, avoiding focal stress on the incision. In contrast, hand milking stresses the surgical incision edges focally. This promotes infiltration of milk in the wound and particularly fatty droplets interfering with the healing process and predisposing to fistula formation. For a period of 1 week, manual handling of the teat should be limited.

Congenital anomalies

Supernumerary teats

Presence of supernumerary teats (hyperthelia or polythelia) is the most frequent congenital anomaly in cattle [40]. The extra teats generally are smaller and harmless. If the extra teats are removed at a young age, however, the udder's appearance is more acceptable. Some extra teats can become a nuisance to milking when they're located near a normal teat; when they produce milk, their secretions are a possible source of contamination.

Generally, extra teats are located along the embryonic ridge, behind the regular teats, or between an anterior and a posterior teat, on the same side. Occasionally, they can be close or even attached to a normal teat; in this case, special attention is required during surgery to keep the good teat, especially if the surgery is performed on calves. The ideal time to perform surgical ablation is between 4 and 6 months of age. Ablation should be done with a sharp scissor, with the section oriented in the cranial-caudal axis to prevent excessive scarring. A normal sterilization and a small amount of local anesthetic injected at the base of the teat to be removed complete the procedure [30,40]. It is important to pay special attention to the sterilization of instruments to avoid the transmission of blood-carried infectious agents.

When two teats are close to each other, selection of the extra teat to be removed is based on size and location. In case of doubt, it is preferable to wait for the development of the mammary gland. Some extra teats can communicate with the lumen of the main teat. It is possible to verify this communication by injecting a coloring agent in the extra teat and looking for its passage in the main teat's secretion [41]. In the adult, excision of extra teats must be completed by appropriate closing of the wound.

Incidence of this anomaly is variable, ranging from 10% to 40%. Its heritability factor is believed to be between 0.2 and 0.3 [42]. Occasionally, discussions arise as to the necessity of this intervention and the withholding of these animals from reproduction because of the hereditary aspect. In rare cases, one or more normally present teats can be rudimentary (oligothelia) or absent. In this situation, the corresponding quarter is usually absent (oligomastia).

Congenital atresia

Atresia is the strangling or the obstruction of an orifice or natural duct. These anomalies can be classified as either congenital or acquired. In the case of congenital atresia, they can be classified as follows:

1. Distal part of the papillary canal, if there are no openings on the skin
2. At the teat's cisterna
3. At the junction of both cisternas, papillary and glandular, at the annular shrinking

Obstruction of the distal part of the papillary canal usually is limited to the cutaneous part. After thorough examination, using a large-caliber needle (No. 12 or 14) or a scalpel blade, the skin is opened, and the papillary canal is reached [30]. Treatment postoperatively consists of rolling the teat between the thumb and forefinger before milking, or inserting for a few days a silicone rod into the canal between milking. Generally, prognosis is excellent.

At the papillary cisterns, anomalies are rare. Occasionally, in a heifer at first calving, a membrane can be seen partially or totally obstructing the distal part of the teat's cisterna. Appearance of the mucosa covering this wall leads the authors to believe that its origin is not due to an inflammatory process. Treatment consists of two approaches: (1) Through the papillary canal, the membrane is pierced, and a cross-shaped opening is created; (2) through the teat's opening (thelotomy), the membrane is removed, the mucosa is sutured, and the teat's wall is closed using the technique previously described. Postoperative treatment is as described earlier. The authors favor thelotomy over intervention through the papillary canal.

The therapeutic approach to the membrane situated at the level of the annular shrinking is the same as the one described earlier—either through the papillary canal or by thelotomy. This membrane easily can have a thickness of 2 to 3 mm. Blind intervention through the papillary canal presents a certain risk, given the thickness of the membrane and the close proximity of the venous ring located around the annular ring. The authors prefer the surgical approach through the teat's lining; in addition, it might be preferable to install a prosthesis at this level [36]. As mentioned by Hull [30], an area of fibrous tissues often is observed in this plane, probably originating from a trauma or an infection. Occasionally, it is possible to observe other congenital anomalies in the organization of the linings of both sinuses [12]. Diagnosis of these conditions is made after a thorough clinical examination, which can be complemented with ultrasound or radiology using a contrast solution.

Acquired atresia

Acquired atresia is a result of infection or trauma. Localization of this fibrosis can be at or to the papillary canal, extending into the gland itself involving both cisternas. In heifers at first calving, this kind of lesion can be observed on one or more quarters. Sucking at a young age by the animal or among the animals seems to be the principal cause of this condition. Contamination spreads this way, and infection sets in. The extent of the damage is not noticed until later.

Accessory mammary gland (web teats, conjoined teats)

A conjoined teat is actually a supernumerary teat adjoined to a main teat. This anomaly is fairly frequent in dairy cows. The ones observed at the veterinary faculty hospital were located mainly at the posterior teats. Supernumerary teats being one of the most common hereditary anomalies, the accessory gland is part of these irregularities. The opening or sphincter of that gland can be located between the distal extremity of the main teat and the base of the corresponding quarter. Occasionally, it is joined to the main teat and is confused with a fistula or extrudes from it, and the whole looks like two joined teats. In some cases, when the opening of the accessory gland is linked intimately to the main teat, a differentiation must be made between this condition and a teat fistula. The fistula can be congenital or acquired: Most of these fistulas are acquired, and they do not possess a papillary canal [43]. One way to differentiate the fistula from the accessory gland is to inject coloring (methylene blue) and to verify the color of the main gland's product. Ultrasound also is an excellent means of differentiation of these two conditions. This accessory gland is independent from the main one in the sense that the secretory tissue is separate, that it has its own glandular cisterna draining in a papillary sinus. The papillary canal can be functional or not, in that it may or may not have an efficient sphincter. In the absence of this structure, milk drips continually [43]. In the presence of this accessory gland, the owner consults for one of the three following reasons:

1. Difficulties can be encountered at milking. Depending on localization on the main teat and importance of the accessory teat, there can be interference at milking.
2. The quarter remains after milking. Even if there is no interference with the teat cup during milking, there is a possibility that the quarter will remain bigger than the others after milking. In this case, the accessory gland is important. The authors have observed cases in which the accessory gland accounted for 50% of the corresponding quarter's total milk production. This difference in production also is reported by Shappell and Schneider [44].
3. The reason can be purely esthetic. For some breeders, presence of this anomaly represents a defect with consequences in the animal's classification.

Diagnosis and prognosis of this condition are based on visual examination, palpation, and measurement of milk produced by this accessory gland. To measure these volumes, a milking probe is placed in each of the papillary canals to measure the volumes of milk produced by each gland during mechanical milking of the other three quarters. Assessment of this accessory gland can be completed by ultrasound or radiology with contrast material (Fig. 8). These two methods allow for visualization of the papillary cisternas and evaluation of the position and thickness of the septum separating them.

To complete the evaluation of an accessory gland, a contrast study is performed. A radiopaque substance (15–20 mL) is injected through a disposable teat cannula into the accessory gland first. This method allows visualization of the volume and positioning (cranial or caudal) of the accessory gland. After this first radiographic view is obtained, a second contrast study is done on the normal teat. The resulting image allows evaluation of the septum's thickness between the two sinuses.

Surgical approach

Intervention should be adapted according to the importance of the accessory gland's production [30,44]. When the milk production is small, the

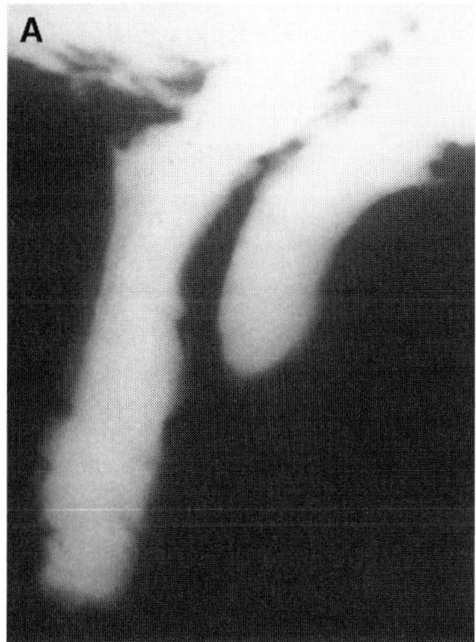

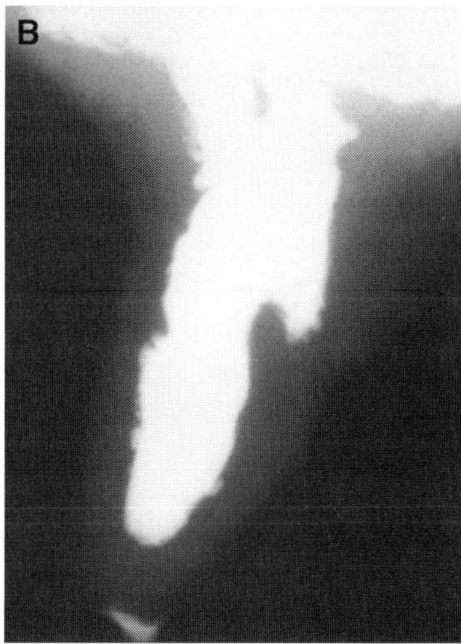

Fig. 8. Contrast radiograph of an accessory mammary gland (webbed teat). (*A*) Before surgery. (*B*) After surgery.

supernumerary teat can be dissected out followed by primary closure of the accessory gland's cisterna. If milk production is significant, it is preferable to anastomose both teats' cisterna (main and accessory).

Closure of the accessory gland

An elliptical incision is performed around the teat of the accessory gland, parallel to the teat's axis. Dissection includes the teat's cisterna, to be removed up to the accessory gland's cisterna, where it is transected. During this dissection, special attention must be paid to avoid perforating the main teat's cisterna. The amount of cutaneous tissue to remove is a function of the importance of the supernumerary teat, after excision and closing, trying to respect symmetry. Closure is done following the approach described earlier. An inverted technique can be used to close the accessory gland's cisterna because some fibrosis reaction is desired to close this gland definitively.

Cisterna anastomosis

The first step of the surgical approach is the same as previously described for teat accessory gland resection and closure. To facilitate identification of the structures, a metal teat cannula is inserted in both papillary canals. An elliptical incision is performed around the accessory gland's cisterna and continued as a longitudinal incision along the teat toward its more proximal aspect. Then the elliptical portion of the incision is deepened to resect completely the accessory gland's cisterna. This approach exposes the septum, the common lining of the cisterna of the supernumerary and the main teat. With the help of the probe inserted in the main teat's papillary canal, the septum is incised 2 to 3 cm. This incision is slightly elliptical, allowing removal of part of this wall. The septum can be 3 to 5 mm thick and is well vascularized. Occasionally, bleeding significantly obscures the surgical field. The hemorrhage has to be controlled before resuming the surgery because the venous ring is usually close, and further dissection can detrimental for the animal (Fig. 9).

Both septa are anastomosed with a simple continuous suture with absorbable material of USP 4-0 or 5-0, on an swaged-on taper needle. During this suture, the authors limit themselves to both mucosae only, to cover completely the subtissue supporting these two mucosae. As reported by Hull [30], this step is important because this tissue band, uncovered or incompletely covered, has a tendency to granulate. Excessive granulation obstructs the opening created. Closure is completed with the method described earlier. The authors prefer to perform this surgery while the cow is in lactation because the continuous presence of milk through the anastomosis prevents unwanted closure of the communication between the glands.

Postoperative care

Mechanical milking is reintroduced quickly, 10 to 12 hours after intervention, at the second milking; the first one is done with a milking probe. Because the product of the accessory gland often is contaminated, a microbiologic culture and sensitivity of the milk is strongly recommended. Because both cisterna communicate, the main gland could be contaminated. Postoperatively, systemic antibiotics are administered for 3 days. Penicillin is the authors' antibiotic of choice, unless sensitivity suggests otherwise.

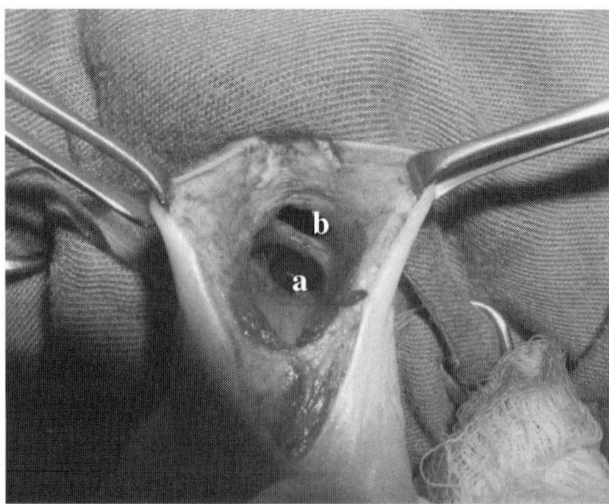

Fig. 9. Surgical exposure of the accessory mammary gland (webbed teat) and anastomosis of the principal (a) to the accessory (b) cisterna.

Antibiotics also can be administered intramammary if mastitis is present. It is advisable to administer nonsteroidal anti-inflammatory drugs (NSAIDs) before surgery to control postoperative inflammation. Sometimes, blood clots from uncontrolled surgery bleeding obstruct the canal and prevent normal mechanical milking. These clots are extracted from the teat using negative pressure with a teat cannula and a syringe. Hand milking and teat manipulation should be avoided unless unavoidable. Teat swelling, if significant, can be controlled with postoperative NSAIDs or simply ice on the teat. Hydrotherapy should be avoided for 48 hours on a fresh surgical wound. The location of the supernumerary teat determines the difficulty of the intervention and consequently the prognosis. The closer the accessory teat's opening is to the main teat's proximal end, the more difficult and delicate the intervention because the septum is deeper and the incision is closer to the vascular ring. Taking these intervention particularities into account and as reported by Schmit et al [43], the authors believe that this corrective surgery is efficient, is esthetic, presents a minimal rate of complications, and does not interfere with milk production.

Traumatic lesions

Internal lesions: tight streak canal (fibrosis of Fürstenberg rosette)

Lesions on the streak canal result in reduced milk flow. The etiology of these conditions is multiple. Cows can traumatize themselves when rising, squeezing their teat several times between the floor and the claw. Inadequate tuning of the milking machine system (eg, excessive vacuum) may be at the origin of the injury and results in a major herd problem. Intervention on the acute injured teat has to be delayed in time to decrease the inflammation. It is crucial at this time to keep the teat at rest and stop milking the quarter with the milking machine until a surgical decision is made [45].

Mucosal default: fibrosis of Fürstenberg rosette

The main complaint of the owner, the reduced milk flow, is the most current clinical sign of a mucosal default. A firm palpation of the streak canal is always present and can be associated with an eversion of the streak canal secondary to a circular rupture of the distal quarter of the streak canal. Ultrasound reveals no abnormality at the distal part of the teat's cistern, but an inflammation at Fürstenberg rosette and an increase in echogenicity of the streak canal. Insertion of a probe is difficult because of the stenosis of the streak canal, but can be performed gently without any sensation of obstruction (Fig. 10).

Until more recently, the treatment of choice consisted of a blunt opening of the streak canal by introduction of a Hug knife. The Hug knife is introduced through the streak canal and gently pulled out at 45°, cutting off a portion of the rosette and the proximal third of the streak canal, but

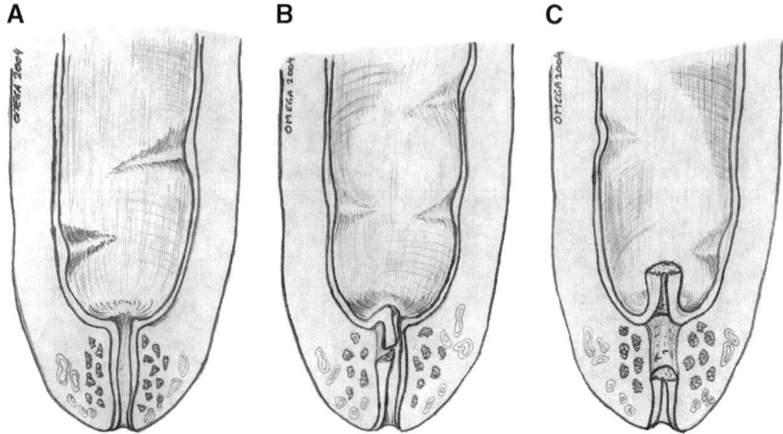

Fig. 10. Milk flow difficulty secondary to papillary canal trauma. (*A*) Normal structures of the papillary canal and the Fürstenberg rosette. (*B*) Partial rupture of the mucosa in the papillary canal resulting in inflammation of the Fürstenberg rosette. (*C*) Complete resection and eversion of the papillary canal.

preserving the external teat sphincter and the skin. Today, this procedure can be performed under theloscopy, allowing precise débridement of the abnormal rosette, as described in a subsequent article. The milk flow can be compared with the contralateral teat after each cut.

Obstruction of the area of Fürstenberg rosette

Obstruction of the milk flow at the area of Fürstenberg rosette is always due to a loss of integrity of the streak canal's mucosa at the level of the proximal third. A partial protrusion (see Fig. 10B) resulting in a complete internal eversion (see Fig. 10C) can occur after a trauma in the streak canal; this creates a mucosal flap that eventually obstructs the canal during the vacuum phase of mechanical milking or increased pressure during manual milking. The palpation of the distal extremity of the teat offers the impression of a rolling mass originating from the area of Fürstenberg rosette. Ultrasound is useful to confirm the diagnosis and establish a treatment plan. With incomplete rupture, a hyperechogenic sessile mass at the level of Fürstenberg rosette is seen, whereas two hyperechogenic lines lifted up the rosette are seen when the inversion of the canal is complete. In this particular situation, a teat cannula should be inserted with great care to avoid taking the wrong path and ending up underneath the cistern mucosa.

Treatment consists of removing the mucosal flap. Three approaches can be considered: (1) blind removal, (2) via thelotomy, and (3) via theloscopy. Many instruments have been described for these problems, but most of them only tear the exuberant tissue without entirely resecting it, predisposing the teat to a recurrent flap. It is the authors' opinion that the Eisenhut stenosis cutter [45] is the best instrumentation for this condition (Fig. 11).

The blind resection of such a mucosal flap is not recommended because of iatrogenic lesions that can occur during the process, especially to the streak canal lining. The complete removal of the injured mucosa and the secondary fibrous tissue is impossible to assess. Recurrence rate with blunt resection is almost 100%. Performing a 1- or 2-cm theliotomy allows good exposure of the rosette and direct control of the mucosal resection. This procedure is safe and quick. It allows a faster return in normal milk flow with low complications. Lateral theloscopy permits good visualization of Fürstenberg rosette allowing excellent control during débridement and limiting unnecessary cutting. Cattle treated by theloscopy have a significant better milk flow during the following milking session compared with cattle treated by thelotomy [46].

The aftercare of these procedures is controversial and depends on the udder health. Current aftercare is to hand milk the quarter every 1 or 2 hours until the following milking to break the adherences in the streak canal. Hand milking is performed whether or not mastitis is present in the quarter. In the authors' opinion, keeping the injured teat at rest and avoiding mechanically milking the quarter for 9 days is a better solution. Mastitis in the affected quarter does not allow such a treatment regimen [45]. A silicone teat stent is introduced during the first 3 days with a complete physical examination of the udder twice a day to detect any sign of inflammation, heat, redness, or pain that may indicate mastitis. After 3 days (or earlier if needed), the quarter is emptied out with a teat cannula. This

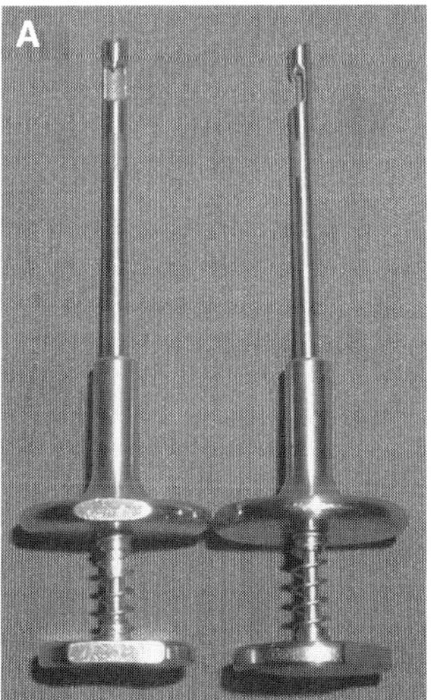

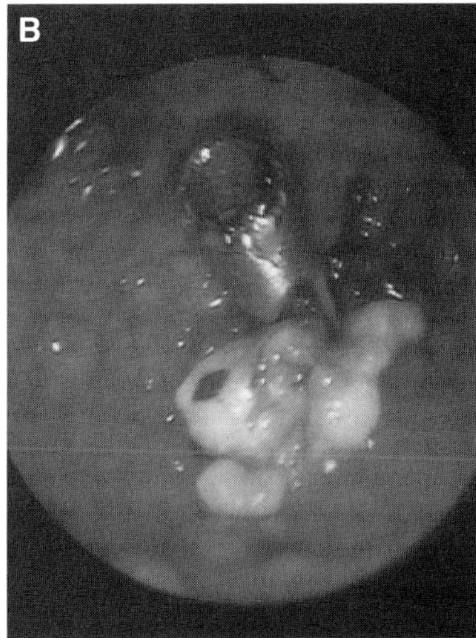

Fig. 11. (*A*) Eisenhut stenosis cutter (Dr Fritz GmbH, Tuttlingen, Germany). (*B*) Intrasurgical view, via lateral theloscopy, of fibrosis tissue resection at the level of the Fürstenberg rosette.

schedule should be repeated three times, allowing time for the streak canal's mucosa to heal without excessive fibrous tissue. Introduction of a melting teat stent in wax after each milking during 1 week after the 9 days of treatment is necessary to avoid any unwanted milk leakage.

Localized hemorrhage

Self-injury to the distal portion of the teat can seriously damage the distal vascular plexus, resulting in a local hematoma. The teat appears painful and swollen, with a red/dark purple color. Conservative treatment should be started promptly; NSAIDs are administered as needed, and cold hydrotherapy is given twice daily for the following 6 days. A temporary dry period is started, and local antibiotics for cows in lactation can be inserted carefully in the teat, followed by a wax stent. After the acute inflammatory phase, if the fibrosis is significant in the distal extremity, a partial apical teat amputation can be performed. The teat is cut transversely from the distal third of the streak canal to the middle streak canal. A silicone teat stent is inserted in the streak canal, and the wound is left to close by second intention (Fig. 12).

Parietal stenosis: mucosal flap

The mucosa can be separated off from the intermediate layer after trauma [28] or by the probe used for the diagnosis of streak canal obstructions when it is passed under the injured streak canal mucosa. Milk flow is mildly decreased in the acute phase, but inflammation is severe, and the teat is painful at palpation and during milking. Ultrasound reveals a white hyperechogenic line floating in the teat cistern. Axial theloscopy allows the visualization of the mucosal flap.

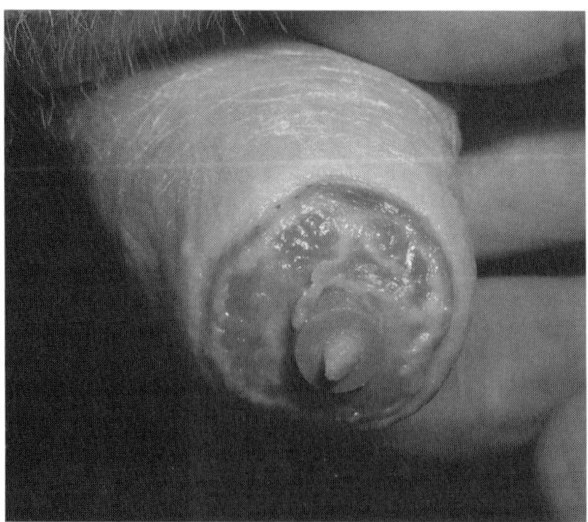

Fig. 12. View of the distal end amputation of the teat, 4 days after surgery, at the proximal third of the papillary canal. A teat wax insert was left in the papillary canal.

Surgery is performed by thelotomy on the opposite side from the injury. The nonviable mucosa is removed. The edges of the wound are separated from the intermediate layer by blunt dissection with Metzenbaum scissors, and the gap is closed by apposition of the mucosa with a simple interrupted suture pattern. The teat wall is closed in a routine fashion (Figs. 13 and 14).

Fibrosis in the teat wall (insertion of a prosthesis)

Fibrosis of the teat wall can originate from the chronic evolution of the teat cistern mucosal flap or from a hematoma in the teat wall resulting from an injury to the linear vessels or from contamination and infection [47,48]. In case of infection, the glandular part of the cisterna can be implicated in the fibrous reaction. Ultrasound of the teat is useful to assess the severity of the fibrosis. The cistern lumen is narrow to almost nonexistent, and a multifocal hyperechogenic teat wall is compatible with fibrous tissue. A contrast radiographic study also can be performed to evaluate patency of the cistern. For contrast radiography, insertion of a teat cannula often is performed without difficulty, but injection of the contrast medium requires positive pressure, and it may be impossible in some cases. Contrast radiographic images show a small lumen in the middle of the teat or laterally

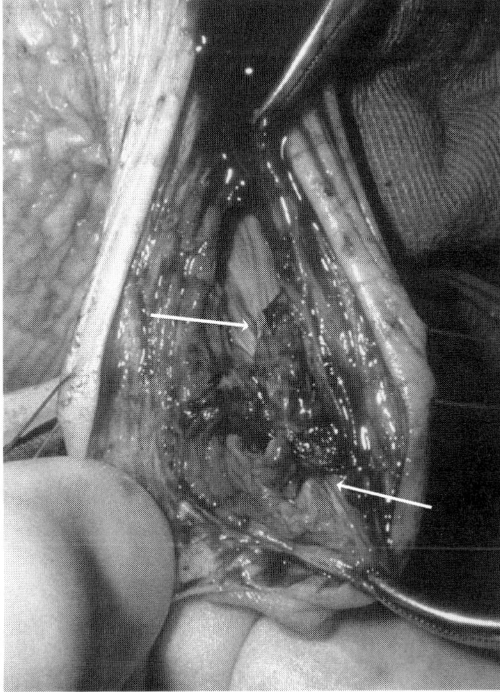

Fig. 13. Intrasurgical view of fibrosis of the teat cistern mucosa, at the middle third of the teat. Normal mucosa (*arrows*) is visible at the proximal and distal level of the scar tissue.

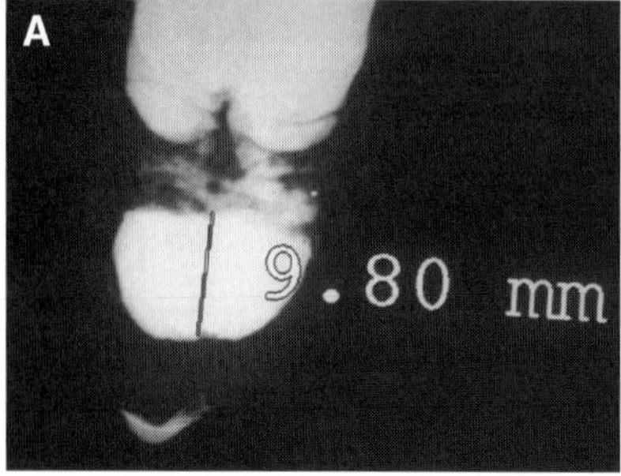

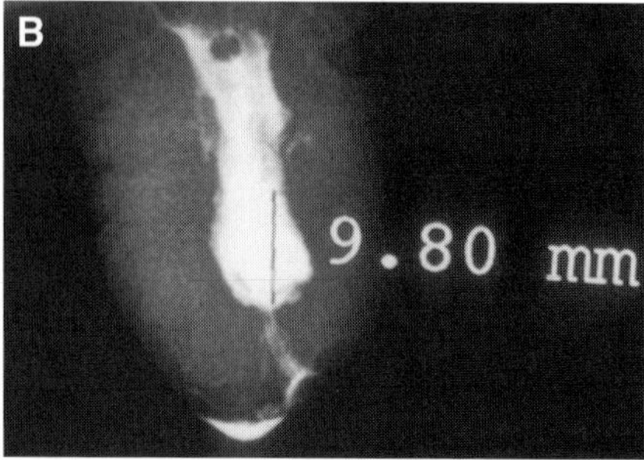

Fig. 14. Preoperative (*A*) and postoperative (*B*) contrast radiographs of the teat cistern with an annular fibrosis of the mucosa.

depending on the localization of the fibrosis. Teat theloscopy through the streak canal may be possible and useful in some situations.

The surgery correction consists of a complete resection of the fibrous tissue through a vertical thelotomy on the opposite side of the fibrosis. If the fibrosis is circular, the incision in made on the lateral side of the teat to facilitate the suture removal. After opening the teat cistern, the fibrous tissue is removed by blunt dissection. Hemorrhages are controlled by clamping the vessels or ligaturing them with a 4-0 absorbable suture material. If the fibrous tissue is localized, it is preferable to separate the normal mucosa from the intermediate layer to cover the defect. If the fibrous tissue is too extensive, a silicone teat prosthesis should be placed to favor reepithelialization of the teat cistern [35,49–52]. Normal mucosa should be present distal and proximal to the lesion; otherwise, the prosthesis may stimulate granulation tissue at its contact point with denuded tissue. Introducing the implant into the glandular cistern is controversial. In the authors' opinion, the morbidity rate does not increase because of the introduction of the implant into the glandular cistern. Prosthesis positioning is important for the success of the surgery. Its distal extremity should not be in contact with Fürstenberg rosette because of mechanical irritation and further inflammation. The implant is attached to the teat wall with three stitches with 2-0 monofilament nonabsorbable suture on a cutting needle. Milking can be performed the following day of the surgery with the milking machine. It is advisable to remove the prosthesis 4 weeks later. After this time, epithelialization should be adequate. If left longer, the prosthesis dislodges from its original position to migrate toward the gland [52]. It may or may not cause damage to the gland. The teat prosthesis is removed through a stab incision on the lateral aspect of the teat.

Reinforced polytetraethylene vascular grafts have been evaluated over 1 year for the treatment of artificial defects of the teat cistern in cattle with a limited issue for the long term [53]. Oral [54,49], peritoneal [55], and vaginal [56] mucosal autografts have been used to replace the injured teat mucosa. Oral mucosal autograft seems to be less effective than the vaginal origin to limit the granulation tissue during the healing process. Molaei et al [56] reported a good adhesion between vaginal autograft and host epithelium border after surgical repair of a large mucosal default limiting the narrowing of the teat cistern. The combination of vaginal autograft and silicone teat prosthesis can be a new avenue for severe teat mucosal fibrosis.

Laceration of the teat

Lacerations can be superficial or deep with involvement of the papillary canal's mucosa, resulting in milk seepage from the wound. These same lesions are more or less linear and vertical or transverse in relation to the teat's axis, or they can be irregularly notched with or without tissue destruction. These observations allow clinicians to establish a prognosis depending on localization, orientation, outline, extent of tissue destruction, and time lapsed since laceration.

Localization

A laceration involving the distal end of the teat and the sphincter has a poor prognosis because fibrosis at this area can interfere with normal milking. Injuries to the base of the teat may result in more hemorrhaging because the lesion is near the venous ring.

Vertical versus horizontal laceration

The teat's blood vessels, mainly found in the submucosa and the median layer, run parallel to the teat's axis. Considering this, horizontal lesions have a worse prognosis than vertical ones. Blood flow to the distal part of the teat can be compromised, leading to a cautious prognosis. For a horizontal laceration involving more than 50% of the teat's circumference, prognosis is poor because of the probability of ischemic necrosis. Because the proximal end of the teat has a better blood flow, prognosis is better than for a laceration located at the distal end of the teat [40].

Linear versus notched laceration

Wherever the laceration is located on the teat, the prognosis is worse for a notched laceration, often the result of a crush injury, compared with a linear one. In this case, the amount of destroyed or damaged tissue is more significant, and blood flow is compromised. During the surgical procedure, tissues are excised, consequently affecting the teat's cisterna diameter.

Intervention time

A small percentage of deep linear lacerations left alone and wrapped in a dressing after the injury can heal by first intention. During an experimental procedure on four animals, Makady et al [37] reported three fistulas for one healing. Most of these lesions are the result of the animal's self-inflicted trauma. These wounds are always contaminated, but the multiplication and proliferation of microorganisms in the surrounding tissues, necessary for infection, are slower to set in; after 12 hours, the infection risk to the surrounding tissue and to the gland is greatly increased. Rapid intervention increases the chances of success for avoiding infection of the laceration and the gland [57].

Even after 24 or 48 hours, it is recommended to suture these wounds, especially if they do not present too much notching, to initiate first intention healing and to reestablish mechanical milking as early as possible [58]. At this time, inflammation being at its peak, hydrotherapy, frequently for 24 hours, is a good choice, with surgery postponed until the next day. For lesions 48 to 96 hours old, infection risk to the wound or the gland is high. Surgical intervention can be attempted anyway, particularly for linear lacerations. For notched lacerations or lesions with lots of surrounding injury, surgical intervention is likely to result in a fistula. Nevertheless, in some circumstances, considering the animal's value, it might be indicated to proceed with surgery; the fistula is smaller, and intervention on it is quicker. More than 96 hours after the accident, first intention healing has little chance of success. With granulation tissue having set in, and the different layers of tissue blending together, surgery is not recommended. It is preferable to let healing proceed by second intention.

These distinctions in time remain general guidelines; regardless of time lapsed, the decision to operate should be based on the animal's value, and the severity, nature, and localization of the injury. The authors have had success with immediate reoperation after a first intervention that had evolved to a fistula. During surgery, the basic principles must be respected: cleansing, irrigation, débridement, and hemostasis. Particularly for older lacerations, débridement is essential; all affected, inflamed, or reactive tissues are removed. The wound can be remodeled at the same time, if need be. These tissues are delicate, and careful handling is in order. Gauzes used for surgery should be soaked with saline. As mentioned before, notched lacerations can be remodeled, but special attention must be paid to the cisterna's mucosa; when sutured, its diameter depends on it. As suggested by Howard et al [59], a pediatric Foley catheter (No. 8, 2.7 mm and 3 mL, or No. 10, 3.3 mm and 3 mL) can be used to maintain a certain diameter during healing of the teat's cisterna. The catheter is inserted in the papillary canal, and the balloon is inflated using saline; it is left in place for 48 to 72 hours; milking is performed through the catheter. The material used and the surgical technique are the same as the ones described earlier.

Superficial lesions

For lacerations not reaching the mucosa, the same general principles apply. Occasionally, if they interfere with mechanical milking, the skin flicks can be removed, and healing by second intention takes its course.

Fistula

When a laceration, surgically repaired or not, heals by second intention, it evolves to the formation of a fistula. This granulation process generally is completed approximately 4 weeks after the original lesions. Surgical repair is accomplished by doing an elliptical incision around the fistula, including the mucosa. Special care is taken to excise the fibrous tissue to free the mucosa of the teat's cisterna. The regular suture techniques used are the ones previously described.

Lymphatic fistula

The authors occasionally have seen a serous discharge coming from the area of the mammary gland's cisterna, mainly from the posterior quarters. Volume output may start with a few drops per minute to a constant leaking that intensifies with the action of milking. The point of leakage originates from a small fistula without surrounding tissue reaction. The liquid's low protein content compared with serum and the absence of coagulation could be of lymphatic origin. To obstruct this fistula, intervention consists of a small elliptical incision at the point of leakage, cauterization, and suturing of the skin.

Teat's lining masses

Occasionally, after a gradual decrease in milking rate, a mass of variable size can be observed on examination of the teat's lining. This condition can be linked to an abscess [60], an evolving hematoma, a fibrous mass, or a venous dilation. Some of these fibrous samples were submitted for histopathologic analysis; they often are polygranulomatous dermatitis and occasionally tuberculoid nodular thelitis. Surgery consists of an elliptical incision around the mass, to isolate it and to excise it, while protecting the teat's cisterna mucosa. Incision is sutured as described before.

Varicose veins

Varicose veins consist of a dilation and deformation of one vein or a branch of the vein from the venous ring, located at the base of the teat. To the authors' knowledge, there is no report of such a condition in the veterinary literature. At the veterinary medicine faculty's hospital, between 1993 and 2004 and particularly in recent years, the authors have observed eight cows presenting venous dilation with deformation of this vessel. The principal complaint for referral was slow and incomplete milking problems of one quarter. The problem seemed to appear gradually and become worse after awhile. Visual examination showed a slightly larger teat with a fleshier proximal third. Palpation was not diagnostic, but gave the indication of the presence of a fluctuating mass of a certain volume. Ultrasound showed important vacuoles or a U-shaped space containing a darker substance than the cisterna at the teat's proximal third. Contrast radiology showed a narrowing, a compression of the teat's cisterna, with smooth linings. This smooth lining led the authors to believe that it is not a fibrous reaction. Angiography of one of these veins allowed the authors to visualize this anomaly. The vein appeared very dilated, its diameter reaching 1.5 cm in some areas, and was U shaped, extending to the proximal half of the teat (Fig. 15). Manual milking is relatively good, in contrast to mechanical milking. The authors believe that the teat cup shell compresses the dilated vein on the teat's cisterna when it reaches this area, slowing down the milk's descent. The vacuum created by the mechanical milking increases blood congestion at the level of this vein, compounding the slow milking.

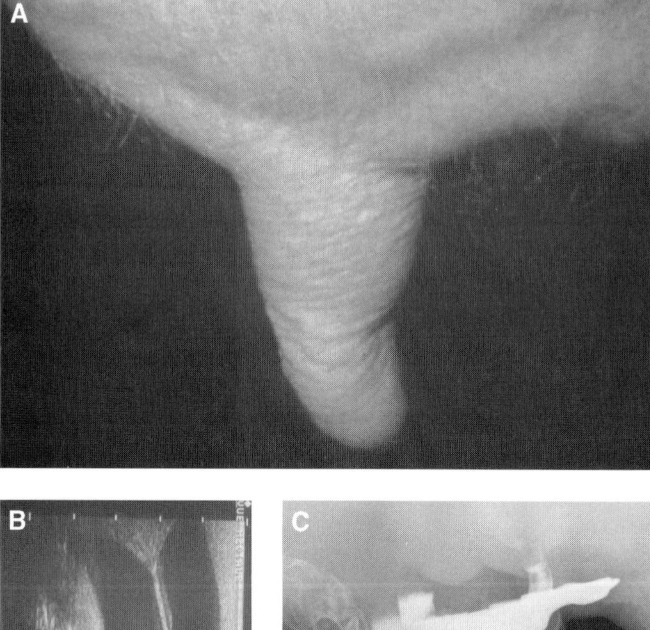

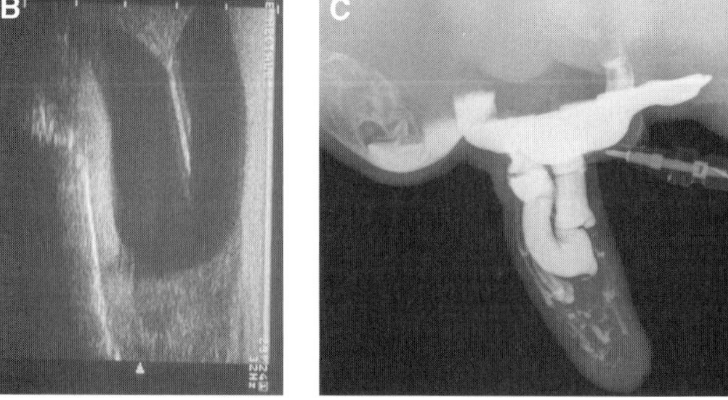

Fig. 15. Varicose vein. (*A*) External conformation. (*B*) Ultrasound. (*C*) Contrast angiography. The varicose vein appears as a large U-shaped hypoechoic tube. Contrast angiography illustrates the vascular ring origin of the vascular problem.

Treatment

In the first case, observation of this fluctuating area led the authors to opt for surgery. During the procedure, it was realized that the intervention was leading the authors to a vein measuring 1 cm in diameter. For three cases, the authors proceeded with a sclerosing substance (dextrose 25%) with average results in one case and a slight improvement in the other two. Twice the authors ligatured at the base of the two branches of the U. This double ligature did not lead to valid results. The ligatures' failure seems to be attributable to the many anastomoses present at the vascular ring. Excision of the vein was performed in two cases; this procedure gave better results than the other two. Excision of the vein is a hemorrhagic procedure; the many veins attached to the varicose vein make hemostasis difficult to attain. There is also an intense local postoperative reaction. Basing the theory on human medical experience with sclerosing products and techniques [61], the authors believe this method is worthy of further investigation.

Summary

Injuries to the end of the teat are frequent and frustrating to treat. Treatment of these injuries evolved from being aggressive using teat knives to a more conservative approach employing rest nonreactive teat inserts. The process of milking seems simple, but it involves fine-tuned mechanics. Teat fibrosis, even when small, has a disastrous effect on the production life of an animal. There is no place for error; any surgical intervention should be precise and aim for perfection. Medical imaging techniques and minimally invasive surgery help the surgeon to make the best decision. Finally, more investigation is needed on teat varicose veins to understand the origin and develop better treatment.

Teat injuries have drawn more attention more recently. Surgical interventions are better planned, and blind treatment with unsuitable teat knives is avoided. Treatment of superficial or full-thickness teat lacerations does not require a high level of anatomic or surgical knowledge, although basic surgical principles should be applied. Hemostasis, delicate débridement and tissue handling, and appropriate suture materials and patterns are key to success. Appropriate sedation, anesthesia, and analgesia are essential to achieve this goal and should never be neglected.

References

[1] Programme d'analyse des troupeaux laitiers du Québec. Rapport annuel. 1998–2003.
[2] Michigan Dairy Herd Improvement Association. Animal summary. Lansing (MI): Michigan DHIA Inc; 1981.
[3] Sieber RL, Farnsworth RJ. Prevalence of chronic teat-end lesions and their relationship to intramammary infection in 22 herds of dairy cattle. J Am Vet Med Assoc 1981;178:1263–7.

[4] Agger JF, Willeberg P. Epidemiology of teat lesions in a dairy herd: II. associations with subclinical mastitis. Nord Vet Med 1986;38:220–32.
[5] Geishauser T, Querengässer K, Nitschke M, Sorbiraj A. Milk yield, somatic cell counts, and risk of removal from the herd for dairy cows after covered teat canal injury. J Dairy Sci 1999; 82:1482–8.
[6] Agger JF, Willeberg P. Epidemiology of teat lesions in a dairy herd: I. description of incidence, location and clinical appearance. Nord Vet Med 1986;38:209–19.
[7] Gourreau JM. Accidents et maladies du trayon. Paris: Édition France Agricole; 1995.
[8] McDonald JS. Radiographic method for anatomic study of the teat canal: characteristics related to resistance to new intramammary infection during lactation and the early dry period. Cornell Vet 1975;65:492–9.
[9] Frémont A, Bergonier D, Berthelot X, et al. Intérêt de l'endoscopie pour le diagnostic et le traitement des sténoses du trayon chez la vache laitière: étude d'un cas clinique. Rev Med Vet 2002;153:40–6.
[10] Bisaillon A. Anatomie des glandes mammaires. Med Vet Québec 2002;32:46–51.
[11] Nickerson SC. Bovine mammary gland: structure and function; relationship to milk production and immunity to mastitis. Agri-Pract 1994;15:8–18.
[12] Irwin DHG. Surgical correction of a congenital mammary abnormality in a heifer. J Am Vet Med Assoc 1957;131:186–7.
[13] Van Der Merwe NJ. Some observations on the morphology of the bovine teat canal (Ductus papillaris mammae). J S Afr Vet Assoc 1985;56:13–6.
[14] Schummer A, Wilkens H, Vollmehaus B, et al. The anatomy of the domestic animals. Vol. 3. The circulatory system, the skin, and the cutaneous organs of the domestic mammals. Berlin: Verlag Paul Parey; 1981.
[15] Modransky P, Welker B. Diagnosing and treating milk flow problems. Vet Med 1993;88: 788–804.
[16] Steiner A, Eicher R. La chirurgie du trayon: dans chirurgie des ruminants: chirurgie génitale, locomotrice, de la tête et du cou. Le Point Vétérinaire, Numéro spécial. Tome II 2001;32: 61–7.
[17] Geishauser T, Querengässer K. Investigations on teat canal length in teats with milk flow disturbances. J Dairy Sci 2000;83:1976–80.
[18] Cartee RE, Ibrahim AK, McLeary D. B-mode ultrasonography of the bovine udder and teat. J Am Vet Med Assoc 1986;188:1284–7.
[19] Takeda T. Diagnostic ultrasonography of the bovine udder. Jpn J Vet Res 1989;37:133.
[20] Stocker H, Battig U, Duss M, et al. Evaluation of teat stenoses in cows by ultrasonography. Tierarztl Prax 1989;17:251–6.
[21] Trostle SS, O'Brien RT. Ultrasonography of the bovine mammary gland. Comp Cont Educ Pract Vet 1998;20:564–71.
[22] Nudda A, Pulina G, Vallebella R, Bencini R, Enne G. Ultrasound technique for measuring mammary cistern size of dairy ewes. J Dairy Res 2000;67:101–6.
[23] Franz S, Hofmann-Parisot M, Baumgartner W, Windischbauer G, Suchy A, Bauder B. Ultrasonography of the teat canal in cows and sheep. Vet Rec 2001;149:109–12.
[24] Babkine M, Couture Y. L'échographie du trayon est un outil diagnostique non invasif. Point Vét 2002;33:16–7.
[25] McDonald JS. Radiographic method for anatomic study of the teat canal: observations on 22 lactating dairy cows. Am J Vet Res 1968;29:1315–9.
[26] McDonald JS. Radiographic method for anatomic study of the teat canal: changes within the first lactation. Am J Vet Res 1973;34:169–71.
[27] McDonald JS. Radiographic method for anatomic study of the teat canal: changes between milking periods. Am J Vet Res 1975;36:1241–2.
[28] Witzig P, Rüsch P, Berchold M. Diagnosis and treatment of teat stenosis in dairy cattle with special reference to radiography and thelotomy. Vet Med Rev 1984;2:122–32.

[29] Hospes R, Seeh C. Endoskopische Operationsverfarhren. In: Sonographie und Endoskopie an der Zitze des Rindes—Atlas und Lehrbuch. Stuttgart: Schattauer; 1999. p. 79–100.
[30] Hull BL. Teat and udder surgery. Vet Clin North Am Food Anim Pract 1995;11:1–17.
[31] Bouisset S. Anesthésie du pis de la vache. In: Le point vétérinaire, chirurgie des bovins et des petits ruminants. Tome II. Paris; 2001. p. 59–60.
[32] Cable CS, Peery K, Fubini SL. Radical mastectomy in 20 ruminants. Vet Surg 2004;33: 263–6.
[33] Grymer J, Watson GL, Coy CH, Prindle LV. Healing of experimentally induced wounds of mammary papilla (teat) of the cow: comparison of closure with tissue adhesive versus non sutured wounds. Am J Vet Res 1984;45:1979–83.
[34] Agger JF. Treatment of surgical teat wounds with tissue adhesive. Dan Vet Tidsskr 1982;16: 778–84.
[35] Ducharme NG, Arighi M, Horney FD, Livesey MA, Hurtig MH, Pennock P. Invasive teat surgery in dairy cattle: 1. surgical procedures and classification of lesions. Can Vet J 1987;28: 757–62.
[36] Noordsy JL. Food animal surgery veterinary learning systems. 3rd edition. Trenton (NJ): VLS Books; 1994. p. 245–58.
[37] Makady FM, Whitmore HL, Nelson DR, Simon J. Effect of tissue adhesives and suture patterns on experimentally induced teat lacerations in lactating dairy cattle. J Am Vet Med Assoc 1991;198:1932–4.
[38] Hartigan P. Some aspects of bovine teat surgery. Ir Vet J 1971;25:179–83.
[39] Ghamsari SM, Taguchi K, Abe N, Acorda JA, Sato M, Yamada H. Effect of different suture patterns on wound healing of the teat in dairy cattle. J Vet Med Sci 1995;57:819–24.
[40] Bristol DG. Teat and udder surgery in dairy cattle—part 1. Comp Cont Educ Pract Vet 1989; 11:868–72.
[41] Steere JH, Moody KM, Nealy J. Open teat sinus surgery for correcting teat occlusions. J Am Vet Med Assoc 1960;136:123–7.
[42] Steiner A. Teat surgery. In: Fubini SL, Ducharme NG, editors. Farm animal surgery. Philadelphia: Saunders; 2004. p. 408–18.
[43] Schmit KA, Arighi M, Dobson H. Postoperative evaluation of the surgical treatment of accessory teat and gland cistern complexes in dairy cows. Can Vet J 1994;35:25–30.
[44] Shappell KK, Schneider T. Surgical treatment of accessory teat and gland cistern complexes in three cows. J Am Vet Med Assoc 1989;195:623–6.
[45] Mösenfechtel S. Lateral endoscopy of the bovine teat. Tuttlingen: Dr Fritz; 1998.
[46] Hirsbrunner G, Eicher R, Meylan M, Steiner A. Comparison of thelotomy and theloscopic triangulation for the treatment of distal teat obstruction in dairy cows—a retrospective study (1994–1998). Vet Rec 2001;148:803–5.
[47] Boddie RL, Nickerson SC, Owens WE, Watts JL. Udder microflora in nonlactating heifers. Agri-Pract 1987;8:22–5.
[48] Edwards JF, Wikse SE, Field RW, Hoelscher CC, Herd DB. Bovine teat atresia associated with horn fly (Haematobia irritans irritans [L.])-induced dermatitis. Vet Pathol 2000;37: 360–4.
[49] Trent AM, Smith DF, Cooley AJ, Beck K, Hoffer RE. Use of mucosal grafts and temporary tube implants for treatment of teat sinus mucosal injuries. Am J Vet Res 1990;51:666–76.
[50] Dzuba LM. Reconstructive teat surgery for complete teat canal obstruction. Bov Pract 1983; 18:209–10.
[51] Ames NK, Coy CH. Placement of drain tubes in obstructed teats. Mod Vet Pract 1984;65: 775–7.
[52] Nassef MT, Coy CH, Watson GL. Method to create and maintain the patency of the bovine mammary papilla. Am J Vet Res 1988;49:1131–3.
[53] Metzger L, Hirsbrunner G, Waldvogel A, Eicher R, Schällibaum M, Steiner A. Permanent implantation of a reinforced polytetraethylene vascular graft for treatment of artificial defect of the teat cistern in cows. Am J Vet Res 1999;60:56–62.

[54] Bristol DG. Treatment of teat obstruction in a cow by transfer of oral mucosa and temporary implantation of an intraluminal tube. J Am Vet Med Assoc 1989;195:492–4.
[55] Bristol DG, Cullen J, Anderson K. Peritoneal autografts do not prevent teat cistern stenosis after circumferential mucosal injury. Proceeding XVI congresso mundial de buiatria 1990; TomoI:282–7.
[56] Molaei MM, Oloumi MM, Maleki M, Abshenas J. Experimental reconstruction of teat mucosa by vestibular mucosal graft in cows: a histopathological and radiographic study. J Vet Med Assoc 2002;49:379–84.
[57] Trent AM. Teat surgery Agri-Pract 1993;14:6–8.
[58] Desrochers A. Quelques particularités du traitement des plaies chez les bovines. Méd Vét Québec 2003;33:104–7.
[59] Howard JL, Filipov M, McTherron TA, Nelson D. A simple technique for repairing teat lacerations and fistulas in cattle. Bov Pract 1978;13:107–8.
[60] Dreyfuss DJ, Madison JB, Reef VB. Surgical treatment of a mural teat abscess in a cow. J Am Vet Med Assoc 1990;197:1629–30.
[61] Green D. Sclerotherapy for the permanent eradication of varicose veins: theoretical and practical considerations. J Am Acad Dermatol 1998;38:461–75.

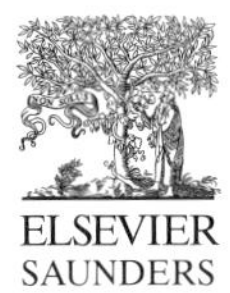
ELSEVIER
SAUNDERS

VETERINARY
CLINICS
Food Animal Practice

Vet Clin Food Anim 21 (2005) 205–225

Teat Endoscopy (Theloscopy) for Diagnosis and Therapy of Milk Flow Disorders in Dairy Cows

Thomas Geishauser, Dr med vet, Dr med vet habil, FTA, MSc[a,*], Klaus Querengässer, Dr med vet[b], Julia Querengässer, Dr med vet[b]

[a]*Department of Population Medicine, Ontario Veterinary College, University of Guelph, Guelph, Ontario, N1G 2W1, Canada*
[b]*Tierärztliche Klinik Babenhausen, Paradiesstraße 34, 87727 Babenhausen, Germany*

Teat injuries keep occurring, although risk factors and means of prevention [1] are known. Average lactational incidence rates were reported at 2% and 3% [2–13], ranging from 0 to 20% between herds [5,12]. Teat injuries cause economical losses because of treatment costs, decreased milk production [14], and increased risks of mastitis [4,15–18] and premature culling [3,19–27].

Teat injuries may be divided into open and covered injuries. In covered teat injuries, the outer teat skin is unaffected—the injury is located inside the teat [28,29]. Covered teat injuries cause teat stenoses and milk flow disorders [29]. In rural veterinary practice, teat canal stenoses accounted for 80% of all teat stenoses [30]. In slaughtered cows, 70% of all teat alterations were located in the teat canal and Fürstenberg rosette area [31]. In the teat canal area, covered injuries were diagnosed without dislocation (Fig. 1) (50%), with inversion (Fig. 2) (49%) or eversion (1%) of teat canal tissue [32].

This article describes a conservative and a surgical approach to restore milk flow, lower the risk of mastitis, and keep the cow in herd after covered teat injury had occurred. Conservative therapy means resting the teat for 3 × 3 days. Surgical therapy means diagnosis and minimally invasive therapy by using teat endoscopy (theloscopy). Conservative therapy may be successful in covered teat canal injuries without tissue dislocation. Inversion

* Corresponding author.
E-mail address: tgeishau@uoguelph.ca (T. Geishauser).

doi:10.1016/j.cvfa.2004.11.003 ***vetfood.theclinics.com***

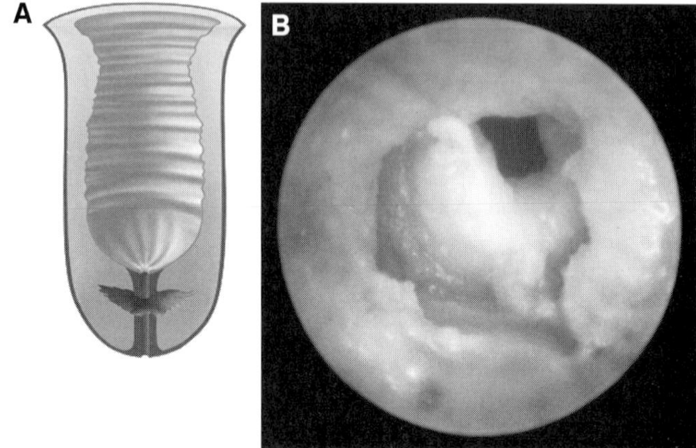

Fig. 1. (*A*) Rupture in the teat canal area (schematic representation). (*B*) Rupture in the teat canal area (canal theloscopy).

of teat canal tissue and other, more complicated injuries require surgery to restore milk flow.

Conservative therapy

Suppose a person hits the tip of his or her finger with a hammer. The finger ends up swollen and black and blue. Would the person treat the finger by massage twice daily and inserting a pipe cleaner into the wound? Or would it be preferable to rest the finger for a couple of days? Conservative therapy means resting and not milking the teat for 3 × 3 days [33,34]. The sooner the teat is rested, the better. Only teats giving normal milk should be

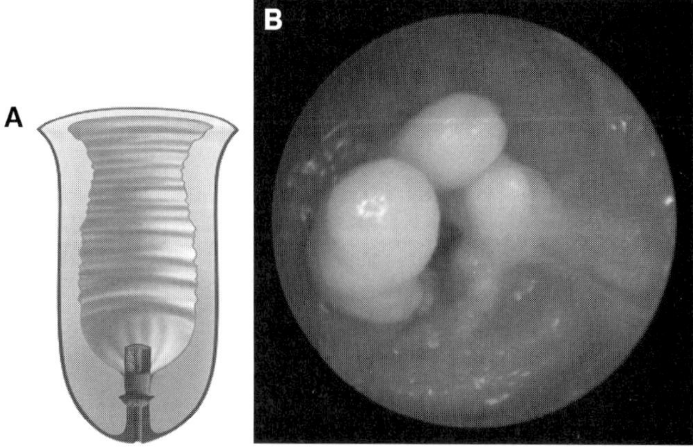

Fig. 2. (*A*) Inversion of teat canal tissue into the teat cistern (schematic representation). (*B*) Three-part inversion of teat canal tissue into the teat cistern (lateral theloscopy).

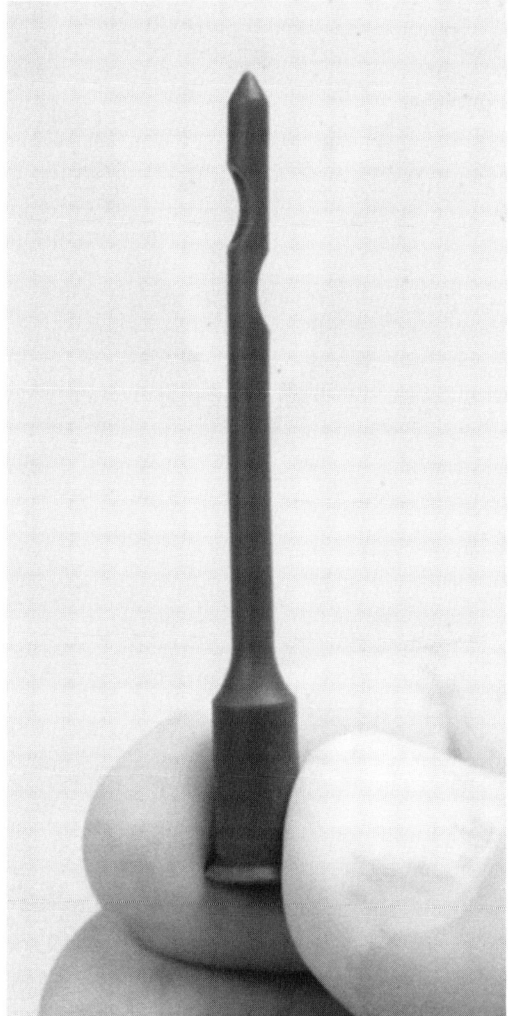

Fig. 3. STERIL—sterile disposable milking tube.

rested. If clinical mastitis is present, the mastitis should be treated first by draining the milk twice daily and administering antibiotics intracisternally. Scrupulous cleanliness is a prerequisite for successful therapy.

Procedure to rest a teat for 3 × 3 days

1. Administer xylazine (0.04 mg/kg) and oxytocin (10 IU) intravenously.
2. Clean the teat with soap and warm water, and disinfect the teat.
3. Drain the milk with a sterile disposable milking tube (eg, STERIL disposable milking tube [www.profs-products.com]) (Fig. 3).

4. Administer an antibiotic intracisternally to treat subclinical mastitis [35] and to prevent clinical mastitis. The antibiotic should be effective against gram-positive and gram-negative bacteria and resistant against penicillinase [36].
5. Insert a sterile silicone implant (SIMPL silicone implant [www.profs-products.com]) (Fig. 4) into the teat canal to prevent adhesions and to keep the teat canal patent. Fewer pathogens were detected after the use silicone implants than after the use of wax inserts [37]. Pipe cleaners ("teat dilators") and teat cannulae caused injuries in the teat (Fig. 5) [38–40], they were contaminated with bacteria [41], and they increased somatic cell count (SCC) and the risk of detecting pathogens in the milk [40,42]. Pipe cleaners slipped into the teat and acted as foreign bodies [43]. The removal of a teat cannula caused rupture and eversion of teat canal skin [40]. (The teat canal skin often has been referred to as *mucosa*; however, this term is not appropriate here with regard to evolution,

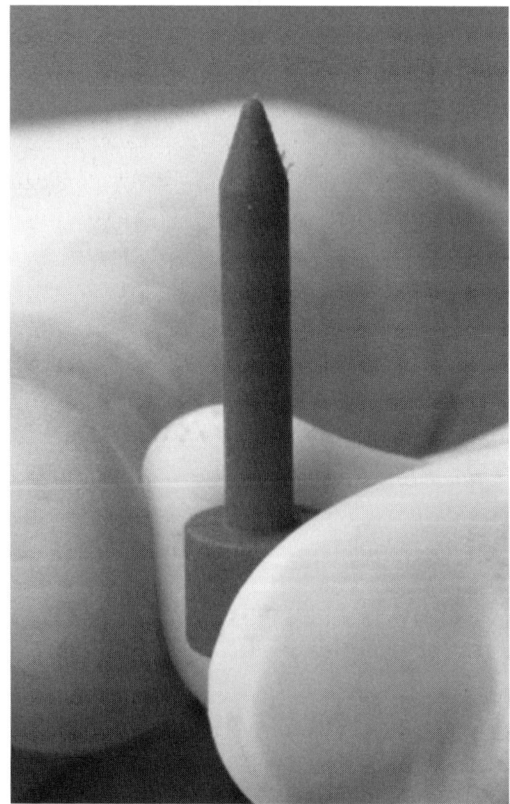

Fig. 4. SIMPL—silicone implant.

structure, and function [44]. The teat canal skin is a part of the outer skin that has been pulled into the inner teat. Its structure is similar to the outer skin: Epidermis and corium make up teat canal skin and outer skin [45].)

6. Bandage the teat with elastic adhesive tape (Teat Bandage [www.kruuse.com]) to prevent the silicone implant from falling out and to indicate to the herdsman not to milk this teat. Apply this procedure on the day the injury occurred (day 0), 3 days later (day 3), and 6 days later (day 6). Rest and do not milk the teat from the day the injury had occurred until 9 days (day 9) thereafter (Table 1).

The milk may appear watery, and milk yield may decrease after resting the teat. Milk appearance returns to normal, however, and milk yield increases after milking is resumed. The earlier in lactation the teat was rested, the better milk yield returned to normal [46]. Resting the teat did not

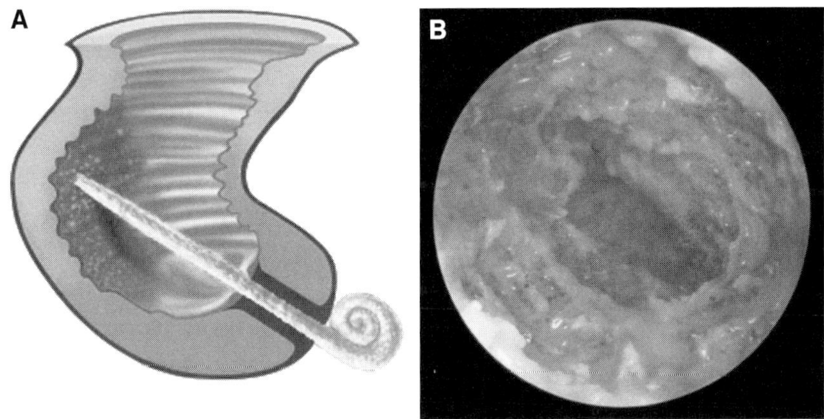

Fig. 5. (*A*) Inflammation of the teat cistern lining—"pipe cleaner disease" (schematic representation). (*B*) Inflammation of the teat cistern lining (canal theloscopy).

Table 1
Resting the teat for 3 × 3 days

Day	0	1	2	3	4	5	6	7	8	9
Administer xylazine and oxytocin	x			x			x			
Clean and disinfect the teat	x			x			x			
Drain the milk	x			x			x			
Administer an antibiotic	x			x			x			
Insert the silicone implant	x			x			x			
Bandage the teat	x			x			x			
Resume milking										x

increase the risk of mastitis [29]. If the teat is not milkable after conservative therapy, surgical therapy may be applied, the teat may be dried off, or the cow may be culled.

Surgical therapy

Precise diagnosis is a prerequisite for successful surgical therapy. In rural veterinary practice, a sufficiently precise diagnosis may be made with the help of theloscopy. Four procedures have been described: classical theloscopy by Medl et al [47–50] (equipment available from www.drfritz.de), theloresectoscopy by Hospes and Seeh [51–55] (equipment available from www.karlstorz.de), triangulation by Hirsbrunner and Steiner [56,57], and wireless theloscopy by Querengässer and Geishauser [58,59] (equipment available from www.eickemeyer.de). A film on wireless theloscopy is available on DVD [60] (www.lehmanns.de).

Procedure

The cow is administered xylazine and oxytocin and properly restrained in a claw trimming chute (Fig. 6) or on a tilt table. After cleaning and disinfection of the teat, a rubber ring is placed at the teat base, an anesthetic

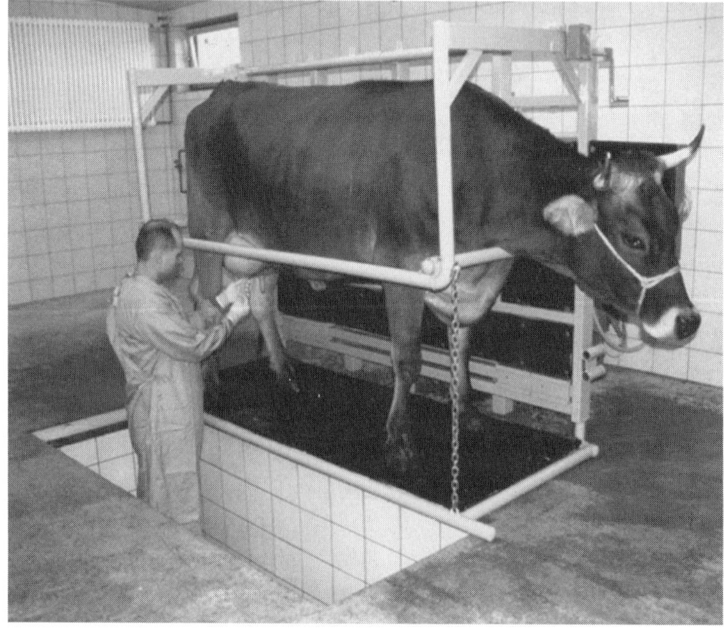

Fig. 6. Fixing the cow in claw trimming chute and examining the teat from a pit.

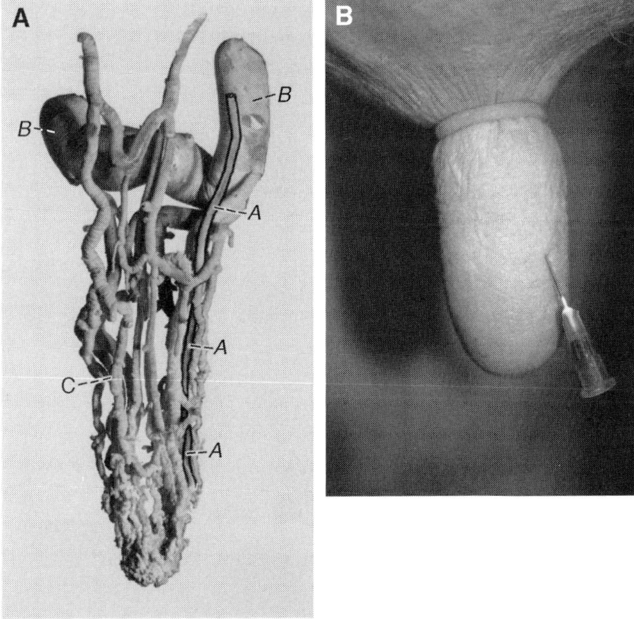

Fig. 7. (*A*) Blood vessels in the teat: artery (A), Fürstenberg vein ring (B), and veins (C), plastoid. (*From* le Roux JMW, Wilkens H. Beitrag zur Gefäßversorgung des Euters der Kuh. Dtsch Tierärztl Wschr 1959;66:429; with permission.). (*B*) Rubber ring around the teat basis: puncture of a teat vein to inject 5 to 10 mL of a 2% lidocaine solution.

is injected into a teat vein (Fig. 7), the milk is drained from the teat (Fig. 8), and the cistern is rinsed with sterile saline. Theloscopy can be performed through either the teat canal (canal theloscopy) or the lateral teat wall (lateral theloscopy) (Figs. 9–11). For lateral theloscopy, an opening is made in the teat wall, and a slide pipe is inserted (Fig. 12). The teat is dilated by pumping air into the teat. When theloscopy is performed through the teat canal, the teat canal (Fig. 13) and the teat cistern (Fig. 14) can be visualized in an upward direction. When theloscopy is performed through the lateral teat wall, the teat cistern, the inner opening of the teat canal, and the Fürstenberg rosette [45] can be visualized in a downward direction (Fig. 15).

Patients presented to the Veterinary Clinic Babenhausen, Germany, were predominantly young Braunvieh cows kept in tie-stall barns and belonging to herds with an average herd size of 38 cows. These patients were at a median of 3 months in milk and mostly pretreated. Predominantly hind teats were affected by an acute milk flow disorder. In 96% of the affected teats, a rupture in the area of the teat canal was diagnosed, 49% with tissue dislocation (see Fig. 2) and 47% without tissue dislocation (see Fig. 1); 4% had other diagnoses, such as ruptures in the teat cistern area or papilloma [61,63]. In 64% of the affected teats, an inflammation of the teat lining ("pipe cleaner

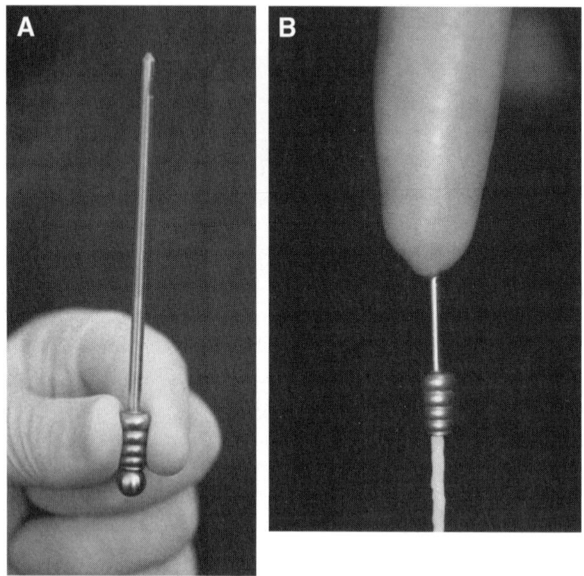

Fig. 8. (*A*) THELOKAL—extra-wide milking tube. (*B*) Draining milk.

disease") was visible (see Fig. 5) [32]. Of the affected quarters, 67% showed the signs of subclinical mastitis (SCC >100,000/mL and pathogens detected). In 67% of the milk samples from affected quarters pathogens were detected: 80% major pathogens (38% *Streptococcus* esculin positive, 24% *Streptococcus* esculin negative, 10% *Staphylococcus aureus*, 7% coliforms, 1% *Streptococcus*

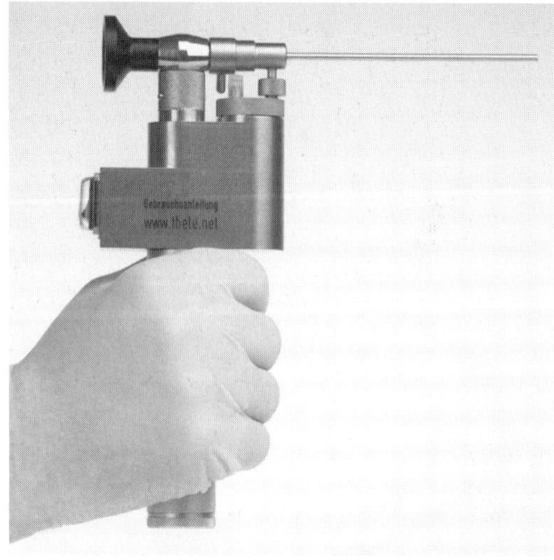

Fig. 9. THELOSCOPE—wireless teat endoscope.

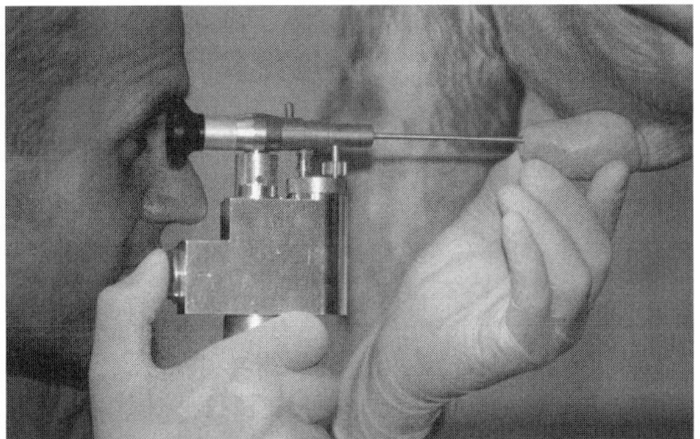

Fig. 10. Theloscopy via the teat canal (canal theloscopy).

agalactiae), 16% minor pathogens (16% *Staphylococcus* species), and 4% uncommon pathogens (4% *Arcanobacter pyogenes*) [35].

Minimally invasive surgical therapy was performed with the help of theloscopy. Ruptured and dislocated tissue was precisely removed by using a teat punch (Fig. 16). Narrowed teat canals were dilated with Hug's teat lancet (Fig. 17) [63,64]. Papilloma were extracted by using teat forceps (Fig. 18) [60]. After surgery, the artificial opening was sutured, the rubber ring was removed, and all milk was drained with an extra-wide milking tube (see Fig. 8). The affected teat was administered a mastitis antibiotic preparation, and a silicone implant was inserted into the teat canal (see Fig. 4). Then the suture was removed again, and the teat was bandaged and rested for several days to speed up healing (see Table 1).

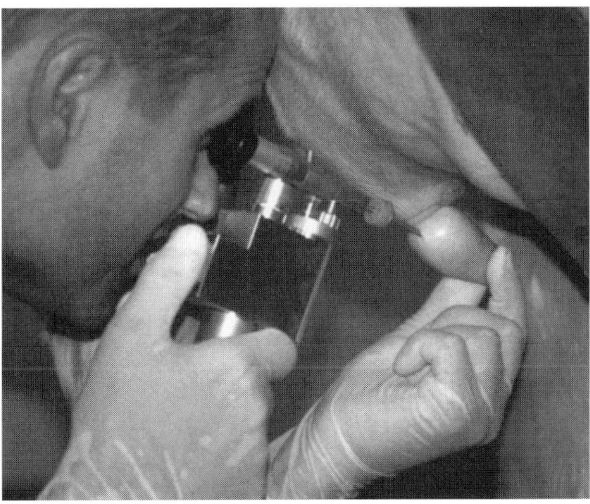

Fig. 11. Theloscopy via the lateral teat wall (lateral theloscopy).

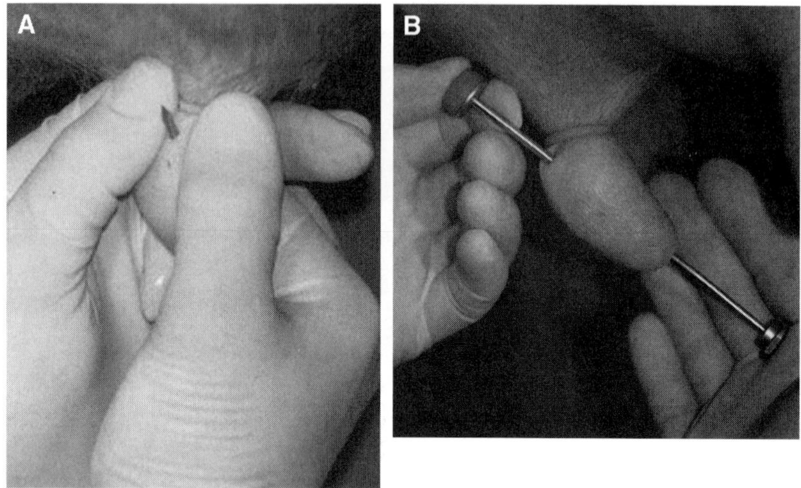

Fig. 12. (*A*) Opening the lateral teat wall using a trocar. (*B*) Insertion of the slide pipe along the trocar.

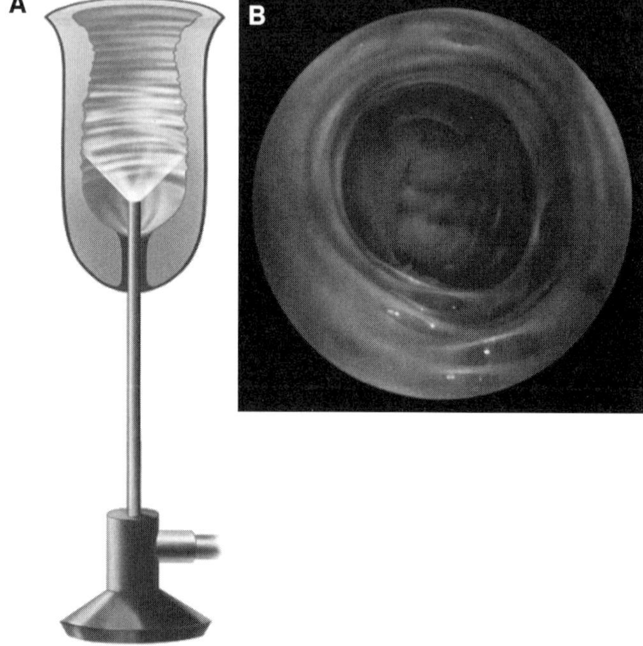

Fig. 13. (*A*) View into the teat cistern via the teat canal (schematic representation). (*B*) Normal teat cistern (lateral theloscopy). Note circular folds.

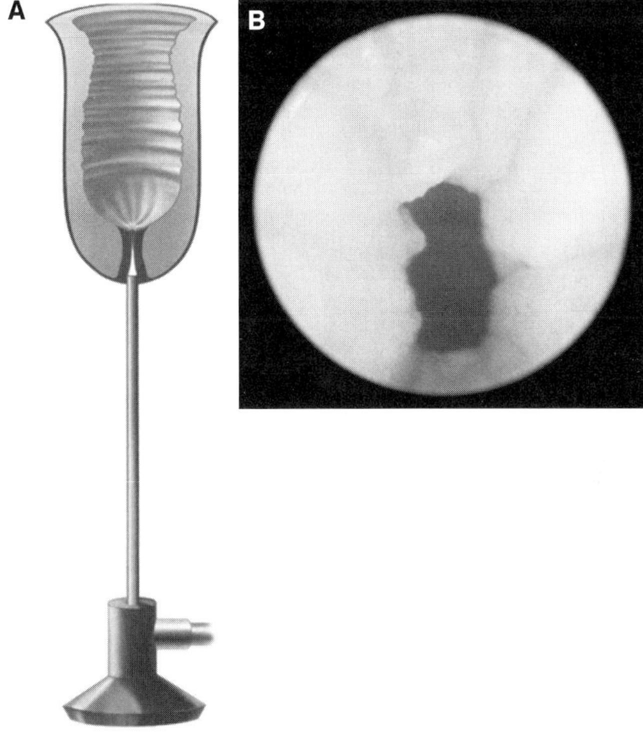

Fig. 14. (*A*) View into the teat canal via the teat canal (schematic representation). (*B*) Normal teat canal (canal theloscopy). Note longitudinal folds.

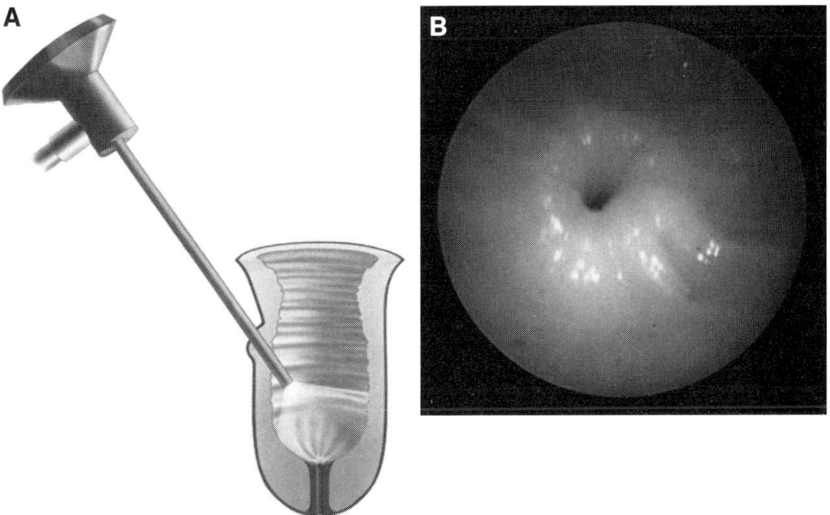

Fig. 15. (*A*) View into the teat cistern via the lateral teat wall (schematic representation). (*B*) Inner opening of the teat canal—Fürstenberg rosette (lateral theloscopy). Note radial folds.

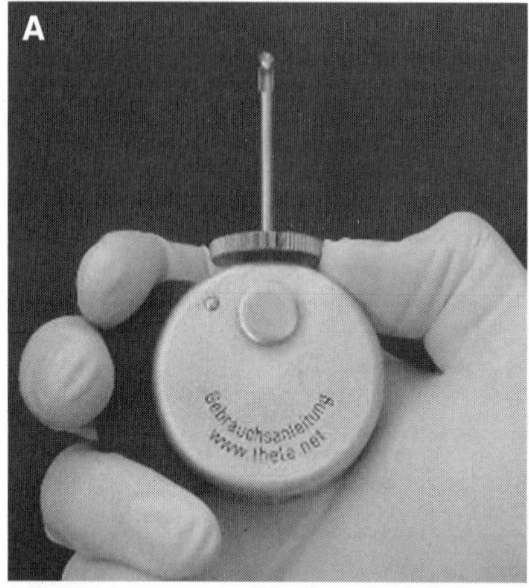

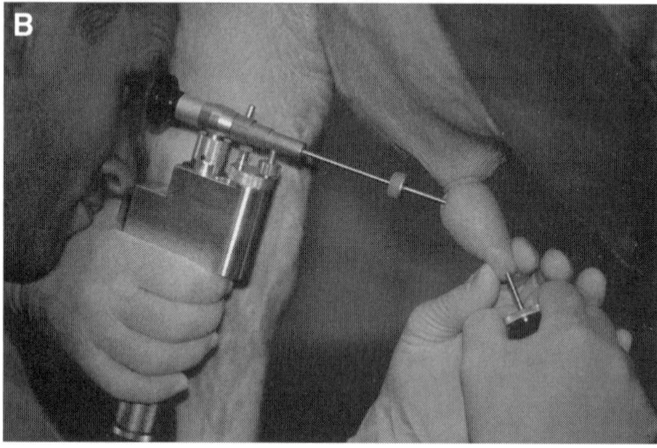

Fig. 16. (*A*) THELOTOME—teat punch. (*B*) Monitoring via lateral theloscopy. (*C*) Removal of inverted tissue (schematic representation). (*D*) Removal of inverted tissue (lateral theloscopy).

Before surgery, peak milk flow from teats with milk flow disorders was on average 24% (22%, 22%) compared with the contralateral (ipsilateral, diagonal) teats; 1 month later, peak milk flow was 73% (68%, 69%); and 6 months later, peak milk flow was 82% (77%, 80%) (Fig. 19). These values may indicate that milk flow from the affected teats was decreased before surgery and increased thereafter. Milkable yield from the affected quarters was minimal before surgery. The milked plus drained yield from the affected teats was on average 115% (106%, 107%), however, compared with the contralateral (ipsilateral, diagonal) teats before surgery; the yield was 67% (69%, 68%) 1 month later; and the yield was 69% (74%, 73%) 6 months later. These values may indicate that milk had congested in the affected quarter before surgery and that the affected quarter did not entirely meet the milk production of not affected quarters after surgery [61,62]. SCC in the

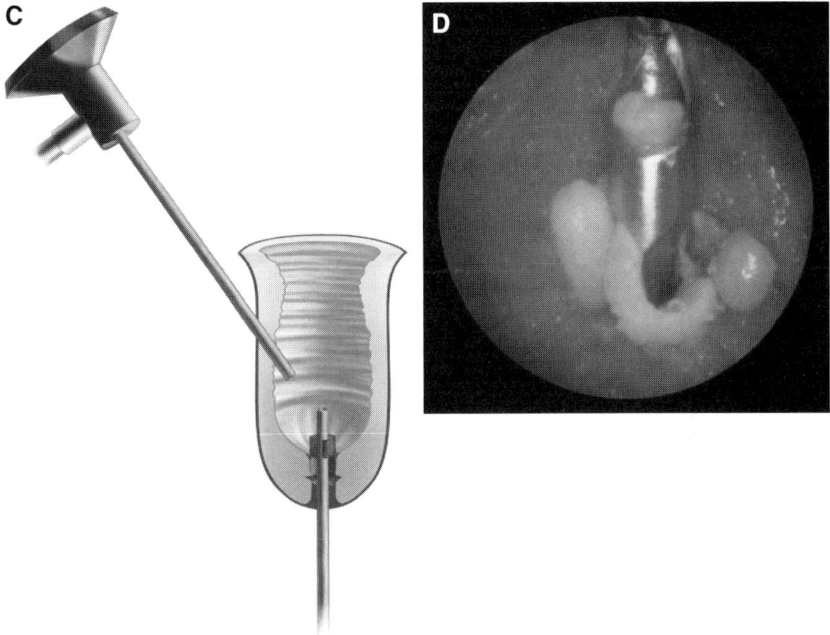

Fig. 16 (*continued*)

milk from affected teats was on average 2.9 million/mL before surgery, 725,000/mL 1 month later, and 426,000/mL 6 months later; SCC in the milk from contralateral (ipsilateral, diagonal) teats was on average 157,000/mL (124,000/mL, 127,000/mL) before surgery, 71,000/mL (49,000/mL, 55,000/mL) 1 month later, and 67,000/mL (45,000/mL, 64,000/mL) 6 months later (Fig. 20). Pathogens were detected in the milk from affected teats in 67% of the cases before surgery, in 69% 1 month later, and in 61% 6 months later; pathogens in the milk from contralateral (ipsilateral, diagonal) teats were found in 17% (13%, 15%)% of the cases before surgery, in 24% (15%, 13%) 1 month later, and in 22% (17%, 10%) 6 months later (Fig. 21). These values may indicate that milk quality from affected quarters was decreased before surgery; SCC decreased significantly after surgery; however, infection with pathogens did not change significantly [35,65].

In the lactation the injury occurred and in the subsequent lactation, affected cows yielded as much milk as nonaffected herdmates on test day (Fig. 22) and throughout lactation. Covered teat injuries increased test day SCC (Fig. 23), however, on average by 128,000/mL. Covered teat injuries that were managed surgically as described did not affect survival in the herd or calving interval (Fig. 24) [14,66].

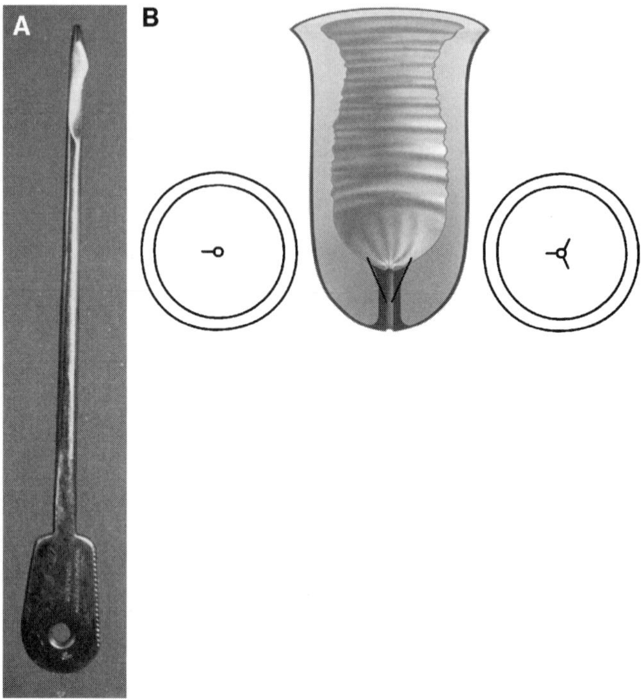

Fig. 17. (*A*) Hug's lancet. (*B*) Widening the teat canal with one, two, or three incisions in the area of the inner teat canal opening (schematic representation).

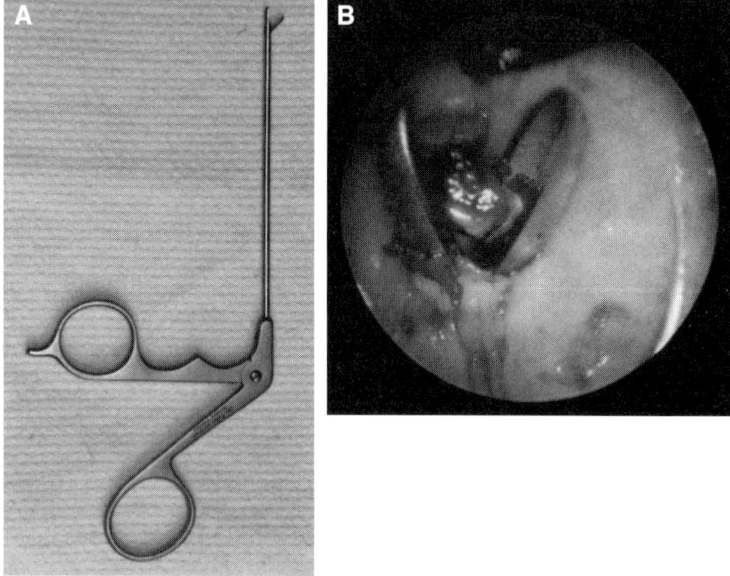

Fig. 18. (*A*) THELAB—teat forceps. (*B*) Removal of tissue with a forceps (lateral theloscopy).

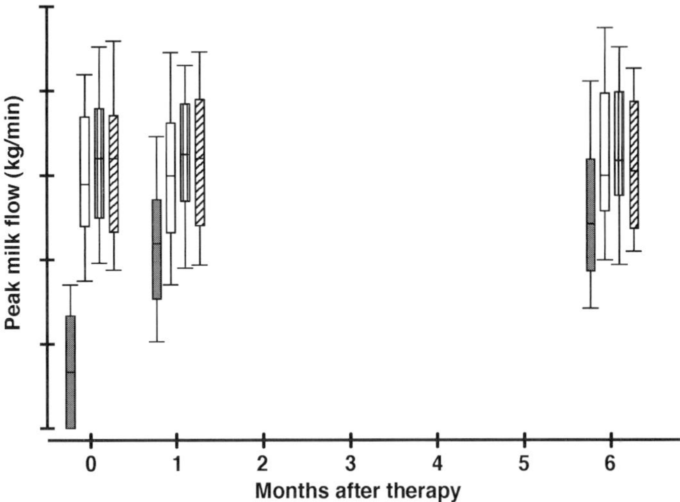

Fig. 19. Peak milk flow from the affected (■), contralateral (□), ipsilateral (◫), and diagonal (▨) teats before treatment, 1 month later, and 6 months later. (*From* Querengässer J, Geishauser T, Querengässer K, et al. Untersuchungen zu Milchfluß und Milchmenge aus Zitzen mit Milchabflußstörungen. Prakt Tierarzt 2002;83:1008; with permission.)

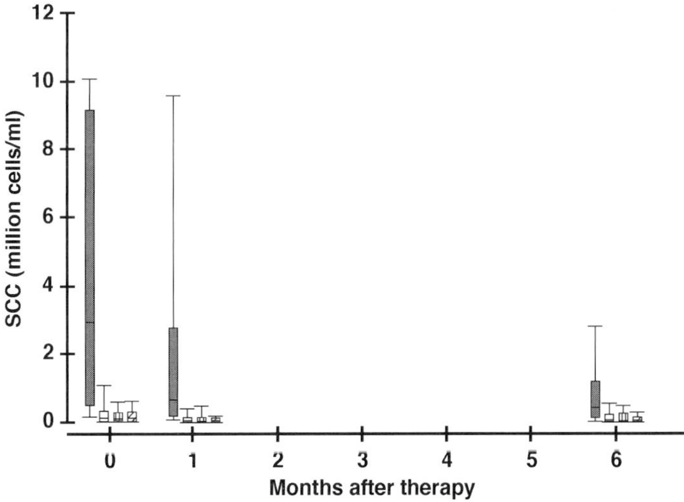

Fig. 20. Somatic cell count in the milk from the affected (■), contralateral (□), ipsilateral (◫), and diagonal (▨) teats before treatment, 1 month later, and 6 months later. (*From* Querengässer J, Geishauser T, Querengässer K, et al. Untersuchungen zur Güte der Milch aus Zitzen mit Milchabflußstörungen. Prakt Tierarzt 2003;84:606; with permission.)

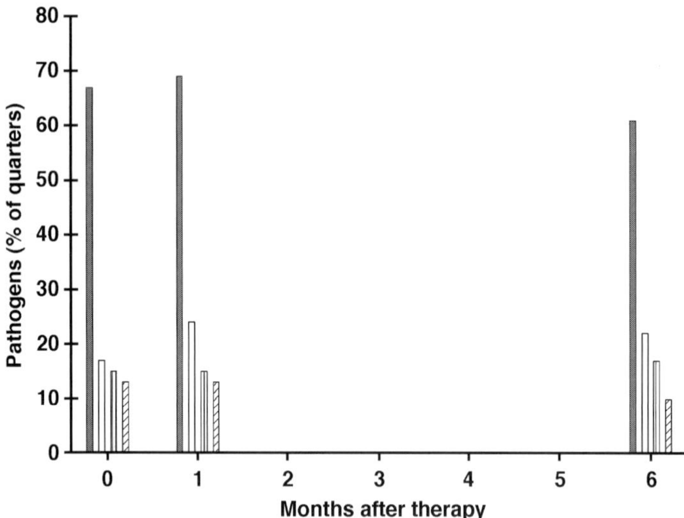

Fig. 21. Detection of pathogens in the milk from the affected (■), contralateral (□), ipsilateral (◫), and diagonal (▨) teats before treatment, 1 month later, and 6 months later. (*From* Querengässer J, Geishauser T, Querengässer K, et al.: Untersuchungen zur Güte der Milch aus Zitzen mit Milchabflußstörungen. Prakt Tierarzt 2003;84:606; with permission.)

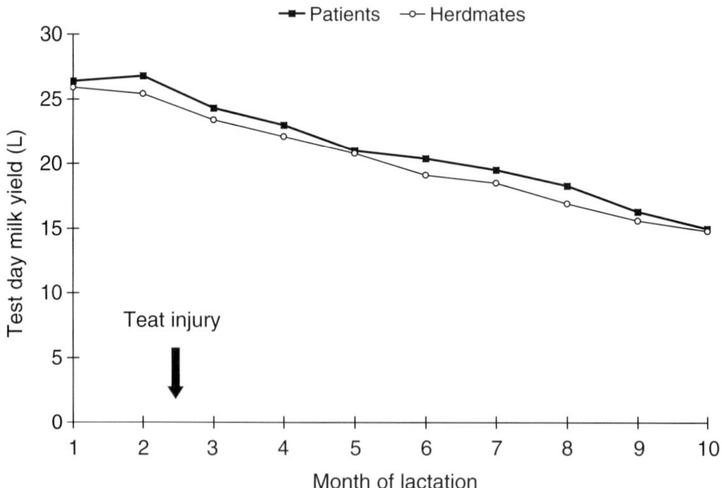

Fig. 22. Test day milk yield in the year the injury had occurred for patients and herdmates. (*From* Geishauser T, Querengässer K, Nitschke M, et al. Milk yield, somatic cell counts and risk of removal from the herd for dairy cows after covered teat canal injury. J Dairy Sci 1999; 82:1482; with permission.)

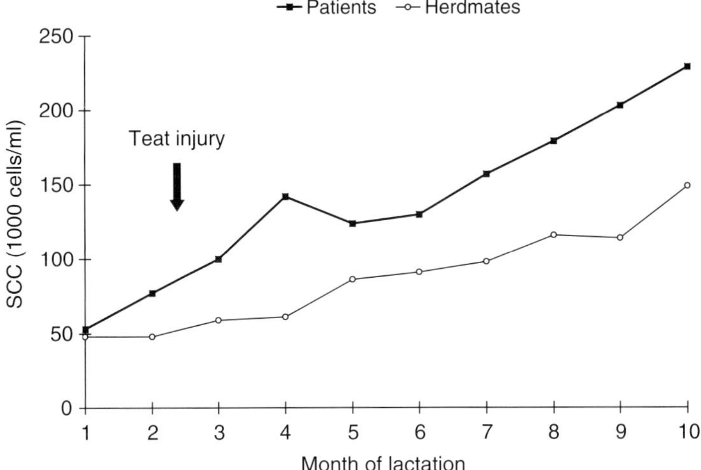

Fig. 23. Somatic cell count in the year the injury had occurred for patients and herdmates. (*From* Geishauser T, Querengässer K, Nitschke M, et al: Milk yield, somatic cell counts and risk of removal from the herd for dairy cows after covered teat canal injury. J Dairy Sci 1999; 82:1482; with permission.)

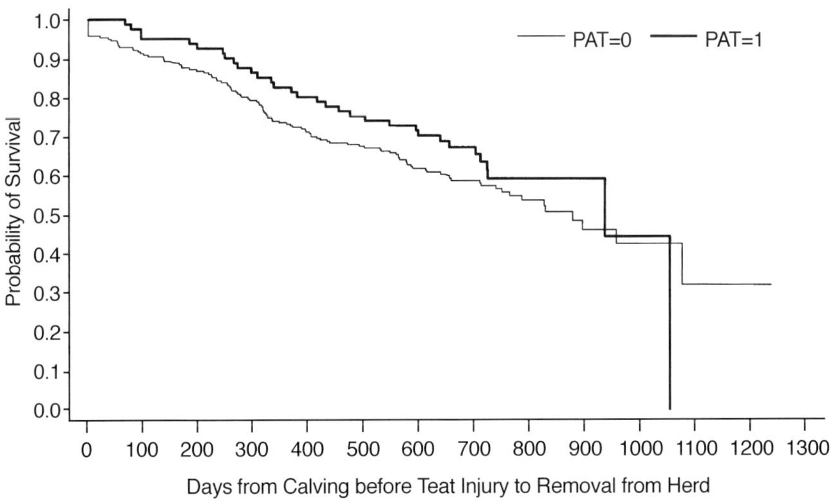

Fig. 24. Survival of patients and herdmates. (*From* Geishauser T, Querengässer K, Nitschke M, et al: Milk yield, somatic cell counts and risk of removal from the herd for dairy cows after covered teat canal injury. J. Dairy Sci 1999;82:1482; with permission.)

Summary

Teat endoscopy (theloscopy) is a useful technique for diagnosis and therapy of covered teat injuries. Minimal invasive theloscopic surgery may help to restore milk flow, milk yield, and SCC of the affected quarter. Infection with pathogens may not change significantly, however. Cows treated as described may yield as much milk as their herdmates at a slightly increased udder SCC and stay as long in the herd as their herdmates. Theloscopy also may be used for diagnosis and therapy of various other teat disorders [32,38–40,42,43,48,49,52,54,67–80].

References

[1] Geishauser T, Querengässer K. Vorbeuge von Zitzenverletzung bei Milchkühen—eine Schriftumsübersicht. Prakt Tierarzt 2002;83:997.
[2] Agger JF, Hesselholdt M. Epidemiology of teat lesions in a dairy herd. I. Description of incidence, location and clinical appearence. Nord Vet Med 1986;38:209.
[3] Beaudeau F, Ducrocq V, Fourichon C, et al. Effect of disease on length of productive life of French Holstein dairy cows assessed by survival analysis. J Dairy Sci 1995;78:103.
[4] Bigras-Poulin M, Meek AH, Martin SW, et al. Health problems in selected Ontario Holstein cows: frequency of occurrences, time to first diagnosis and associations. Prev Vet Med 1990; 10:79.
[5] Distl O. Genetische Analyse von Krankheitshäufigkeiten mit dem Schwellenmodell bei südbayerischen Milchviehherden. Züchtungskunde 1992;64:1.
[6] Dohoo IR, Martin SW, Meek H, et al. Disease, production and culling in Holstein Freisian cows. I. The data. Prev Vet Med 1983;1:321.
[7] Ekesbo J. Disease incidence in tied and loose housed dairy cattle. Acta Agric Scand Suppl 1966;15:1.
[8] Gröhn Y, Saloniemi H, Syväjärvi Y. An epidemiological and genetic study on registered diseases in Finnish Ayrshire cattle. I. The data, disease occurrence and culling. Acta Vet Scand 1986;27:182.
[9] Matzke P, Holzer A, Deneke J. Ein Beitrag zum Einfluß von Umweltfaktoren auf das Vorkommen von Eutererkrankungen. Tierarztl Prax 1992;20:21.
[10] Osteras O, Ronningen O, Sandvik L, et al. Field studies show associations between pulsator characteristics and udder health. J Dairy Res 1995;62:1.
[11] Saloniemi H, Roine K. Field observations on the incidence of bovine clinical mastitis and teat diseases. Nord Med Vet 1981;33:297.
[12] Sargeant J, Scott HM, Leslie KE, et al. Clinical mastitis in dairy cattle in Ontario: Frequency of occurrence and bacteriological isolates. Can Vet J 1998;39:33.
[13] Koskiniemi K. Observations on the incidence of teat injuries in different cowsheds. Nord Med Vet 1982;34:13.
[14] Querengässer K, Geishauser T, Nitschke M. Untersuchungen zu Milchleistung, Milchgüte und Verbleib von Kühen nach gedeckter Zitzenverletzung. Prakt Tierarzt 1999;29:52.
[15] Agger JF, Hesselholdt M. Epidemiology of teat lesions in a dairy herd. II. Association with subclinical mastitis. Nord Vet Med 1986;38:220.
[16] Pyörälä S, Jousimies-Somer H, Mero M. Clinical, bacteriological and therapeutic aspects of bovine mastitis caused by aerobic and anaerobic pathogens. Br Vet J 1992;148:54.
[17] Witzig P, Rüsch P, Berchtold M. Wesen, Diagnose und Behandlung von Schleimhautabrissen im Bereich des Strichkanals. Dtsch Tierärztl Wschr 1984;91:219.
[18] Zähner M. Eutergesundheit nach Zitzenoperationen. Dissertationsschrift, Universität, Vet Med Fak, Zürich, 1989.

[19] Beaudeau F, Fourichon C, Frankena K, et al. Impact of udder disorders on culling of dairy cows. Vet Res 1994;25:223.
[20] Bendixen PH, Vilson B, Ekesbo I, et al. Disease frequencies in dairy cows in Sweden. VI. Tramped teat. Prev Vet Med 1988;6:17.
[21] Dohoo IR, Martin SW. Disease, production and culling in Holstein Friesian cows. V. Survivorship. Prev Vet Med 1984;2:771.
[22] Duffield TF, Leslie KE, Sandals D, et al. Effect of a Monensin-controlled release capsule on cow health and reproductive performance. J Dairy Sci 1999;82:2377.
[23] Milian-Suazo F, Erb H, Smith RD. Descriptive epidemiology of culling in dairy herd cows from 34 herds in New York State. Prev Vet Med 1988;6:243.
[24] Rayala-Schultz PJ, Gröhn YT. Culling of dairy cows. Part I. Effects of diseases on culling in Finnish Ayrshire cows. Prev Vet Med 1999;41:195.
[25] Rayala-Schultz PJ, Gröhn YT. Culling of dairy cows. Part II. Effects of diseases and reproductive performance on culling in Finnish Ayrshire cows. Prev Vet Med 1999;41:279.
[26] Rayala-Schultz PJ, Gröhn YT. Culling of dairy cows. III. Effects of diseases, pregnancy status and milk yield on culling in Finnish Ayrshire cows. Prev Vet Med 1999;41:295.
[27] Sol J, Stelwagen J, Dijkhuizen AA. A three year herd health and management program on thirty Dutch dairy farms. II. Culling strategy and losses caused by forced replacement of dairy cows. Vet Q 1984;6:149.
[28] Kubicek J. Die gedeckten Zitzenverletzungen beim Rind. Tierarztl Umsch 1975;30:59.
[29] Rüsch P. Die gedeckten Zitzenverletzungen beim Rind. Habilitationsschrift, Universität, Veterinär-Medizinische Fakultät, Zürich, 1988.
[30] Roine K. Observations on teat stenosis. Nord Vet Med 1975;27:107.
[31] Alacam E, Dinc DA, Güler M, et al. Vorkommen und röntgenololgische Untersuchungen verschiedener Zitzenveränderungen bei Milchkühen. Dtsch Tierärtl Wschr 1990;97:523.
[32] Querengässer K, Geishauser T, Querengässer J, et al. Milchabflußstörung beim Rind—Befunde von 244 Fällen. Prakt Tierarzt 2001;82:816.
[33] Burkhardt H. Auswirkungen des partiellen Trockenstellens eines Euterviertels beim Rind auf Milchmenge und Milchqualität. Dissertationsschrift, Universität Vetererinär-Medizinische Fakultät, Zürich, 1985.
[34] Weichselbaum H, Baumgartner W, Schoder G. Einfluß der Dauer des temporären Trockenstellens eines Euterviertels bei Kühen auf Milchmenge und Milchqualität. Dtsch Tierärztl Wschr 1995;102:353.
[35] Querengässer J, Geishauser T, Querengässer K, et al. Investigations on milk quality from teats with milk flow disorders. J Dairy Sci 2002;85:2582.
[36] Weigt U, Agthe O, Bleckmann E, et al. Anwendung eines penicillinasefesten Langzeit-penicillins (Bayer 9035 NS) bei Zitzenverletzungen der Rinder. Prakt Tierarzt 1971;52:559.
[37] Querengässer J, Geishauser T, Querengässer K, et al. Comparative evaluation of SIMPL silicone implants and NIT natural teat inserts to keep the teat canal patent after surgery. J Dairy Sci 2002;85:1732.
[38] Bleul U, Seeh C, Teifke JP, et al. Resultate endoskopischer, sonographischer und histologischer Untersuchungen an der Zitzenzisternenschleimhaut des Rindes nach Behandlung mit Wollzitzenstiften. Prakt Tierarzt 2000;81:590.
[39] Höptner C. Documentazione sugli effetti collaterali nell'applicazione di stiloidi e cateteri mammari nella bovina. Tesi di Laura, Universitá Milano, 1994.
[40] Querengässer K, Geishauser T, Höptner C, et al. Effects of teat dilators and teat cannulas on udder health. Bov Practitioner 1999;33:130.
[41] Geishauser T, Querengässer K. Untersuchungen zur Sterilität von Zitzenstiften. Prakt Tierarzt 2001;82:367.
[42] Seeh C, Schlenstedt R, Stengel KH, et al. Prüfung eines neuartigen Strichkanalstabes zur Behandlung von Strichkanalwunden unter besonderer Berücksichtigung der endoskopisch dokumentierten Schleimhautverträglichkeit im Vergleich zu konventionellen Zitzenstiften und Verweilkanülen. Dtsch Tierärztl Wschr 1997;104:277.

[43] Querengässer K, Geishauser T, Querengässer J, et al. Teat dilators as free foreign bodies in the bovine teat. Bov Practitioner 2000;34:41.
[44] Michel G. Zum Bau der Zitze des Rindes. Tierhygiene-Info 5 (Sonderheft) 1973;103.
[45] Fürstenberg MHF. Milchdrüsen der Kuh. Leipzig: Verlag Engelmann; 1868.
[46] Heidrich HJ, Gehring W. Untersuchungsergebnisse über die Beeinflussung der Involution eines einzelnen Euterviertels beim Rind durch zeitlich begrenztes Unterlassen des Melkens. Berl Münch Tierärztl Wschr 1958;71:86.
[47] Medl M, Querengässer K. Die Endoskopie der Zitze des Rindes. Veterinär Spiegel 1994;3:4.
[48] Medl M, Querengässer K, Wagner C, et al. Zur Abklärung und Behandlung von Zitzenstenosen mittels Endoskopie. Tierarztl Prax 1994;22:532.
[49] Querengässer K. Diagnose und Therapie von Zitzenstenosen beim Rind mittels Endoskopie. Dissertationsschrift, Universität, Veterinär-Medizinische Fakultät, Zürich, 1998.
[50] Querengässer J. Studies on milk flow, milk yield and milk quality from teats with milk flow disorders. Dissertationsschrift, Universität, Veterinär-Medizinische Fakultät, Bern, 2002.
[51] Hospes R, Seeh C. Untersuchungen zu den Operationsergebnissen nach theloresektoskopischen Eingriffen an der Zitze des Rindes. Tierarztl Umsch 1998;53:420.
[52] Hospes R, Seeh C. Sonographie und Endoskopie der Zitze des Rindes. Stuttgart: Verlag Schattauer; 1999.
[53] Seeh C, Hospes R. Erfahrungen mit einem Theloresektoskop im Vergleich zur konventionellen Zitzenendoskopie bei der Diagnose und Therapie gedeckter Zitzenverletzungen. Tierarztl Prax 1998;26:110.
[54] Seeh C, Hospes R, Bostedt H. Einsatz bildgebender Verfahren zur Diagnose der Beizitze beim Rind. Tierarztl Prax 1995;24:438.
[55] Zulauf M, Steiner A. Kurz- und Langzeitresultate nach operativer Behandlung von Zitzenstenosen im Bereich der Fürstenberg'schen Rosette mittels Theloresektoskopie (1999–2000). Schweiz Arch Tierheilkd 2001;143:593.
[56] Hirsbrunner G, Steiner A. Use of a theloscopic triangulation technique for endoscopic treatment of teat obstruction in cows. J Am Vet Med Assoc 1999;214:1668.
[57] Hirsbrunner G, Eicher R, Meylan M, et al. Comparison of thelotomy and theloscopic triangulation for the treatment of distal teat obstructions in dairy cows—a retrospective study (1994–1998). Vet Rec 2001;148:803.
[58] Geishauser T, Querengässer K. Using teat endoscopy (theloscopy) to diagnose and treat milk flow disorders in cows. Bov Practitioner 2001;35:156.
[59] Querengässer K, Geishauser T. Zitzenspiegelung (Theloskopie) beim Rind—Ausrüstung und Vorgehen. Prakt Tierarzt 2001;82:527.
[60] Querengässer K, Geishauser T, Querengässer J. Theloskopie beim Rind—ein Film (DVD), Theloscopy in cows—a film (DVD), Théloscopie chez la vache—un Film (DVD). Berlin: Verlag Lehmanns; 2003 Available at: www.lehmanns.de.
[61] Querengässer J, Geishauser T, Querengässer K, et al. Investigations on milk flow and milk yield from teats with milk flow disorders. J Dairy Sci 2002;85:810.
[62] Querengässer J, Geishauser T, Querengässer K, et al. Untersuchungen zu Milchfluß und Milchmenge aus Zitzen mit Milchabflußstörungen. Prakt Tierarzt 2002;83:1008.
[63] Hug JJ. Zur operativen Behandlung der Zitzenanomalien. Schweiz Arch Tierheilk 1903; 45:235.
[64] Hug JJ. Beiträge zur pathologischen Anatomie und Therapie der Zitzenstenose des Rindes. Dissertationsschrift, Universität, Zürich, 1906.
[65] Querengässer J, Geishauser T, Querengässer K, et al. Untersuchungen zur Güte der Milch aus Zitzen mit Milchabflußstörungen. Prakt Tierarzt 2003;84:606.
[66] Geishauser T, Querengässer K, Nitschke M, et al. Milk yield, somatic cell counts and risk of removal from the herd for dairy cows after covered teat canal injury. J Dairy Sci 1999;82:1482.
[67] Dümmer N. Vergleichende palpatorische, sonographische und endoskopische Untersuchungen der Zitzen eutergesunder und euterkranker Tiere. Dissertationsschrift, Tierärztliche Hochschule, Hannover, 1988.

[68] Hospes R, Seeh C. Behebung von Milchabflußstörungen unter endoskopischer Kontrolle. Tierarztl Umsch 1998;53:674.

[69] Inzumisawa Y, Kobayashi T, Nagahata A, et al. Endoscopic appearance of the papillary duct and lacitferous sinus in cows (Japanese). J Jap Vet Med Assoc 1995;48:175.

[70] John H, Hässig M, Gobet D, et al. A new operative method to treat high teat stenoses in dairy cows. Br J Urol 1998;82:906.

[71] John H, Sicher D, Berger-Pusterla J, et al. Videoassistierte theloskopische Elektroinzision einer hohen Zitzenstenose. Schweiz Arch Tierheilk 1998;140:282.

[72] Kiossis E, Riedl J, Daffner BL, et al. Untersuchungen zur Eutergesundheit und Melkbarkeit nach endoskopisch kontrollierter Behandlung von Zitzenstenosen des Rindes. Prakt Tierarzt 2002;83:60.

[73] Melle T. Vergleichende Studie zu diagnostischen Möglichkeiten bei tiefen Zitzenstenosen des Rindes mittels Ultraschall und Endoskopie. Dissertationsschrift, Universität, Fachbereich 18, Gießen, 1998.

[74] Querengässer K, Geishauser T. Untersuchungen zur Zitzenkanallänge bei Milchabfluß-störungen. Prakt Tierarzt 1999;80:796.

[75] Querengässer K, Geishauser T. An evaluation of teat canal length in teats with milk flow disturbances. J Dairy Sci 2000;83:1976.

[76] Querengässer K, Geishauser T, Querengässer J, et al. Vorfall von Zitzenkanalhaut beim Rind—drei Fallberichte. Prakt Tierarzt 2001;82:288.

[77] Riedl J, Kiossis E, Daffner BL, et al. Auswirkung der endoskopisch kontrollierten Therapie von Zitzenstenosen auf Milchmenge und Milchfluss betroffener Viertel. Prakt Tierarzt 2003; 84:302.

[78] Shakespeare AS. Use of endoscopy to investigate abnormalities within the bovine udder and teat. Vet Rec 1998;142:672.

[79] Tulleners E, Hamir A. Effects of teat cistern mural biopsy and teatoscopy stab versus longitudinal incision with or without tube implant on incisional healing in lactating cattle. Am J Vet Res 1990;51:1257.

[80] Wilhelm U, Schebitz J. Diagnose und Therapie proliferativer Wucherungen in der Zitzenzisterne unter Sichtkontrolle mit einem Miniaturresektoskop. Tierarztl Prax 1979; 7:305.

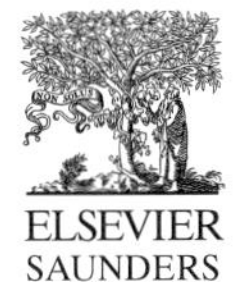

ELSEVIER
SAUNDERS

Vet Clin Food Anim 21 (2005) 227–249

VETERINARY
CLINICS
Food Animal Practice

General Principles of Laparoscopy

Ludovic Bouré, Méd Vét, MSc, DES

Large Animal Surgery, Department of Clinical Studies, Ontario Veterinary College, University of Guelph, Guelph, Ontario, N1G 2W1, Canada

Laparoscopy is a minimally invasive surgical technique using an endoscope inserted transabdominally to observe organs within the abdominal and pelvic cavities. During laparoscopy, the surgeon can inspect the viscera and peritoneal surfaces visually for evidence of disease and perform surgical procedures [1,2].

In 1901, Kelling first reported the examination of the abdominal cavity of a dog with a cystoscope inserted through a small cutaneous incision [3,4]. Jacobeus performed the first exploratory laparoscopy in a human in 1910 [3,4]. Since then, with the development of microtechnology, the use of laparoscopy has increased dramatically, and laparoscopy has gained the favor of human and veterinary surgeons [3–5]. The use of laparoscopy in cattle has been described since the mid-1930s; however, until the late 1970s, laparoscopy in cattle was used mainly to observe the reproductive tract and explore its physiology [1,6]. Since the early 1990s, several surgical techniques performed under laparoscopic guidance have been described in neonatal calves and mature cows [7–9].

Equipment

The equipment used during laparoscopy includes an optical system, an insufflation system (Fig. 1), and adapted surgical instruments for increased length (Fig. 2). The optical system provides the surgeon with a live picture of the inside of the abdominal cavity, and the insufflation system is used to create pneumoperitoneum, which improves the observation of the abdominal organs [2,3,6,10]. The laparoscope and laparoscopic surgical instruments are introduced into the abdominal cavity through cannulas, which are placed through the body wall using sharp trocars [2,3,6,10].

E-mail address: lboure@ovc.uoguelph.ca

doi:10.1016/j.cvfa.2004.12.002 ***vetfood.theclinics.com***

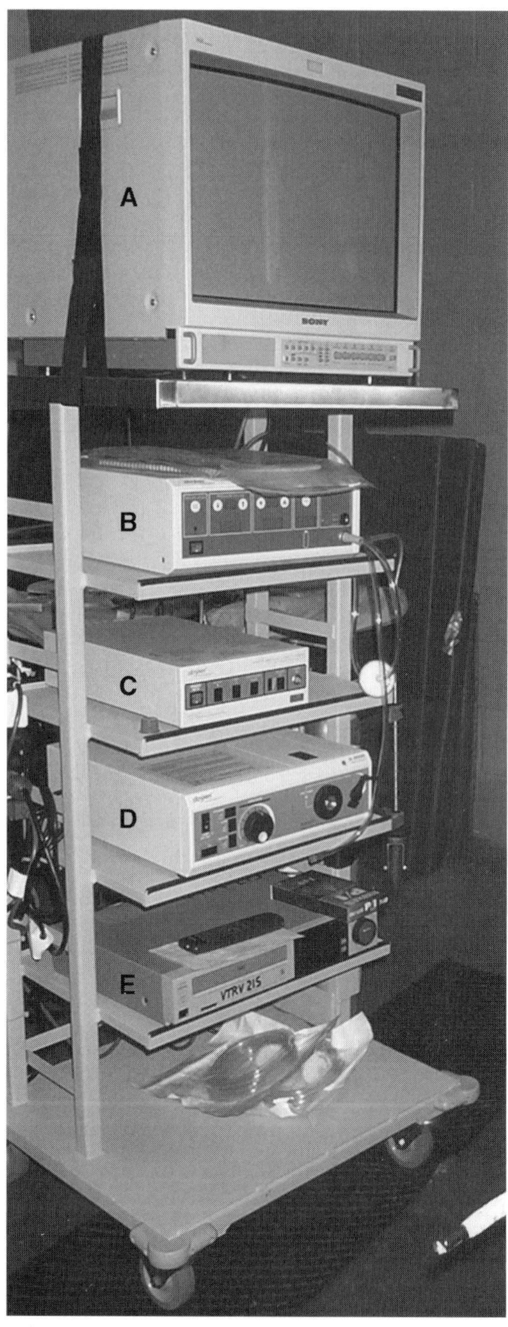

Fig. 1. Laparoscopic tower used for bovine laparoscopy. (*A*) Television monitor. (*B*) CO_2 insufflator. (*C*) Video camera. (*D*) Light source. (*E*) VCR.

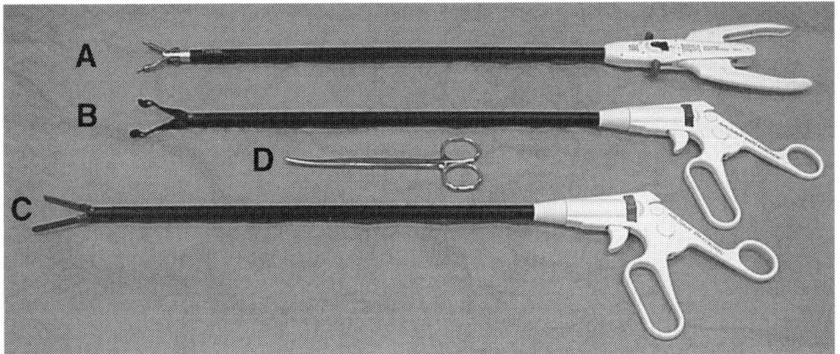

Fig. 2. Laparoscopic surgical instruments (*A–C*) compared with conventional surgical instrument (*D*).

Optical system

The optical system consists of an endoscope, a light source, and a light cable. Endoscopes can be either flexible or rigid. Although the use of flexible endoscopes has been described to explore the bovine abdomen [11], rigid endoscopes are used more commonly because they provide the most light, the largest field of view, and the greatest clarity of vision. Rigid endoscopes used in the abdominal cavity are called *laparoscopes*. They allow the observation of abdominal contents without creating a large incision in the body wall.

Laparoscope

Laparoscopes are composed of an external metal tube, an optical channel, and optical fibers (Fig. 3) [2,12]. The optical channel is composed of a series of high-resolution optical lenses, which transmit the images to an eyepiece [2,12]. In cattle, laparoscopy can be performed either under direct visualization or using a video camera and television monitor [6,8,11,13 15]. Direct visualization is used for exploratory laparoscopy or simple laparoscopic surgical procedures [6,8,14,16,17]. When available, a video camera connected to a television monitor is attached to the laparoscope eyepiece, allowing the surgeon and assistants to follow the procedure on the television monitor screen. The use of a video camera and television monitor is mandatory when complex surgical procedures requiring two surgeons are performed [1,7,15,18]. The optical fibers, which are the light-carrying portion of the laparoscope, are wrapped around the optical channel, and when coupled to a powerful light source, they illuminate the intra-abdominal structures [2,12]. There are two broad categories of laparoscopes: diagnostic and operating laparoscopes [2,12]. Diagnostic laparoscopes are built exactly as previously described and are used most frequently because they permit a wide range of diagnostic and surgical procedures (see Fig. 3) [2,12]. Operating laparoscopes have an additional open channel for the insertion of instruments such as biopsy forceps. Operating laparoscopes are

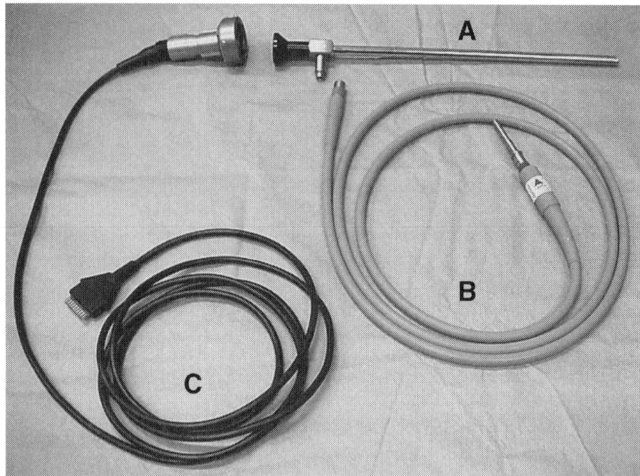

Fig. 3. Diagnostic laparoscope (*A*), light cable (*B*), and video camera (*C*) used for bovine laparoscopy.

ideal for limited access techniques using a single entry site and usually are used to obtain biopsy specimens [9,19].

Laparoscopes are described by their outer diameter and viewing angle. They are manufactured in 5-, 8-, and 10-mm outer diameter. When a video camera and television monitor are used, laparoscopes with a 10-mm outer diameter are recommended because they are large enough to provide an adequate amount of light into the bovine abdomen. The length of the laparoscope most frequently used varies between 35 cm and 40 cm and is sufficient to allow visualization of organs situated on the ipsilateral side of the laparoscope [8,14,15,18,19]. The most popular laparoscopes have either a 0° or 30° viewing angle. A 0° laparoscope provides the surgeon with a visual field that is in line with the true field [2,12,20]. This type of laparoscope makes orientation and manipulation of instruments easier [2,12,20]. It also maximizes light transmission compared with laparoscopes with an offset viewing angle (30° laparoscope). By rotating a 30° laparoscope along its longitudinal axis, the surgeon is able to view a wider area of the abdominal cavity [2,12,20].

One advantage of laparoscopy is that the laparoscope magnifies the images of the intra-abdominal structures. By definition, the distance of unity magnification of a laparoscope is the distance between the laparoscope and an object when the image of this object has the exact same dimensions as the object itself (Fig. 4) [20,21]. When the laparoscope and an object are placed at a different distance than the distance of unity magnification, the image magnification is the reciprocal ratio of that distance to the distance of unity magnification (ie, if the distance of unity magnification of a particular laparoscope is 25 mm, the magnification of the images provided by this

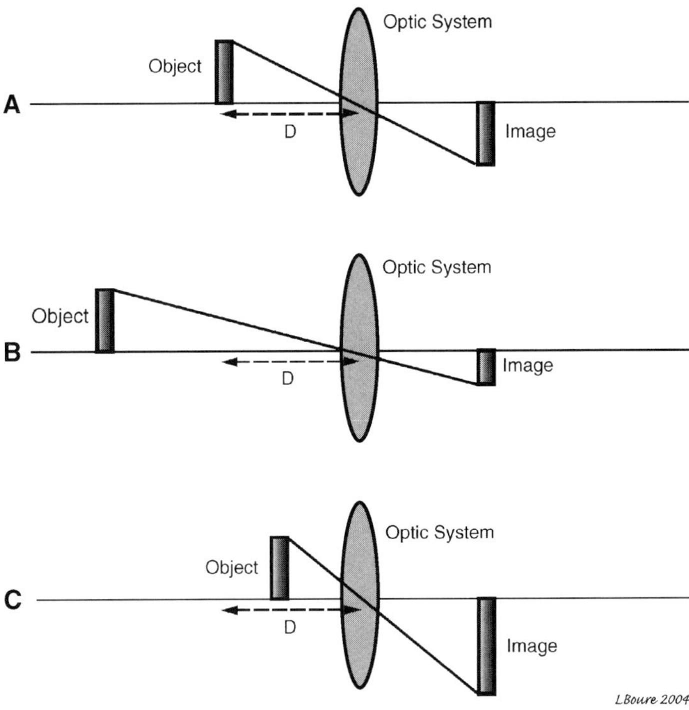

Fig. 4. (*A*) By definition, the distance of unity magnification (D) of a laparoscope is the distance between the laparoscope and an object when the image of this object has the exact same dimensions as the object itself. When the laparoscope and an object are placed at a different distance than the distance of unity magnification, the image magnification is the reciprocal ratio of that distance to the distance of unity magnification. (*B*) When the distance between the laparoscope and an object is longer than the distance of unity magnification (D) of the laparoscope, the image of the observed object has smaller dimensions than the object itself. (*C*) When the distance between the laparoscope and an object is shorter than the distance of unity magnification (D) of the laparoscope, the image of the observed object has larger dimensions than the object itself.

laparoscope placed 10 mm from a particular abdominal structure is 2.5 times, or 25/10) [20,21]. The bigger the distance of unity magnification is, the more magnification capacity the laparoscope has (see Fig. 4).

Light source

The abdominal cavity must be illuminated for laparoscopy to be performed [2,12]. Because of the large abdominal cavity of most cows, a high-wattage light source is required to perform laparoscopy in this species [6,15,18]. Currently available light sources have outputs ranging from 3% to 14%. These light sources transform at best 14% of the electric energy they receive into light; the remainder of the electric energy dissipates in the form of heat [2,12]. Extracorporeal light sources are used in laparoscopy, and a cold light–carrying cable connects the light source and the laparoscope (see Fig. 3).

Tungsten, halogen, and xenon light sources are available. Xenon sources provide the best quality of light. Xenon light is close to natural light, and the colors of anatomic structures are reproduced more accurately [2,12]. A 300-W xenon light source is recommended to perform laparoscopy in cattle, especially if recording of the procedure is intended [6]. Light sources of less wattage (150 W), although not ideal, can be used to perform laparoscopic procedures under direct visualization. Halogen light sources cannot be compared with xenon light sources because halogen produces significantly fewer lumens per watt [12].

Most light sources have a bulb life meter. Newer versions of equipment have built-in spare bulbs that can be switched on if the primary bulb burns out during the procedure. Without this feature, an extra light bulb always should be readily available during any laparoscopic procedure; otherwise a sudden loss of the light would require the conversion of the laparoscopy to a laparotomy and potentially could place the patient at risk if it should occur at a crucial moment in the procedure [2,12].

Light cable

Light cables connect the light source and the laparoscope (see Fig. 3). They bring cold, high-intensity light into the abdominal cavity [20,21]. Light cables are made of bundles of optic fibers assembled and set in epoxy resin. Each optic fiber is made of a thin quartz rod, optically isolated with a layer of low refraction index quartz [20,21]. They transmit a light beam through their entire length with minimal loss of light intensity [20,21]. They also transport the light produced by an incandescent light bulb without transporting the heat it generates. For maximal illumination of the abdominal cavity, a large-diameter (minimum 6 mm) light cable should be used for bovine laparoscopy. A smaller diameter (4.5 mm) light cable, although not ideal, can be used to perform laparoscopic procedures under direct visualization. Optic fibers are fragile, and the light cable should be handled with care. With time and use, optic fibers break, and the light cable should be replaced. Broken optic fibers do not transmit light, and black "holes" appear in the light the cable projects onto a white surface. If more than 20% of the optic fibers appear to be broken, the light cable should be replaced because visualization becomes compromised [2,12].

Video camera and television monitor

Although the surgeon can look directly through the eyepiece of the laparoscope, a video camera attached to the laparoscope is used on modern equipment for bovine laparoscopy (see Fig. 3). Cameras with video feed ensure proper visibility with high-quality images, free up the head and both hands of the surgeon, and prevent contamination of the laparoscope eyepiece. Single-chip or three-chip cameras are commonly used. Three-chip cameras provide the best picture resolution, which is important when high-precision procedures, such as adhesiolysis, are performed [2,12].

Insufflation system

The insufflation system permits the creation of pneumoperitoneum. Pneumoperitoneum separates the body wall from the abdominal organs so that the surgeon can observe the abdominal organs and work inside the abdominal cavity [10]. Some authors do not recommend the use of insufflation and pneumoperitoneum and report that they can be associated with intraoperative discomfort, restlessness, and even collapse of the patient. In the author's opinion, when used correctly, pneumoperitoneum is useful and even mandatory when complex laparoscopic procedures, such as laparoscopic ovarian tumor removal, adhesiolysis, or resection of the apex of the bladder and umbilical structures, are performed [7]. The author has never observed any major intraoperative complications with intra-abdominal pressures of 15 mm Hg.

Automatic, high-flow insufflators (>10 L/min) usually are used to insufflate the bovine abdomen. These insufflators allow careful regulation of gas flow and intra-abdominal pressure and monitoring of the amount of gas left in the gas supply tank. Some authors use open cannulas or a medical pump for the insufflation of the bovine abdomen [6]. When the insufflator system used is not equipped with a manometer, some authors monitor the insufflated gas volume and use 5 to 35 L of gas, depending on the animal size and the extent of gastrointestinal filling, to obtain an adequate pneumoperitoneum [6,8,15]. Other authors insufflate gas until slight distention of the flank hollows is evident if the procedure is performed in standing animals [19] or until the craniad abdominal organs are visible and the abomasum is no longer in contact with the parietal peritoneum if the procedure is performed in dorsally recumbent cattle [22]. When an insufflation system is used, it is connected to one of the laparoscopic cannulas, through a tubing system. Carbon dioxide (CO_2) is the most widely used gas for insufflation because it is inexpensive and is the least likely to cause gaseous emboli compared with nitrous oxide, air, and helium. The primary disadvantage of CO_2 is the production of postoperative discomfort when it turns into carbonic acid on the moist peritoneal surfaces. This complication is reported frequently in people [23–25] and has been observed in horses [26–30]. The author has not observed this complication in calves or mature cows. Some insufflators use filtered ambient air as insufflating gas, which is an inexpensive and practical solution for field laparoscopy in cattle [8].

Trocar-cannula system

A trocar-cannula system is used to penetrate the body wall and allow introduction of the laparoscope and surgical instruments into the abdominal cavity (Figs. 5 and 6) [10]. Cannulas have a lateral Luer-Lok connector for the attachment of the insufflation tubing system (see Figs. 5 and 6). They also contain a one-way valve that allows for entry and exit of instruments with maintenance of the pneumoperitoneum. Disposable (see Fig. 5) and nondisposable (see Fig. 6) trocar-cannula systems can be used. The trocar preferred by the author is equipped with a security mechanism: It has a pyramid cutting edge and a spring-loaded safety shield. When it penetrates the abdominal wall, the safety shield is pushed back into the cannula (Fig. 7). As soon as the pyramid cutting edge of the trocar enters the abdominal cavity, the spring pushes out the safety shield with an audible click (Fig. 8). The risk of traumatizing intra-abdominal structures is minimized. In the author's experience, the most common complications associated with laparoscopy in cattle occur during the placement of the first trocar/cannula unit. This part of the procedure should be performed with great care and attention to detail and after having mastered the technique.

The total width of the body wall of a cow is relatively thin compared with that of a horse; 10-cm-long cannulas are usually adequate to perform laparoscopic procedures in cattle. The laparoscope and most laparoscopic instruments used in bovine laparoscopy are 10 mm in diameter; 10/12 mm trocar-cannula units are used. The internal diameter of the cannula is slightly larger than the outer diameter of the laparoscopes and instruments so that gas can be insufflated into the abdomen through one of the cannulas. Cattle have a relatively compliant body wall, and peritoneum tenting is a frequent complication during the insertion of the trocar-cannula units. To avoid this complication, the author recommends that trocar-cannula units be inserted with a slow pressing-drilling action. The drilling action aids trocar penetration of the body wall. In addition, manual compression on the abdomen during the maneuver increases the resistance to the advancing trocar and facilitates safe introduction.

Surgical instruments

Because the surgical site is far from the operator during laparoscopy, adapted surgical instrumentation is necessary [10]. A multitude of surgical

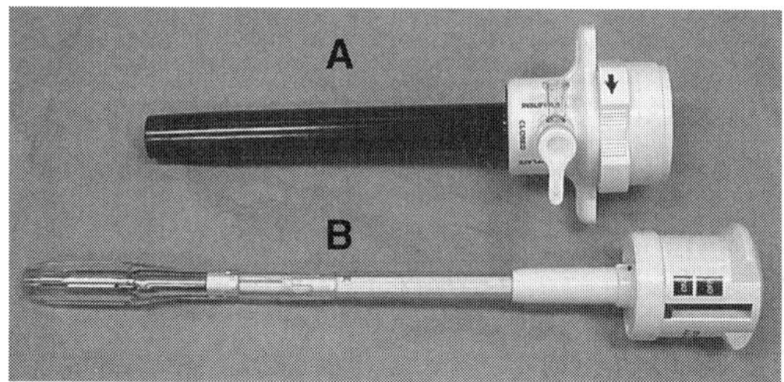

Fig. 5. Disposable cannula (*A*) and trocar (*B*) used for bovine laparoscopy.

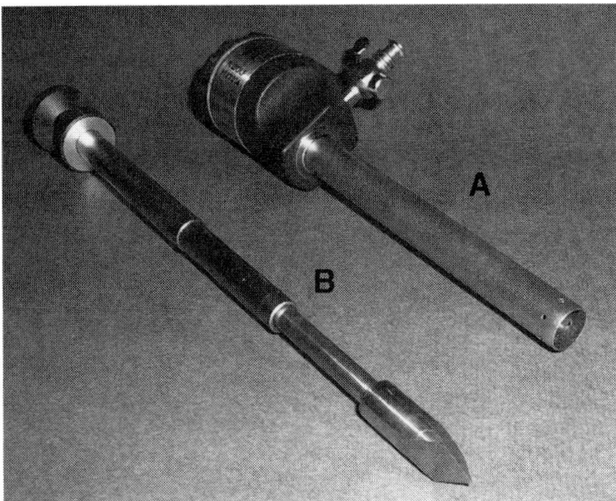

Fig. 6. Nondisposable cannula (*A*) and trocar (*B*) used for bovine laparoscopy.

instruments of a minimum 40 cm length exist for human laparoscopy and should be used when performing laparoscopy in cattle. The large size of abdominal organs in mature cows often requires the use of instruments of 10-mm diameter, especially when organs are manipulated, grasped, or retracted. The use of atraumatic forceps, such as laparoscopic Babcock forceps, or palpation probes for visceral manipulation are recommended to improve the quality of the examination in exploratory laparoscopy [10]. In most exploratory and simple laparoscopic surgical procedures, 10-mm diameter laparoscopic Babcock forceps, Kelly forceps, and Metzenbaum scissors are used (Fig. 9). For more complex procedures, endoscopic surturing devices, needle drivers, clips applicators, automatic staplers, pretied loop ligatures, and electrosurgical instrumentation are available.

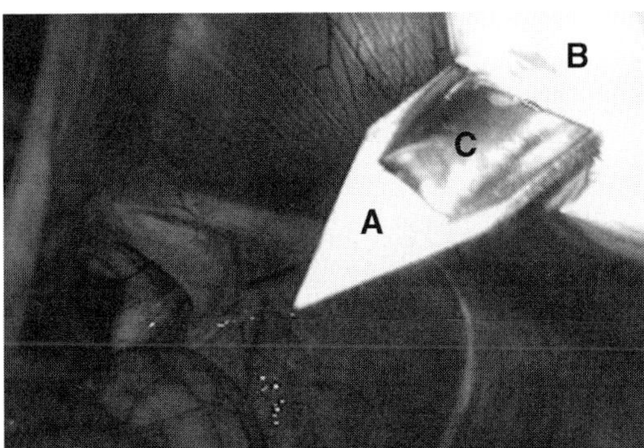

Fig. 7. Trocar-cannula unit with a safety mechanism used by the author. When the pyramid cutting edge (*A*) of the trocar penetrates the body wall (*B*), the safety shield (*C*) is pushed back into the cannula.

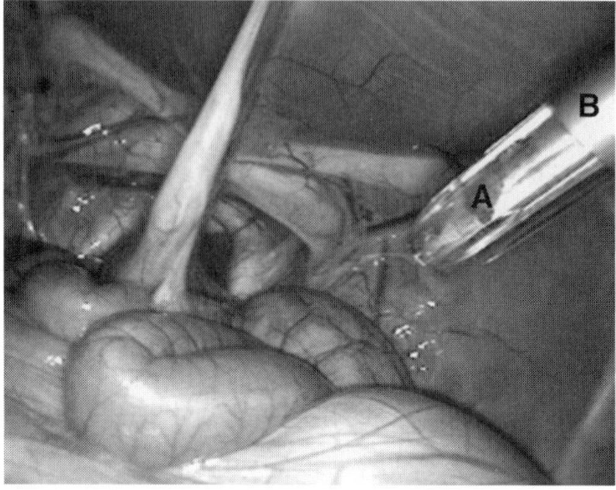

Fig. 8. Trocar-cannula unit with a safety mechanism used by the author. As soon as the trocar enters the abdominal cavity, the spring pushes the safety shield (*A*) out of the cannula (*B*) so that it covers the trocar pyramid cutting edge.

Disposable (see Fig. 9) and nondisposable (Fig. 10) laparoscopic instruments are available on the market. Disposable instruments are always sharp and do not need reassembling, but they increase significantly the cost of laparoscopic procedures if they are used as single-use instruments. Nondisposable instruments are durable and cost-effective in the long-term, but they require good maintenance, need to be reassembled after sterilization, and are expensive. The author prefers to use disposable laparoscopic instruments because they are convenient and can be used at least five times without loss of sharpness. Reusing disposable instruments, although not recommended by manufacturers, considerably decreases the cost of laparoscopic instruments.

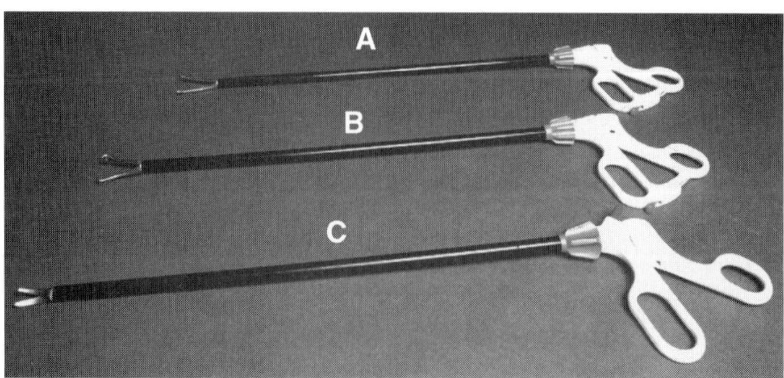

Fig. 9. Disposable laparoscopic Kelly forceps (*A*), Babcock forceps (*B*), and Metzenbaum scissors (*C*).

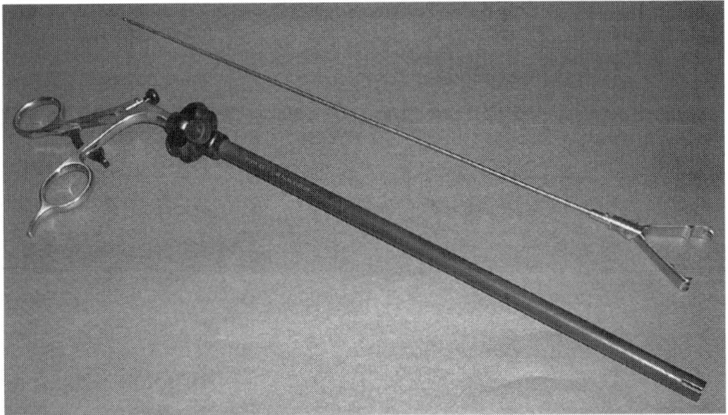

Fig. 10. Nondisposable disassembled laparoscopic claw forceps.

Patient preparation

Presurgical fasting is mandatory before any laparoscopic procedure [6,15]. The rumen and large intestine decrease in content and the intestinal peristalsis reduces during fasting. This reduces the risk of organ penetration during trocar introduction and improves the observation of the abdominal structures. In the author's experience, 24-hour fasting (water and food) is adequate in most mature dairy cows and thin beef cows. Roughage is withheld for 72 hours from heavy cows; they may receive concentrated feed up to 24 hours before the surgery. Calves less than 4 weeks old are not fasted before the surgery.

It is paramount to perform a rectal examination before a laparoscopic procedure is done through the paralumbar fossae. This examination helps to assess the thickness of the body wall, localize the abdominal structures and the portal sites, and empty the rectum. During this examination, the abdominal cavity also is assessed for any abnormalities, such as adhesions, masses, or dilated abdominal organs.

When the laparoscopy is performed standing, it is recommended that the cow be bathed before it is walked into the operating room. Bathing prevents gross contamination of the operating room and improves sterility of the surgical procedure itself; this is particularly important if the cow is coming straight out of the field for surgery. Some authors do not recommend the use of perioperative medication for laparoscopy in cattle [8]. The author still administers routine perioperative medication (antibiotics and nonsteroidal anti-inflammatory drugs) before and for 24 hours after the surgery.

Patient restraint

In preparation for standing laparoscopy, although docile animals can be placed in stocks, aggressive animals should be placed in a squeeze chute

(Fig. 11). Exploratory standing laparoscopy on docile animals commonly is accomplished with minimal animal stress using only physical restraint and local anesthesia of the portal sites (8–10 mL of 2% mepivacaine solution) [6]. Sedation is used when dealing with aggressive animals or when complex laparoscopic surgical procedures are performed [8,15]. The combination of xylazine (0.01 mg/kg intravenously) and butorphanol tartrate (0.02 mg/kg intravenously) is used for chemical restraint and analgesia.

When laparoscopy is performed on sedated animals placed in dorsal recumbency, nasal oxygen supplementation (15 L/min) is recommended [18,22]. If the procedure is performed under general anesthesia, it is mandatory to place an orotracheal tube immediately after induction and use a positive-pressure ventilator to ventilate the animal before creating the pneumoperitoneum.

Basic laparoscopic surgical technique

Historically, two insertion sites have been described for entry of the laparoscope during standing laparoscopy in cattle: the vaginal fornix and the paralumbar fossa [1,6,9,15,18,19]. The author's preferred technique for standing laparoscopic examination in cattle is direct insertion of the laparoscope and instruments in the paralumbar fossa.

Before preparation of the surgical sites, the animal's tail is tied to its hock or neck on the opposite side of the surgery. One or both paralumbar fossae are clipped and prepared for aseptic surgery. The abdominal wall is infiltrated with a local anesthetic (8–10 mL of 2% mepivacaine solution per site) at the portal sites. A pneumoperitoneum can be created before or after

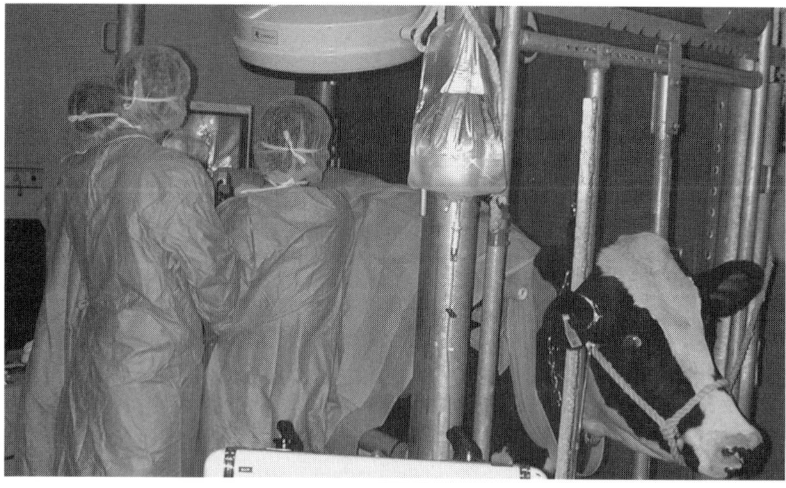

Fig. 11. Standing right flank laparoscopy performed on a dairy cow.

the insertion of the laparoscopic cannula into the abdomen. If the pneumoperitoneum is created first, a 1-cm skin incision is made, and a 120-mm-long Veress needle (Figs. 12 and 13), teat cannula, or 12F catheter is inserted into the abdominal cavity. The instrument is attached to an insufflator, and the insufflation begins. If the pneumoperitoneum is created after insertion of the laparoscopic cannula, the gas source is connected directly to this cannula as soon as it is in place. The author prefers the latter option and places the laparoscopic cannula using an open laparoscopy technique. A 1-cm minilaparotomy incision is made at the portal site, and the first cannula is introduced bluntly in the abdomen. This technique dramatically decreases the risk of penetrating an abdominal viscus during

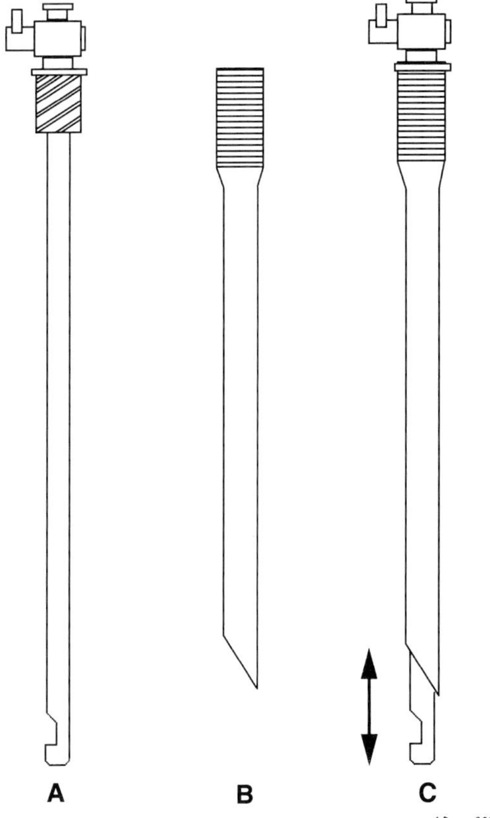

Fig. 12. Veress needles have a sharp cutting tip and contain a spring-loaded blunt obturator. When the Veress needle penetrates the abdominal wall, the spring-loaded blunt obturator is pushed back into the needle. As soon as the cutting tip of the needle enters the abdominal cavity, the spring pushes out the blunt obturator and protects the abdominal organs from injury by the sharp tip of the needle. (*A*) Spring-loaded blunt obturator of the Veress needle. (*B*) Sharp tip of the Veress needle. (*C*) Veress needle.

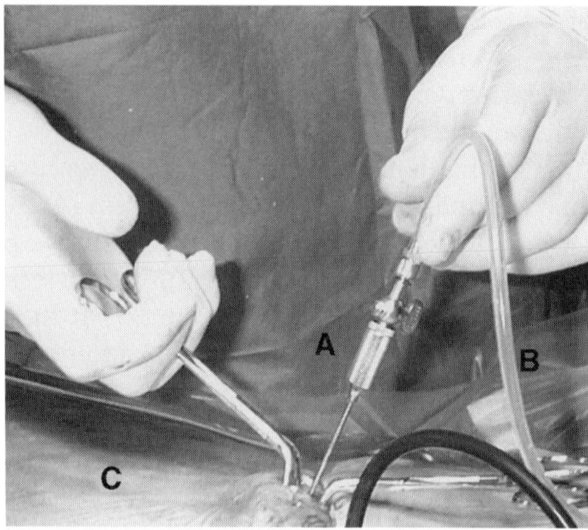

Fig. 13. Veress needle (*A*) connected to an insufflator by a tubing system (*B*) is inserted through the body wall (*C*) to create a pneumoperitoneum before the laparoscopic cannula is inserted.

the insertion of the laparoscopic cannula. When the first cannula is placed through the body wall, the trocar is replaced with a 10-mm, 0° or 30° laparoscope with a video camera and fiberoptic light cable attached. A rapid examination of the surrounding intra-abdominal structures is performed to determine if trauma caused by the cannula insertion had occurred. Tubing connected to the insufflator is attached to the cannula. The intra-abdominal pressure is increased to 8 to 12 mm Hg, which requires 15 to 35 L of CO_2 for a mature dairy cow depending on its size. If intra-abdominal pressure or volume outflow could not be monitored, insufflation is stopped when organs are visualized, and the laparoscope can move freely in the abdomen. Excessive abdominal distention may increase the distance between the abdominal wall and the affected organs sufficiently to prevent any adequate manipulation with conventional laparoscopic instruments.

For an exploratory laparoscopy, the procedure starts with a right paralumbar approach (see Fig. 11). The laparoscopic cannula is inserted in the middle of the fossa, dorsally to the crus of the internal oblique muscle. The particular interests of the surgeon determine the entry sites for the palpation probes or laparoscopic surgical instruments. The sites are determined using the triangulation principle and generally are located 4 to 6 cm to the right or left of the laparoscope portal site. To avoid injury to the abdominal structures, instrument cannulas are introduced under laparoscopic guidance. Instruments never are introduced blindly into the cannula because severe injuries to peritoneal structures may occur. Before introducing an instrument into a particular cannula, the laparoscope is positioned so that the end of the cannula is visible inside the optical field. The instrument is pushed slowly in the cannula and enters the abdominal cavity under laparoscopic guidance. If forceps or scissors are used, the jaws are kept closed until the instrument reaches the surgical site.

After the exploration of the right abdomen is completed, the left paralumbar fossa is entered. This approach provides a more limited exploration of the abdominal cavity because the rumen generally occupies most of the left side of the animal. With the left paralumbar fossa approach, it is crucial that the animal is fasted for at least 24 to 48 hours to reduce the rumen size. The laparoscopic cannula is introduced in the caudodorsal aspect of the left paralumbar fossa to avoid penetrating the rumen lumen. If by accident a cannula is introduced in the rumen lumen, it is left in situ, the portal site is enlarged dorsally and ventrally using sharp instruments, and a pair of Babcock forceps is used to grasp the rumen wall ventral and dorsal to the cannula. The rumen wall and the cannula are exteriorized by applying traction on both Babcock forceps. The cannula is removed, and the rumen wall routinely is closed with a two-layer closure technique using a closure surgical kit. The site is lavaged with sterile 0.9% sodium chloride solution and placed back in the abdomen. After changing sterile gloves, the surgeon can continue with the laparoscopy using an open laparoscopic technique.

For a thorough exploration of the abdomen, a cranioventral midline laparoscopy can be performed with the animal placed in dorsal recumbency [18]. The laparoscopic cannula is inserted on the linea alba, 10 cm caudal to the xiphoid process [18].

When the laparoscopic examination is complete, the endoscope is removed, and the surgeon releases the CO_2 gas/air via the open cannulas. The portal sites are not sutured until the end of the procedure, after all gas has been evacuated; this limits subcutaneous emphysema around the surgical sites and allows the maximal amount of CO_2 to escape and helps prevent postoperative discomfort.

The cannulas are removed, and closure of the portal sites is performed. The external sheath of external abdominal oblique muscles or the linea alba is closed using one or two simple interrupted sutures, ensuring that the omentum or part of the intestine is not incorporated in the closure; this prevents hernia formation and results in incisions with excellent cosmetic appearance. Skin and subcutaneous tissues are closed in a routine manner. Normal feed is reintroduced within hours after the surgery. If the procedure is performed without complications, systemic antibiotics and nonsteroidal anti-inflammatory drugs are required for only 24 hours after the surgery.

Advanced laparoscopic surgical technique

Exploratory laparoscopy or simple laparoscopic surgical procedures, such as laparoscopic biopsy collection, are performed using basic laparoscopic techniques [1,6,13,15,18,31]. It is beyond the scope of this article to describe complex laparoscopic procedures, such as laparoscopic adhesiolysis, laparoscopic abomasopexy, and laparoscopic resection of the umbilical structures and apex of the bladder [7,8,22]. These procedures all are performed using advanced laparoscopic surgical techniques and skills. During complex procedures, the primary surgeon uses both hands to handle laparoscopic instruments, and the assistant surgeon drives the laparoscope (Fig. 14). Skills such as the ability to focus on a two-dimensional field, receive tactile input from both hands, and apply tension and counter-tension with laparoscopic instruments are required to perform complex laparoscopic procedures. These skills are gained with practice and experience.

Tissue handling and retraction

Techniques for handling tissue during laparoscopic surgery are difficult to teach and learn [32]. For the novice laparoscopist, it is initially hard to determine how tightly tissue can be grasped and manipulated. These techniques are learned most often by trial and error. Training on cadaver tissues in training boxes and during terminal surgical exercises is paramount to develop laparoscopic tissue handling skills.

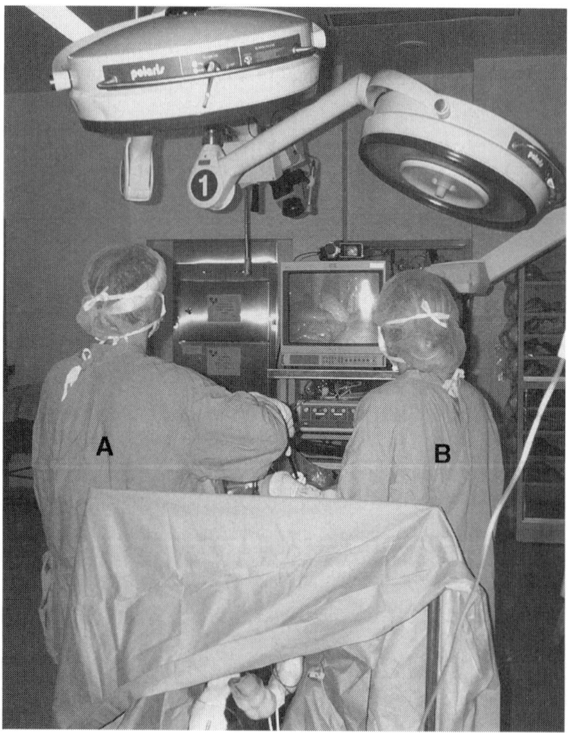

Fig. 14. During advanced laparoscopic surgical procedures, the primary surgeon (*A*) uses both hands to handle laparoscopic instruments, and the assistant surgeon (*B*) drives the laparoscope.

Most often at the beginning of a laparoscopic procedure, the surgical site is not readily visible or accessible. Retraction of the surrounding tissue and organs is required to improve observation of the operative site and to gain good access. Tilting and rotating the animal are effective methods of retraction during laparoscopy performed under general anesthesia [32]. Specialized instrumentation, such as laparoscopic retractors and bowel clamps, also are available (Fig. 15). They are introduced at the beginning of the procedure and used to manipulate the surrounding tissue and organs away from the surgical site. During the procedure, these instruments also can be applied directly to the tissue to aid in the retraction and exposure of the operative site. An additional portal site sometimes is required to introduce the laparoscopic retractor in the abdomen. The assistant surgeon is usually in charge of maintaining adequate retraction so that the primary surgeon can perform the procedure with good visibility [32].

Dissection

As in open surgery, blunt and sharp dissections can be performed during laparoscopic surgery. Conventional (open) and laparoscopic dissections follow the same rules. Dissections ideally follow tissue plans and depend on traction and countertraction, and blunt dissection is performed in relatively avascular areas [32]. Blunt dissection is performed using grasping forceps, such as Babcock forceps, and atraumatic instruments, such as palpation probes, atraumatic Kelly forceps, or Cherry dissectors (Fig. 16). Grasping forceps and Metzenbaum scissors usually are used for sharp dissection (Fig. 17). During dissection, the tissue is grasped and elevated with the grasping forceps held in the surgeon's nondominant hand, and the dissection is performed with the dissecting instruments held in the surgeon's dominant hand [32]. The magnification provided by the laparoscope permits precise and complex dissection, such as that required during laparoscopic adhesiolysis [33,34].

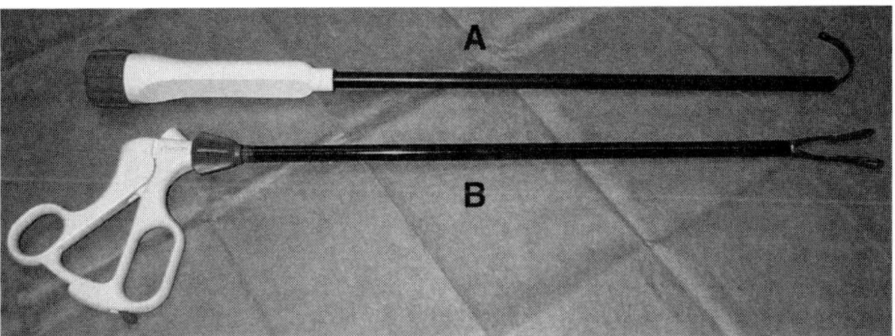

Fig. 15. During a laparoscopic procedure, laparoscopic retractors (*A*) and bowel clamps (*B*) are used to manipulate the surrounding tissue and organs away from the surgical site.

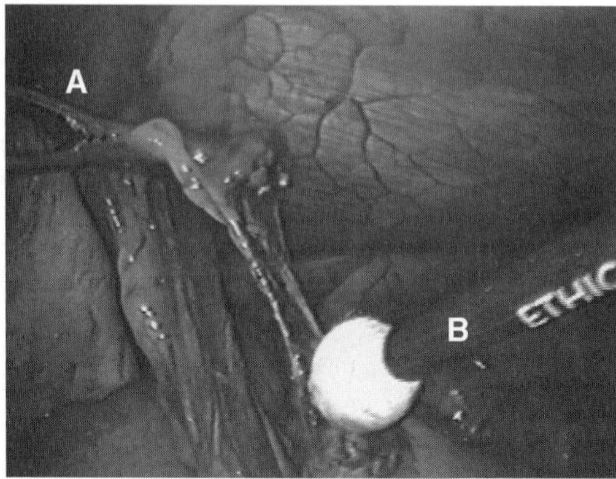

Fig. 16. Blunt dissection is performed using grasping forceps, such as Babcock forceps (*A*), and atraumatic instruments, such as a Cherry dissector (*B*).

Hemostasis

Anticipation and control of intraoperative bleeding is paramount during laparoscopic surgery. A small amount of blood can obscure the laparoscopic surgical site because it absorbs the light and can cover the lens of the laparoscope [32]. Transected blood vessels may retract into the tissue, which makes the source of the bleeding difficult to identify and isolate under laparoscopic conditions. Similar to in open surgery, several techniques can be used to control intraoperative bleeding during laparoscopy. Minor bleeding can be contained by applying pressure using a palpation probe or a Cherry dissector (see Fig. 16). Temporary control also can be achieved by clamping the tissue with grasping forceps. Major bleeding usually is

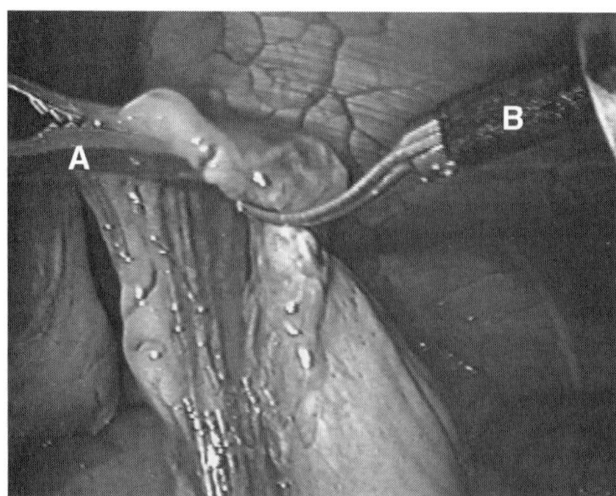

Fig. 17. Sharp dissection is performed using grasping forceps, such as Babcock forceps (*A*) and Metzenbaum scissors (*B*).

controlled using monopolar or bipolar electrosurgery, hemostatic clip appliers (Fig. 18), pretied loop ligatures, or automatic staplers. Uncontrolled intraoperative hemorrhage is an indication for prompt conversion to laparotomy [32].

Tissue approximation

Extirpative techniques, such as ovariectomy and cryptorchidectomy, are the most frequently reported laparoscopic surgical techniques in large animals [28,30,35]. The use of reconstructive laparoscopic surgery is still limited in these species mainly because of difficult, time-consuming, or expensive methods of intra-abdominal tissue approximation. Automatic laparoscopic staplers are available but expensive. Laparoscopic suturing can be performed using either extracorporeal or intracorporeal knots techniques [36]. Extracorporeal knots are tied outside the abdominal cavity and advanced into the abdomen using a knot push rod. The extracorporeal knots usually are used for hemostasis, pedicle ligation, collection of biopsy specimens, and tissue approximation [36]. Extracorporeal knots are inconvenient for the closure of large defects. Laparoscopic surgeons can tie extracorporeal knots or use pretied sutures (Endoloop ligatures) [36]. Excellent descriptions and reviews of extracorporeal knot–tying techniques have been published [36,37]. Intracorporeal knots are created entirely within the abdominal cavity [36]. These knots allow for ligature and simple interrupted or continuous suture patterns to be performed within the abdomen. Intracorporeal suturing can be performed using either two laparoscopic needle drivers or a special endoscopic suturing device [36,37]. Intracorporeal suturing is the most challenging technique used during laparoscopic surgery [36,37]. There is a steep learning curve associated with gaining proficiency in laparoscopic suturing using two laparoscopic needle holders, but an endoscopic suturing device that can be used to tie intracorporeal square knots, surgeon's knots, and a variety of slipknots during laparoscopic surgery in large animals is commercially available (Figs. 19 and 20) [7]. The main advantage of this endoscopic suturing device is that the learning curve associated with gaining proficiency is short.

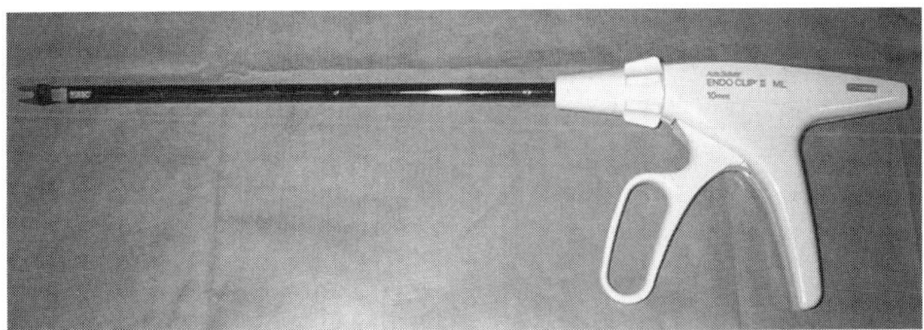

Fig. 18. Laparoscopic clips applier.

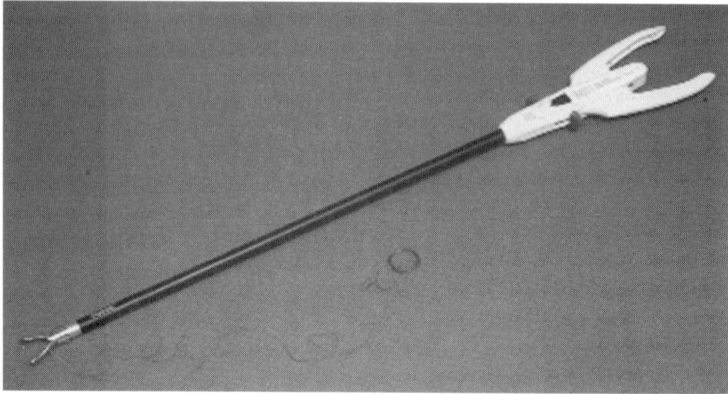

Fig. 19. An endoscopic suturing device that can be used to tie intracorporeal square knots, surgeon's knots, and a variety of slipknots during laparoscopic surgery in large animals; this item is commercially available.

Tissue removal

Removal of diseased tissue isolated or dissected during laparoscopic surgery often requires abdominal incisions larger than the one used for the cannulas (Fig. 21). In the author's opinion, conventional open techniques require the abdominal incision size to be determined more by the location rather than the size of the tissue to be removed. One of the advantages of laparoscopic surgery is that the diseased tissue can be accessed and dissected through only three 10-mm portal sites. The tissue can be removed through an abdominal incision just large enough to pull the diseased tissue through (usually much smaller than a laparotomy incision would be). This abdominal incision usually is made extending the incisions between two cannula portal sites. Infected or tumoral tissue may be removed in specimen retrieval bags. These bags are introduced in the abdomen through a cannula.

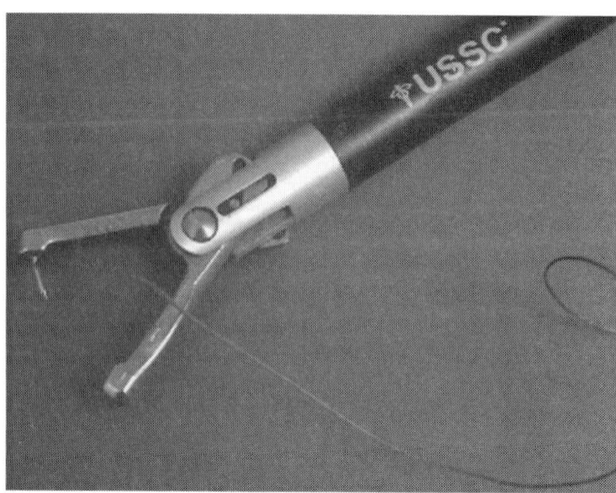

Fig. 20. Close-up view of the jaws of the endoscopic suturing device.

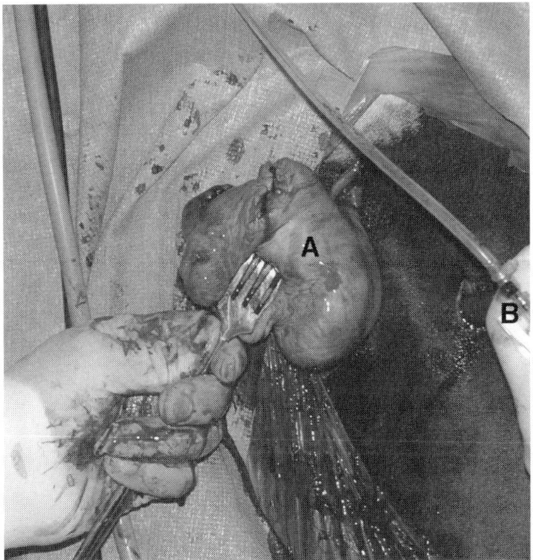

Fig. 21. Extending the incisions between two laparoscopic portal sites allows the removal of a large bovine ovarian tumor (*A*) after its pedicle has been ligated and sectioned under laparoscopic guidance. Laparoscopic cannula (*B*).

The specimen is placed under laparoscopic guidance in the introduced open bag. The cannula is removed, the portal site is enlarged, and the bag is pulled out of the abdomen through the enlarged portal site. With the help of laparoscopic scissors and under laparoscopic guidance, it is possible to morcellate the specimen within the bag to decrease its size.

Summary

Laparoscopic surgery is minimally invasive and minimally traumatic in cattle. It allows the animal to return rapidly to production. These techniques are destined to develop further, especially in the dairy and show cattle industries, where recovery periods must be as short as possible. Although it is important to remain skeptical about new procedures if they do not offer advantages over open techniques, in many cases laparoscopy is clearly superior. Laparoscopy is not an easy surgical technique. It requires a good knowledge of anatomy and abdominal topography and rigorous training. It must be performed with great care and delicacy because complications, such as perforated organs, can occur. Laparoscopy also requires the use of sophisticated and costly technology.

References

[1] Traub-Dargatz J. Laparoscopy, endoscopy, and surgical biopsy in large animals. In: Anderson DE, editor. Veterinary gastroenterology. Malvern (PA): Lea & Febiger; 1992. p. 61–9.

[2] Freeman L. Operating room set-up, equipment, and instrumentation. In: Freeman L, editor. Veterinary endosurgery. St. Louis: Mosby; 1999. p. 3–23.
[3] Nord H. Technique of laparoscopy. In: Sivak M, editor. Gastroenterologic endoscopy. Philadelphia: WB Saunders; 1987. p. 994–1029.
[4] Berci G, Cuschieri A. Historical notes. In: Berci G, Cuschieri A, editors. Practical laparoscopy. London: Balliere Tindall; 1986. p. 1–2.
[5] Klohnen A. History of laparoscopy in animals and humans. In: Fischer AT, editor. Equine diagnostic and surgical laparoscopy. Philadelphia: WB Saunders; 2002. p. 3–5.
[6] Maxwell D, Kraemer D. Laparoscopy in cattle. In: Harrison RM, Wildt DE, editors. Animal laparoscopy. Baltimore: Williams & Wilkins; 1980. p. 133–57.
[7] Boure L, Foster RA, Palmer M, et al. Use of an endoscopic suturing device for laparoscopic resection of the apex of the bladder and umbilical structures in normal neonatal calves. Vet Surg 2001;30:319–26.
[8] Janowitz H. Laparoscopic reposition and fixation of the left displaced abomasum in cattle. Tierarztl Prax 1998;26:308–13.
[9] Santl B, Wenigerkind H, Schernthaner W, et al. Comparison of ultrasound-guided vs laparoscopic transvaginal ovum pick-up (OPU) in simmental heifers. Theriogenology 1998; 50:89–100.
[10] Fischer AT. Basic laparoscopic techniques and training. In: Fischer AT, editor. Equine diagnostic and surgical laparoscopy. Philadelphia: WB Saunders; 2002. p. 29–35.
[11] Wilson A, Ferguson J. Use of flexible fiberoptic laparoscope as a diagnostic aid in cattle. Can Vet J 1984;25:229–34.
[12] Chamness C. Nondisposable instrumentation for equine laparoscopy. In: Fischer AT, editor. Equine diagnostic and surgical laparoscopy. Philadelphia: WB Saunders; 2002. p. 37–49.
[13] Guay P, Bedoya M. A study of the equivalence between rectal palpation, laparoscopy, laparotomy and ovarian dissection for evaluation of the ovarian response of PMSG-superovulated cows. Can Vet J 1981;22:353–5.
[14] Lambert R, Bernard C, Rioux J, et al. Endoscopy in cattle by paralumbar route: technique for ovarian examination and follicular aspiration. Theriogenology 1983;20:149–61.
[15] Steiner A, Zulauf M. Diagnostic laparoscopy in the cow. Schweiz Arch Tierheilkd 1999;141: 397–406.
[16] Seeger K. Laparoscopic investigation of the bovine ovary. Vet Med Small Anim Clin 1977; 72:1037–44.
[17] Sirard M, Lambert R, Beland R, et al. The effects of repeated laparoscopic surgery used for ovarian examination and follicular aspiration in cows. Anim Reprod Sci 1985;9:25–30.
[18] Anderson DE, Gaughan EM, St-Jean G. Normal laparoscopic anatomy of the bovine abdomen. Am J Vet Res 1993;54:1170–6.
[19] Reichenbach HD, Wiebke NH, Modl J, et al. Laparoscopy through the vaginal fornix of cows for the repeated aspiration of follicular oocytes. Vet Rec 1994;135:353–6.
[20] Prescott R. Optical principles of laparoscopy. In: Harrison R, Wildt D, editors. Animal laparoscopy. Baltimore: Williams & Wilkins; 1980. p. 15–29.
[21] Prescott R. Optical principles of endoscopy. J Med Primatol 1976;5:133–47.
[22] Babkine M, Desrochers A, Bouré L, et al. Ventral laparoscopic abomasopexy on adult cattle. Méd Vét Québec 2004;34:154.
[23] Van Glabeke E, Mandron E, Desrez G, et al. Review on the use of CO_2 in laparoscopy surgery. Prog Urol 1998;8:586–9.
[24] Sharp JR, Pierson WP, Brady CE 3rd. Comparison of CO_2- and N_2O-induced discomfort during peritoneoscopy under local anesthesia. Gastroenterology 1982;82:453–6.
[25] Holthausen UH, Nagelschmidt M, Troidl H. CO_2 pneumoperitoneum: what we know and what we need to know. World J Surg 1999;23:794–800.
[26] Fischer AT Jr, Lloyd KC, Carlson GP, et al. Diagnostic laparoscopy in the horse. J Am Vet Med Assoc 1986;189:289–92.

[27] Fischer AT Jr. Standing laparoscopic surgery. Vet Clin North Am Equine Pract 1991;7: 641–7.

[28] Fischer AT Jr, Vachon AM. Laparoscopic cryptorchidectomy in horses. J Am Vet Med Assoc 1992;201:1705–8.

[29] Bouré L, Marcoux M, Laverty S. Laparoscopic abdominal anatomy of foals positioned in dorsal recumbency. Vet Surg 1997;26:1–6.

[30] Bouré L, Marcoux M, Laverty S. Paralumbar fossa laparoscopic ovariectomy in horses with use of Endoloop ligatures. Vet Surg 1997;26:478–83.

[31] Naoi M, Kokue E, Takahashi Y, et al. Laparoscopic-assisted serial biopsy of the bovine kidney. Am J Vet Res 1985;46:699–702.

[32] Kolata R, Freeman L. Access, port placement and basic endosurgical skills. In: Freeman L, editor. Veterinary endosurgery. St. Louis: Mosby; 1999. p. 44–60.

[33] Bouré LP, Pearce SG, Kerr CL, et al. Evaluation of laparoscopic adhesiolysis for the treatment of experimentally induced adhesions in pony foals. Am J Vet Res 2002;63:289–94.

[34] Bouré L, Marcoux M, Lavoie JP, et al. Use of laparoscopic equipment to divide abdominal adhesions in a filly. J Am Vet Med Assoc 1998;212:845–7.

[35] Walmsley JP. Review of equine laparoscopy and an analysis of 158 laparoscopies in the horse. Equine Vet J 1999;31:456–64.

[36] Pasic R, Levine RL. Laparoscopic suturing and ligation techniques. J Am Assoc Gynecol Laparosc 1995;3:67–79.

[37] Palmer S. Selected laparoscopic suturing and knot-tying techniques. In: Fischer AT, editor. Equine diagnostic and surgical laparoscopy. Philadelphia: WB Saunders; 2002. p. 91–101.

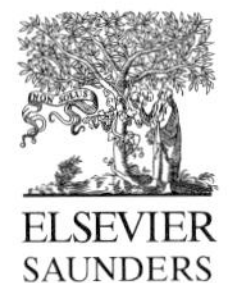

ELSEVIER
SAUNDERS

Vet Clin Food Anim 21 (2005) 251–279

VETERINARY
CLINICS
Food Animal Practice

Laparoscopic Surgery in Adult Cattle

Marie Babkine, DMV, DES*,
André Desrochers, DMV, MS

Department of Clinical Sciences, Faculté de Médecine Vétérinaire, Université de Montréal, 3200, Sicotte, St Hyacinthe, Québec, J2S 6K9, Canada

Laparoscopy or celioscopy is a minimally invasive technique that permits the observation of the abdominal organs. Laparoscopy has been used routinely in human medicine since the 1980s [1,2]. The development of this technique has not been limited to diagnosis and has benefited from advances in surgical techniques using laparoscopy [3,4]. The many advantages of this technique have been recognized rapidly. Minimal invasion of the abdominal cavity is not only esthetically advantageous, but also therapeutically beneficial. Because this technique causes little pain, patients are hospitalized for shorter periods and return to normal activity levels quickly [5–7].

Several authors have used laparoscopy in cattle [8] to describe normal anatomy [9], to evaluate the different structures of the reproductive system [10], to use as a guide for renal biopsy [11], to help diagnose traumatic reticuloperitonitis [12], and to describe a method of bladder and umbilical structure resection in the calf [13]. In 1998, Janowitz [14] described a laparoscopic technique for the correction and fixation of a left displaced abomasum.

Laparoscopy in cattle permits the visualization of the different abdominal organs. It may be performed via a ventral, right, or left flank approach. It is important to master the basics of laparoscopic anatomy because the abdomen cannot be explored in entirety via one port of entry. For example, the reticulum can be explored only by a ventral approach.

* Corresponding author.
E-mail address: marie.babkine@umontreal.ca (M. Babkine).

doi:10.1016/j.cvfa.2004.12.003 ***vetfood.theclinics.com***

Laparoscopic technique

Equipment

Standard equipment is used. A rigid, 0° laparoscope measuring between 30 cm (Richard Wolf GmbH, Knittlingen, Germany) and 42 cm (Dr Fritz GmbH, Tuttlingen, Germany) in length and having a diameter between 8 mm (Dr Fritz GmbH, Tuttlingen, Germany) and 10 mm (Richard Wolf GmbH, Knittlingen, Germany) is used. The light source consists of a 150-W halogen bulb. Depending on the company, abdominal insufflators use either carbon dioxide (Richard Wolf GmbH, Knittlingen, Germany) or filtered ambient air (Dr Fritz GmbH, Tuttlingen, Germany) and may possess a pressure control system (Richard Wolf GmbH, Knittlingen, Germany).

To obtain a pneumoperitoneum, it is recommendable to use a 15-cm Veress needle (Richard Wolf GmbH, Knittlingen, Germany). In certain animals, such as overly conditioned or muscular beef cattle, the use of a longer Veress needle (24 cm; Richard Wolf GmbH, Knittlingen, Germany) is preferable so that penetration of the peritoneal space is ensured.

The trocar/cannula units used by the authors are standardized. The 8-mm (internal diameter) trocar measures 12 cm in length (Dr Fritz GmbH, Tuttlingen, Germany). It allows the entry of an 8-mm (external diameter) laparoscope (Dr Fritz GmbH, Tuttlingen, Germany). The 10-mm (internal diameter) trocar measures 10 cm, 12.5 cm, or 15 cm (Richard Wolf GmbH, Knittlingen, Germany). It allows for the passage of a 10-mm (external diameter) (Richard Wolf GmbH, Knittlingen, Germany) laparoscope or instruments measuring 10 mm in diameter (eg, grasping forceps). In the case of obese animals, the 15-cm trocar may be preferential. The 5.5-mm (internal diameter) trocar measures 10 cm (Richard Wolf GmbH, Knittlingen, Germany) to 12 cm (Dr Fritz GmbH, Tuttlingen, Germany) in length and allows for the passage of instruments that are 5 mm in diameter (eg, needle holders, scissors).

Preparation and anesthesia of subjects

Whenever possible, the animal should be off feed for 24 to 48 hours. For interventions requiring dorsal recumbence, this preventive method may help to diminish risks related to this positioning and the chances of rumen perforation during the insertion of the primary trocar.

The flank or ventral abdomen is surgically prepared—shaved, washed, and scrubbed. If the intervention is performed on the left or right flank, a paravertebral anesthesia of T13, L1, and L2 is done. Other authors perform only local anesthesia at the site of the trocar insertion [14,15]. For ventral interventions, the animal is sedated with xylazine (0.05–0.1 mg/kg intravenously) or acepromazine (0.1 mg/kg intramuscularly 30 minutes before laying the animal down) and placed and maintained in dorsal recumbency with the use of cables on the limbs. After surgical preparation, insertion sites of the trocar/cannula units are anesthetized with a local infiltration of 2% lidocaine.

Surgical technique

Right flank

Pneumoperitoneum is obtained after the introduction of the Veress needle into the abdominal cavity [16] or after the direct insertion of the trocar into the abdominal cavity without prior pneumoperitoneum [15,17,18]. The authors are more comfortable with the use of the Veress needle because there are fewer chances of penetration of digestive organs or other possible negative consequences with this technique.

The site of entry of the Veress needle or the primary trocar varies depending on the author. According to Anderson et al [15], a cutaneous incision approximately 2 cm in length is executed 5 cm behind the caudal aspect of the last rib and 8 cm ventral to the extremity of the transverse processes. Guidoni et al [16] propose two possible entry sites depending on the observations that are required. For visualization of the abdominal organs, the same incision site as Anderson described is used. A more caudal entry site, 5 cm below the point of the hip in the hollow of the flank, is proposed for visualization of the pelvic organs. The authors suggest an entry site 10 cm below the transverse processes and in the middle of the flank to ensure access to the abdominal and the pelvic cavities. If the animal is too large, or the laparoscope is too small, a second trocar may be inserted to allow access to the desired area. The Veress needle or the primary trocar is introduced via an incision in the abdominal cavity and is oriented caudally at a 45° angle in relation to the sagittal plane of the cow. As soon as the needle or trocar pierces the abdominal wall, air should be heard entering the abdomen. To ensure that a digestive organ has not been perforated, the air escaping the abdomen must be odorless. The insufflator may be attached, and a pneumoperitoneum is induced. At this time, a possible complication besides the accidental penetration of a digestive organ would be the detachment of the peritoneum because of an insufficiently long or incorrectly positioned needle. If during insufflation the intra-abdominal pressure increases too quickly, or if the abdomen does not distend uniformly, it is preferable to stop insufflation and check for retroperitoneal distention by transrectal examination. In the case in which the peritoneum is slightly detached, it is preferable to restart the insufflation through the left flank and insert a trocar in the right flank only after the pneumoperitoneum has been established.

Insufflation of the cow's abdomen by means of the left flank has been recommended [16] because the peritoneum is less prone to detachment on this side; this is probably due to the fact that the rumen takes up more space on the left flank and keeps the peritoneum against the abdominal wall. More recently, the authors used a 5-mm trocar directly inserted through the left flank, avoiding any peritoneal tenting, even if the laparoscopy itself is performed in the right flank. (Dr Hans Janowitz, personnal communication, 2004). After previously incising the skin, the trocar is inserted 5 cm ventral to the transverse process and 5 cm cranial to the ilium. The trocar is oriented caudally with an angle of 45° in relation to the sagittal plan of the cow. The trocar itself is removed, and the valve is kept open to let the air penetrate the abdominal cavity freely. By removing the top portion of the cannula, the air moves a lot faster into the abdomen. This technique precludes the use of an insufflator in some situations (Fig. 1).

Insufflation is done when all organs are sufficiently separated, without exceeding a pressure of 20 mm Hg, as suggested by Anderson [19]. Exploration of the abdominal cavity may begin by orienting the laparoscope cranially.

Left flank

A pneumoperitoneum is induced in the same manner as for the right flank. The Veress needle is introduced through a 1-cm incision in the middle of the left flank (or 5 cm behind the caudal aspect of the last rib according to Anderson [19]), 8 to 10 cm beneath the transverse processes, oriented caudally with a 45° angle in relation to the sagittal plane of the cow. In such a way, perforation of the rumen is avoided. The trocar is inserted in the same direction.

Ventral

Anderson et al [15,19] proposes a medial, cranioventral path. After a standard preparation, a 2-cm-long, full-thickness body wall incision is performed 10 cm caudal to the xyphoid process. The examination of the cranioventral abdomen begins with the central portion of the diaphragm.

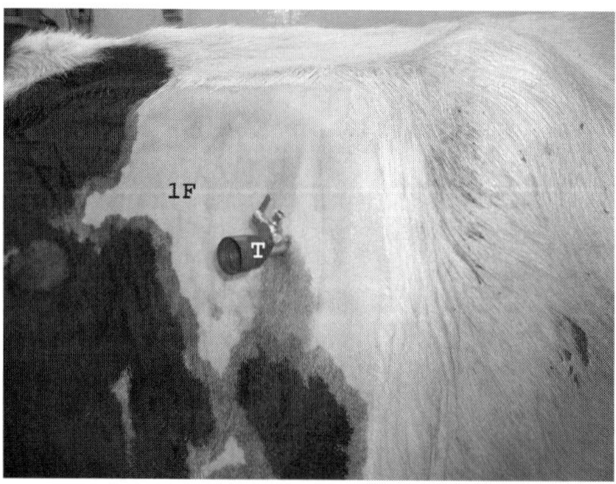

Fig. 1. Visualization of a pneumoperitoneum was obtained after the insertion of a 5-mm trocar into the abdominal cavity. The cannula is open to let air go into the abdomen freely. lF, left flank; T, open cannula.

The authors propose a more caudal approach, especially if a ventral laparoscopic abomasopexy has to be performed. After a standard preparation of the site, a full-thickness abdominal wall incision is made left of the umbilicus. Perforation of the dilated abomasum is avoided. The 8-mm trocar/cannula unit is inserted into the abdomen and is directed cranially at a 45° angle with respect to abdomen. Insufflation is achieved directly through the cannula. Of 10 cows that underwent ventral laparoscopy, the authors reported no major complications on the introduction of the trocar, although in 4 cows there was accidental penetration of the omental leaves. When insufflation begins, the laparoscope is introduced into the abdomen by the cannula to ensure that it is in the right position. A left-to-right abdominal exploration provides a good view of the cranioventral abdomen.

Normal anatomy

After extensive use of different laparoscopes, light sources, and cameras, the authors have noted that the abdominal organs take on different tints and hues, and that the image quality may vary. Among the following anatomic descriptions, more emphasis is placed on the identifiable structures and their localization using pictures and diagrams than on the aspect that these structures may have.

Right flank

The laparoscope is oriented cranially in the abdominal cavity (Fig. 2). The identifiable organs are the caudal lobe and part of the principal lobe of the liver (Figs. 3 and 4), part of the diaphragm, part of the cranial duodenum and the descending duodenum (Figs. 3 and 4), part of the greater and lesser omentum, and the right kidney surrounded by adipose tissue in

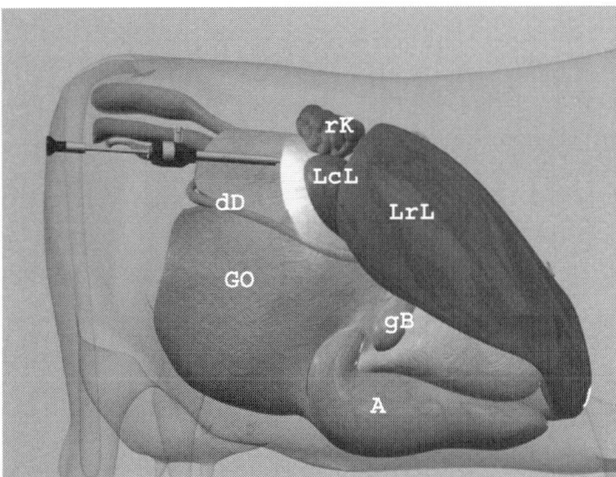

Fig. 2. Right flank laparoscopy. The laparoscope is oriented cranially. The light source highlights the visible organs from this position. A, abomasum; dD, descending duodenum; gB, gallbladder; GO, greater omentum; LcL, caudate lobe of the liver; LrL, right lobe of the liver; rK, right kidney in the retroperitoneal space.

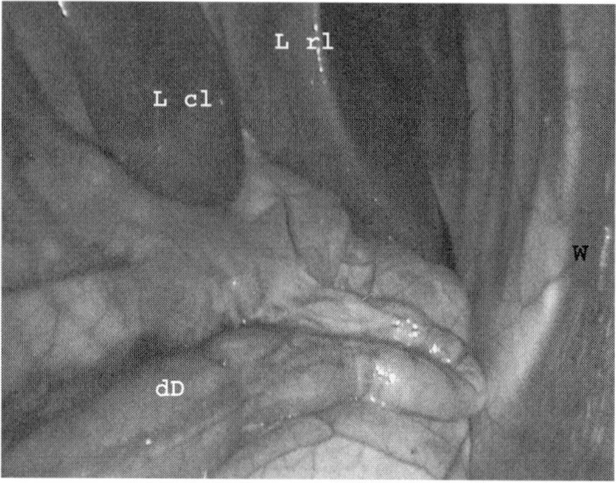

Fig. 3. Right flank laparoscopy, cranial view. dD, descending duodenum; Lcl, caudate lobe of the liver; LrL, right lobe of the liver.

the retroperitoneal space (Fig. 5). Anderson [19] also has reported that the pancreas always can be identified. In the authors' experience, it was more difficult to find the pancreas in overly conditioned cattle (see Fig. 3). When the abomasum is dilated on the right, it is identifiable between the abdominal wall and the liver.

A caudal orientation of the laparoscope (Fig. 6) allows the identification of part of the descending duodenum and the greater omentum, where it forms the supraepiploic bursa (Fig. 7). If the laparoscope is long enough or if it is inserted more caudally, it is possible to view the genital system of the cow, part of the rumen, the cecum, the intestines, and the descending colon (Figs. 8–10). It also is possible to see the bladder if the uterus is raised by an assistant doing a rectal palpation (Fig. 11). The ovarian structures also can

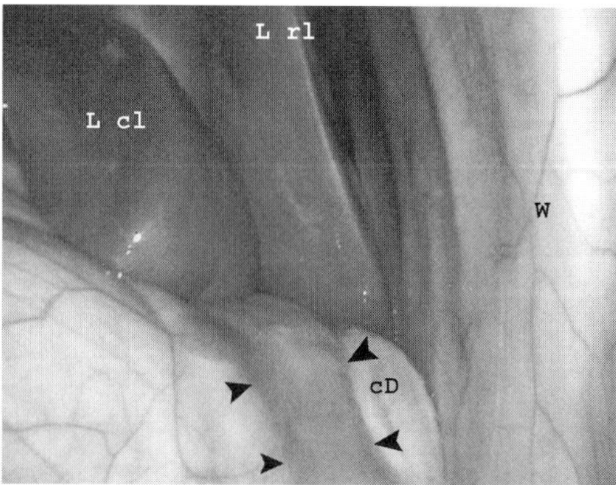

Fig. 4. Right flank laparoscopy, cranial view. On this view, the pancreas is visible. Arrowheads point to the right lobe of the pancreas. cD, cranial part of the duodenum; Lcl, caudate lobe of the liver; LrL, right lobe of the liver; W, right abdominal wall.

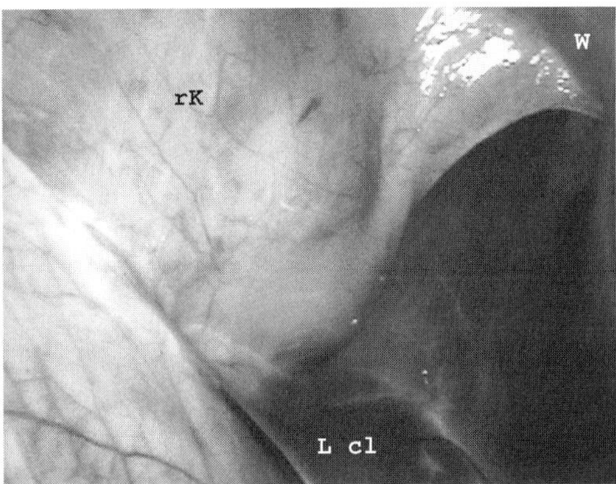

Fig. 5. Right flank laparoscopy. Lcl, caudate lobe of the liver; rK, right kidney in the retroperitoneal space; W, right abdominal wall.

be identified using this technique. An assistant performing a rectal palpation, lifting the rectum, and manipulating the reproductive system of the cow permits a better visualization of the right caudal abdomen of the cow.

Left flank

The exploration of the left side of the abdominal cavity is achieved by orienting the laparoscope caudally (Fig. 12). The dorsal sac of the rumen, the left kidney covered in retroperitoneal fat, the rectum, part of the intestines, possibly a portion of the spiral colon, and the uterus are visible (Fig. 13). According to Anderson et al [15], the bladder occasionally is

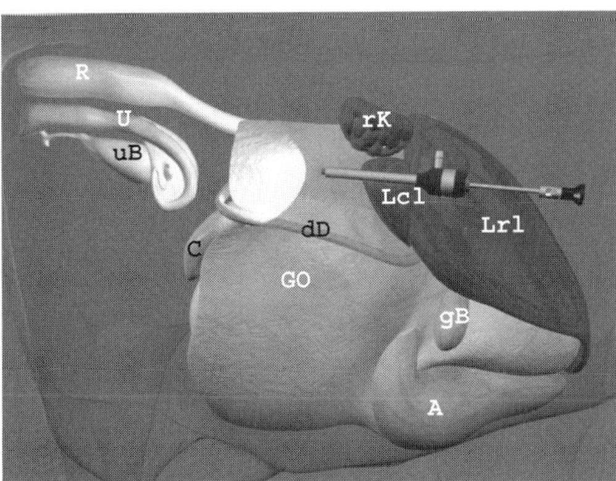

Fig. 6. Right flank laparoscopy. The laparoscope is oriented caudally. The light source highlights the visible organs from this position. A, abomasum; C, cecum; dD, descending duodenum; gB, gallbladder; GO, greater omentum; LcL, caudate lobe of the liver; LrL, right lobe of the liver; R, rectum; rK, right kidney in the retroperitoneal space; U, uterus; uB, urinary bladder.

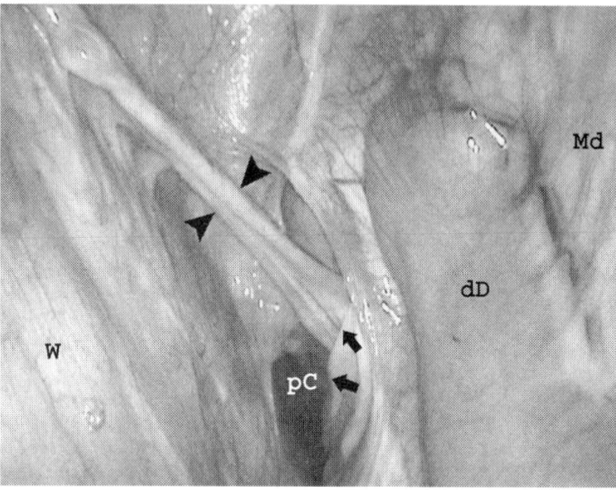

Fig. 7. Right flank laparoscopy, caudal view. Arrowheads point to mesovarium, and arrows point to omental fold. dD, descending duodenum; Md, mesoduodenum; pC, pelvic cavity; W, right abdominal wall.

identifiable on the left side (one case out of six), and the left lobe of the pancreas is seen situated cranially to the left kidney, near the rumen's attachment to the dorsal abdominal wall (one case out of six). The spiral colon, uterus, and left ovary are visualized more easily by manipulating the rectum during a transrectal palpation. A cranial orientation of the laparoscope (Fig. 14) permits the observation of part of the diaphragm, the spleen, the rumen, and possibly the greater omentum's attachment on the rumen (Fig. 15). If there is a left displaced abomasum, it is identified easily between the abdominal wall and the rumen.

Wilson and Ferguson [12] reported that it is possible to diagnose a traumatic reticuloperitonitis in a cow that shows clinical signs of the

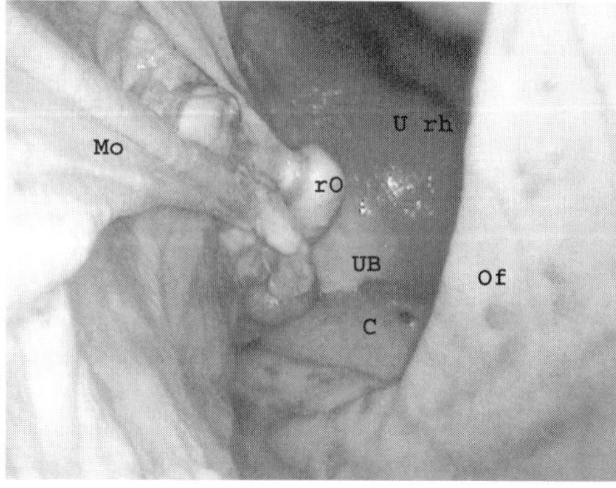

Fig. 8. Right flank laparoscopy, caudal view. C, cecum; Mo, mesovarium; Of, omental fold; rO, right ovary; UB, urinary bladder; Urh, right horn of the uterus.

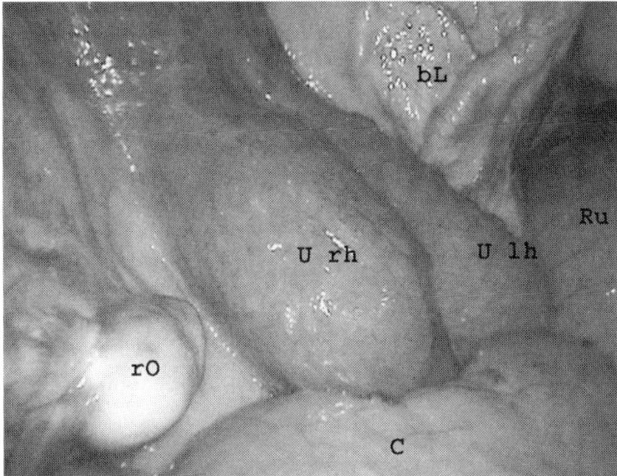

Fig. 9. Right flank laparoscopy, caudal view. bL, broad ligament, ovarian artery and vein; C, cecum; rO, right ovary; Ru, rumen; Ulh, left horn of the uterus; Urh, right horn of the uterus.

disease with the help of a colonoscope inserted through the left flank. Consequently, these lesions were detected and characterized in all cases.

Ventral

The laparoscope is inserted to the left of the umbilicus and is oriented toward the left cranial portion of the abdomen (Fig. 16). The diaphragm, the spleen, and the rumen are identified easily (Fig. 17). By manipulating the laparoscope left to right in the cranial portion of the abdomen, the diaphragm, the reticulum, sometimes part of the liver, and the omentum covering the rumen are visible (Fig. 18). The reticulum is recognizable by its regular contractions. If the abomasum is dilated, it is visible against the right ventral abdominal wall. When it is in its physiologic position, the laparoscope must be maneuvered to the right to be able to identify it. The

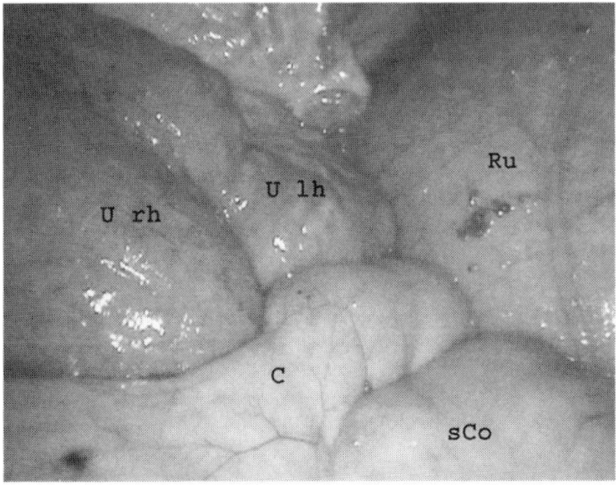

Fig. 10. Right flank laparoscopy, caudal view. C, cecum; Ru, rumen; sCo, spiral colon; Ulh, left horn of the uterus; Urh, right horn of the uterus.

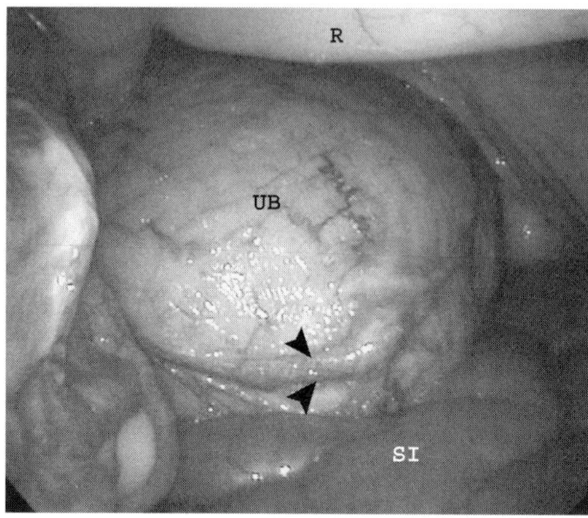

Fig. 11. Right flank laparoscopy, caudal view. Bladder is visible. The rectum is elevated by an assistant palpating per rectum. Arrowheads indicate lateral vesicular ligament. R, rectum; SI, small intestine; UB, urinary bladder.

abomasum is recognized by its serosa and its attachment to the greater omentum that creates a contrast with the smooth portion of the serosa. The reticuloabomasal ligament sometimes can be identified (Fig. 19). A portion of the pyloric part of the abomasum may be identified against the right abdominal wall by moving the laparoscope the most dorsally possible, in the same axis as the umbilicus (Fig. 20). On an adult cow, the ventral caudal part of the abomasum is not visible by this entry site because of interference of the greater omentum.

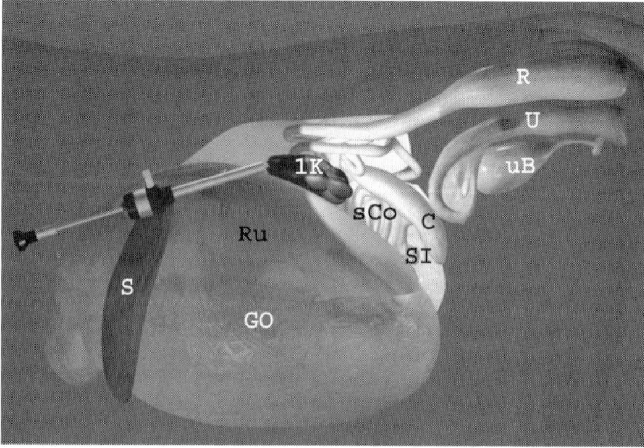

Fig. 12. Left flank laparoscopy, caudal view. The light source highlights visible organs from this position. C, cecum; GO, greater omentum at its insertion on the rumen; lK, left kidney from the retroperitoneal space; R, rectum; Ru, rumen; S, spleen; sCo, spiral colon; SI, small intestine; U, uterus; uB, urinary bladder.

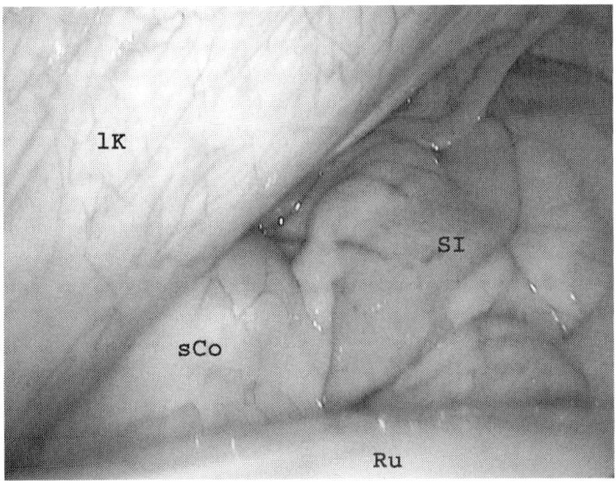

Fig. 13. Left flank laparoscopy, caudal view. lK, left kidney from the retroperitoneal space; Ru, rumen; sCo, spiral colon; SI, small intestine.

Effects of laparoscopy on the complete blood count, biochemical analysis, and peritoneal fluid

Studies by Wilson and Ferguson [12] and Anderson et al [15] have shown that laparoscopic examinations on normal, healthy cattle have no influence on the complete blood count results. Anderson et al [15] also stated that biochemical analyses and peritoneal fluid likewise were unaltered before and 72 hours after the laparoscopic examination. In a study by Carter et al [20] performed on five adult beef cows, it was shown that repeated use of laparoscopy did not alter the reproductive cycle or function of these animals.

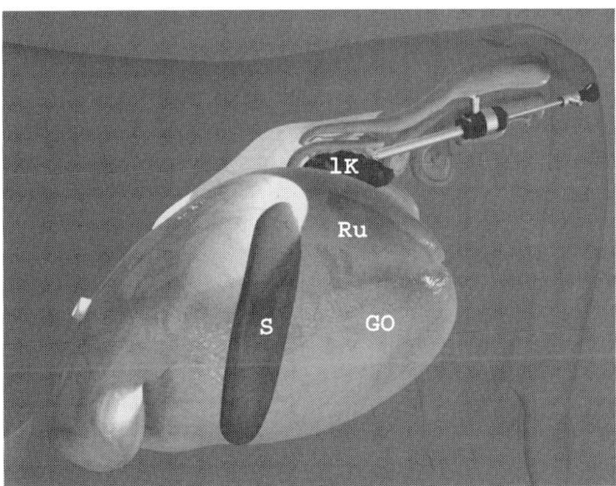

Fig. 14. Left flank laparoscopy, cranial view. The light source highlights the visible organs from this position. GO, greater omentum; lK, left kidney from the retroperitoneal space; Ru, rumen; S, spleen.

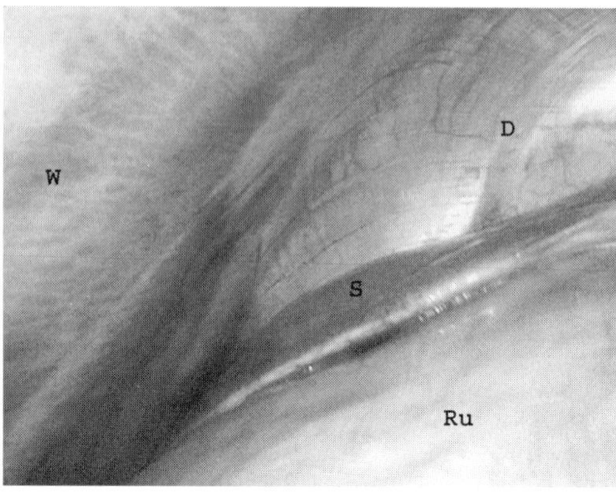

Fig. 15. Left flank laparoscopy, cranial view. D, costal part of the diaphragm; Ru, rumen; S, spleen; W, left abdominal wall.

Effects of pneumoperitoneum

There are no reports or studies that discuss the secondary effects on cattle of induced pneumoperitoneum using either carbon dioxide or ambient air. The only reports concerning ruminants involve the effects of a carbon dioxide–induced pneumoperitoneum on pregnant ewes [21]. In this study, the creation of a pneumoperitoneum with a pressure greater than 15 mm Hg in pregnant ewes caused an increase in uterine pressure, caused a decrease in uterine blood flow, and induced acidosis in the mother and fetus. Despite these effects, the ewes' gestations were brought to term favorably.

In human surgery, the most commonly used gas is carbon dioxide because it is the most inert. In the past, ambient air was used successfully to induce a pneumoperitoneum during interventions on the reproductive

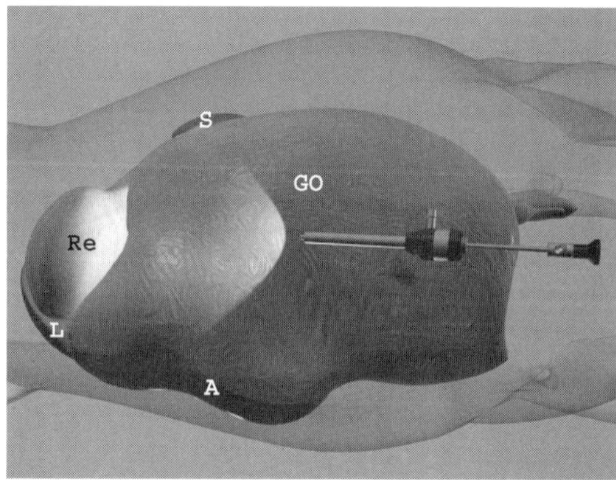

Fig. 16. Ventral laparoscopy, cranial view. The light source highlights the visible organs from this position. A, abomasum; GO, greater omentum; L, part of the right lobe of the liver; Re, reticulum; S, spleen.

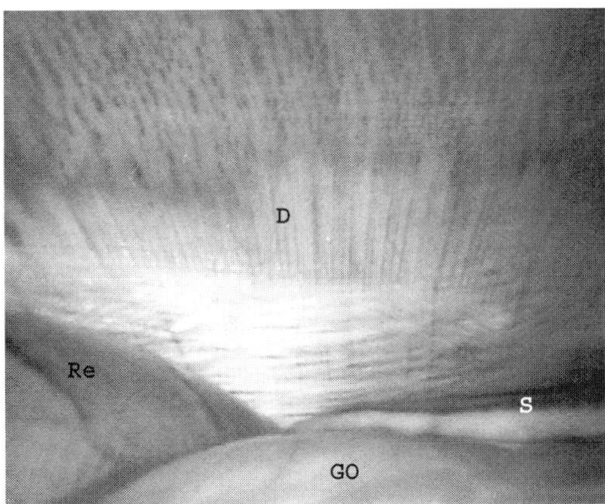

Fig. 17. Ventral laparoscopy, cranial view. D, central tendinous portion of diaphragm; GO, greater omentum; Re, reticulum; S, spleen.

system. No particular problems, such as pain, emboli, infection, or death, were reported after the use of ambient air on 400 patients [22]. Nevertheless, in a study on mice, Tung and Smith [23] revealed an exaggerated interleukin-6 response in the serum and intestinal mucosa after the exposure of the abdominal cavity to ambient air compared with that of carbon dioxide. According to Tung and Smith [23], cytokine measurements may be a good indication of the response to the stress of surgeries. The conclusion of Tung and Smith was that the beneficial effects of laparoscopy might be the exclusion of ambient air from the peritoneal cavity. In more recent studies [24], it has been suggested that the use of carbon dioxide in creating a pneumoperitoneum during laparoscopy possibly could cause ultrastructural, metabolic, and immunologic alterations at the peritoneal surface.

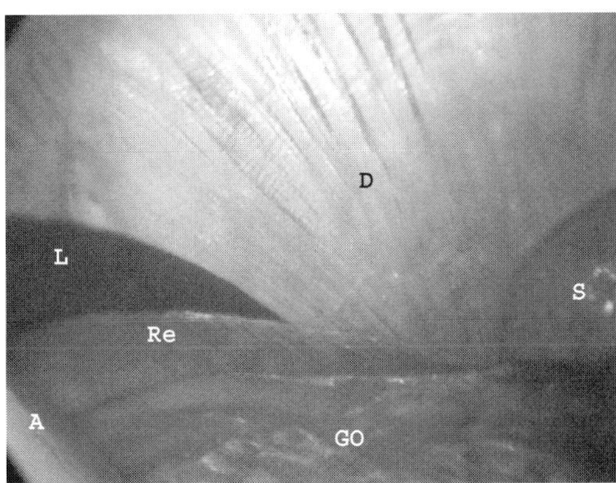

Fig. 18. Ventral laparoscopy, right cranial view. A, abomasum filled with gas; D, central tendinous portion of diaphragm; GO, greater omentum; L, right lobe of the liver; Re, reticulum; S, spleen.

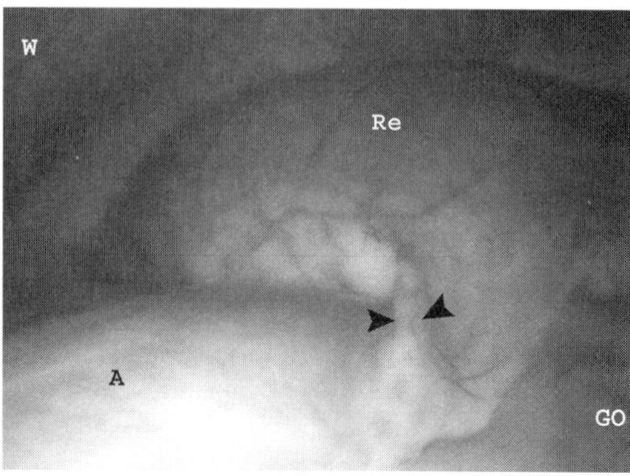

Fig. 19. Ventral laparoscopy, cranial view. The laparoscope is redirected to the right. Arrowheads point to reticuloabomasal ligament. A, abomasum; Re, reticulum; W, ventral abdominal wall.

These alterations could favor tumor implantation in the peritoneal cavity and would affect its capacity to eliminate peritoneal infections. As a result of these controversies, and fact that the use of ambient air does not seem to cause any harm to cattle [14], the authors believe that its use in cattle is a safe, economical way to induce a pneumoperitoneum.

Indications

Reproductive system

The first reports on bovine laparoscopy involve the reproductive system. Lambert [25] described an endoscopic technique through the right flank to

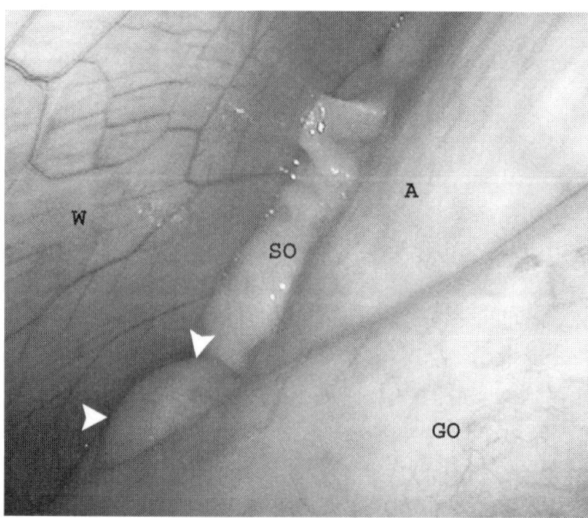

Fig. 20. Ventral laparoscopy, right ventral view. Arrowheads point to pylorus. A, abomasum; GO, greater omentum; SO, smaller omentum; W, abdominal wall.

examine the ovaries and perform follicular aspiration; Bernard et al [26] used laparoscopy to observe ovulation in heifers. Following these studies, several authors described different techniques of follicular aspiration [27–32]. Today in reproduction, these techniques are used mainly for the insemination of small ruminants [33,34] and embryo transfer collections [35,36].

Biopsies

The advantages of the use of laparoscopy-guided biopsy techniques are the direct visualization of the target organ and the selection of the exact biopsy site. In this way, obtaining biopsy specimens of the wrong organ is avoided, and possible hemorrhages are identified and controlled. The direct view of the target organ can provide additional information concerning the condition and eventually its prognosis.

In horses, biopsy techniques are described for the liver, kidneys, spleen, lymphatic nodes, and other masses [37]. Similarly in cattle, the first reports on organ biopsy by laparoscopy guidance involved the kidney [17]. In this technique, the laparoscope is introduced in the middle of the right paralumbar fossa after the site has been surgically prepared (local anesthesia and a 2-cm cutaneous incision). A Franklin-Silverman biopsy needle is used and is introduced 5 cm below the transverse processes, behind the last rib. The biopsy is completed using the sharp part of the needle. It allows one to take a biopsy specimen that is on average 1.5 mm in diameter and 16 mm in length.

Klein et al [38] described an intestinal biopsy technique. This technique is described on calves and sheep placed under general anesthesia in dorsal recumbency. The biopsy is performed outside of the abdominal cavity after the intestine is caught and held laparoscopically with grasping forceps.

Abdominal exploration

Abdominal exploration via laparoscopy can be extremely useful in the diagnosis and prognosis of certain conditions.

Postoperative uterine torsion

Significant ischemias of the uterine blood vessels often result after severe torsion of the uterus. Despite successful interventions to correct this condition, the uterus may remain devitalized and undergo necrosis, explaining slow recovery after the torsion reduction. Early clinical diagnosis of this condition is not easy, and the prognosis is uncertain. Consequently, laparoscopic exploration by the right flank to view the state of the uterus can be beneficial in complicated cases. The laparoscopist should evaluate the color of the uterus, swollen ovaries, and presence of thrombosis.

Incorrect positioning of the abomasum

After a standard surgical procedure for the replacement of a displaced abomasum, it is possible that adequate, normal digestive functions do not return because of an inadequate fixation. Although the abomasum still can be attached, functional stenosis may occur from malpositioning or suturing errors. Laparoscopy allows visualizing in situ the position of the faulty organ. Attention should be paid to the pyloric antrum position. A suture placement can be placed inadvertently through the cranial duodenum creating a kink and causing the digestive transit to slow down and an abomasal reflux toward the rumen (Fig. 21). This condition can be corrected by excising the suture through laparoscopy.

Perforated abomasal ulcer or cranioventral adherence

Exploration of the cranioventral abdomen by laparoscopy using a ventral approach allows for a good view of the abomasum and the reticular region without massively invading the abdomen. This exploration can be advantageous when there is suspicion of a localized problem in the cranioventral region of the abdomen not involving traumatic reticuloperitonitis (Fig. 22).

Postsurgical adhesions

Postoperative evolution can be slow in some animals. Diagnosis of adhesions or local peritonitis is difficult to confirm without performing a second laparotomy. Without knowing exactly which organs are involved and where the possible lesions are, it can be hazardous to perform a laparotomy. A second look can be done by laparoscopy with less stress on the animal. The surgeon then can decide whether or not he or she should intervene with few consequences for the animal (Fig. 23).

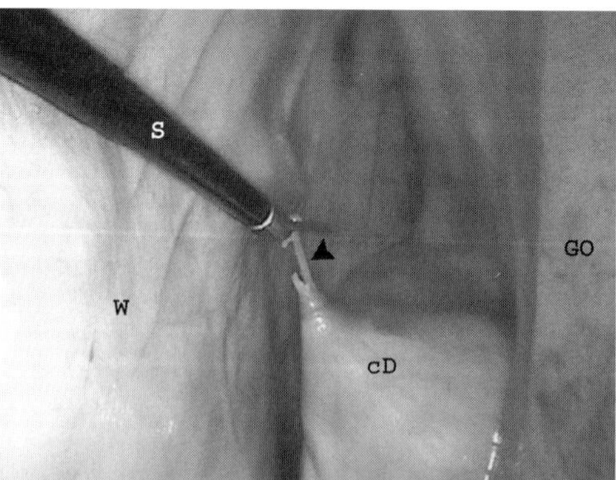

Fig. 21. Right flank laparoscopy. The laparoscope is inserted through the 11th intercostal space and oriented caudally toward the flank. A suture was inadvertently placed through the cranial duodenum creating a kink. The suture was cut with scissors through laparoscopy. Arrowhead indicates where the suture is cut. cD, cranial part of the duodenum; GO, greater omentum; S, laparoscopic scissors; W, right abdominal wall.

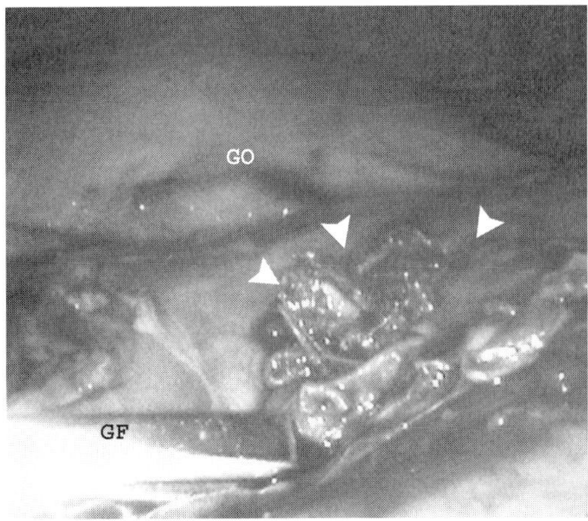

Fig. 22. Ventral view. Perforated ulcer of the abomasum and local peritonitis. Arrowheads point to digestive content and fibrin. GF, grasping forceps; GO, greater omentum.

Pedagogic interests: transrectal examination and surgical manipulation of a left displaced abomasum

If the laparoscope is long enough or if it is inserted in the caudal portion of the right flank, it allows for a good view of the reproductive tract. In this way, a transrectal examination of the genital tract may be performed under laparoscopic guidance, allowing direct identification of the structures palpated. This exercise can be used to explain the examination to students or to test a student's ability to identify the different structures being palpated (Fig. 24).

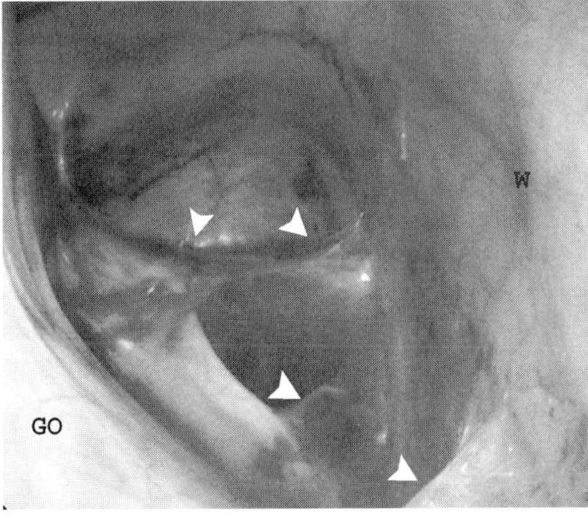

Fig. 23. Right flank laparoscopy, cranial view. Postsurgical adhesions. Arrowheads point to adhesions. GO, greater omentum; W, right abdominal wall.

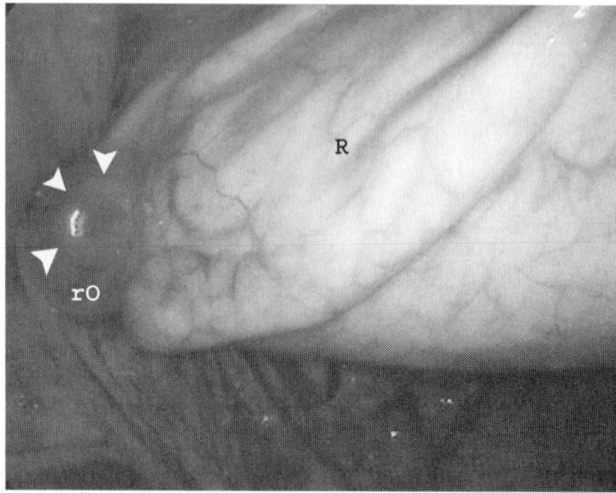

Fig. 24. Right flank laparoscopy, caudal view. Reproductive tract examination. Arrowheads point to corpus hemorrhagicum. R, rectum; rO, right ovary.

In the case of a left displaced abomasum, the explanations given to students on how to put the abomasum back into its place are not always easy to understand. By filming this manipulation via left flank laparoscopy, the positioning of the hand and the work exerted on the left displaced abomasum are explicit.

Laparoscopic limitations

The limitations of laparoscopy are related to the incomplete exploration of the abdomen in cattle, to the innovative personality of the surgeon, and to the limited usable material for animals of greater dimensions.

Surgical techniques using laparoscopy

Three surgical techniques have been reported to correct displaced abomasum by laparoscopy. The first technique, described by Janowitz [14], permits the correction and fixation of a left displaced abomasum. The second technique, described by the authors (unpublished data, 2004), allows the correction and fixation of a left displaced abomasum [39] in addition to allowing the preventive fixation of the abomasum. The latter may be useful in the case of a recurring left displaced abomasum. Abdominal ultrasound of these cases often reveals an extreme ventral positioning of the pylorus, suggesting ongoing displacement. The third technique, described by Barisani [40], allows standing laparoscopic fixation of the displaced abomasum.

Technique for correction and fixation of a left displaced abomasum

The Janowitz technique [14] is a laparoscopy-guided toggle pin fixation. The first step of the procedure is performed through the left flank of the standing animal. The surgical site on the animal is prepared following standard procedure, and the points of entry for the trocar/cannula units are infiltrated with lidocaine (Fig. 25). The entry site for the 8-mm trocar (portal site 1) gives access to the laparoscope through the left paralumbar fossa behind the ribs and beneath the transverse processes. The point of entry of the 5-mm trocar (portal site 2) that gives access to the long trocar used for the placement of the toggle and for emptying the air from the abomasum is situated in the dorsal third of the 11th intercostal space.

A Veress needle is introduced through a cutaneous incision 1 cm in length at portal site 1, and a pneumoperitoneum is induced. The 8-mm trocar/cannula unit is inserted into the abdominal cavity. Next, the 8-mm laparoscope (Dr Fritz GmbH, Tuttlingen, Germany) is introduced by the cannula into the abdominal cavity. The abdominal cavity is explored to ensure that there are no abnormalities that could prevent the continuation of the procedure. Next a 5-mm trocar/cannula unit is inserted in the 11th intercostal space under laparoscopic guidance. The long 5-mm trocar is passed through this cannula and into the abdominal cavity, where it is inserted into the greater curvature of the abomasum (Fig. 26). The modified toggle (toggle with two suture materials; Dr Fritz GmbH, Tuttlingen, Germany) is introduced into this cannula (of the long trocar/cannula unit) and is pushed into the left displaced abomasum with a blunt-ended trocar. The two suture materials are left in place in the abdomen, and the air is emptied form the abomasum through the trocar (Fig. 27). All instruments are then removed, and the incisions are closed in a routine manner.

The second half of the surgery is performed when the animal has been sedated with xylazine (40 mg intravenously) and is placed in dorsal recumbency. The right paramedian region of the abdomen is prepared for

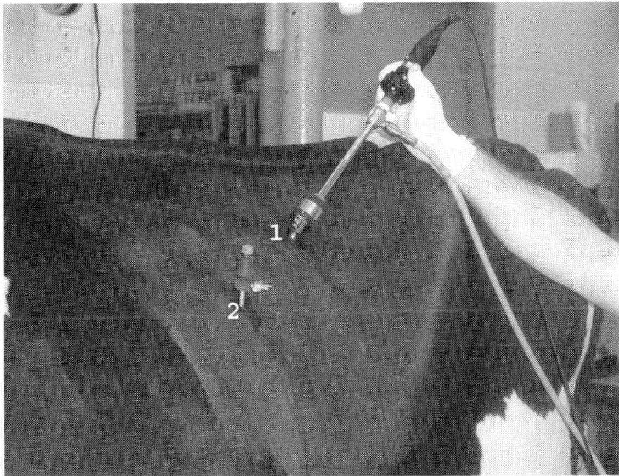

Fig. 25. First part of Janowitz technique of laparoscopic abomasopexy on a standing animal through the left flank. Trocar positioning: 1, portal site 1 (laparoscope); 2, portal site 2 (5-mm trocar).

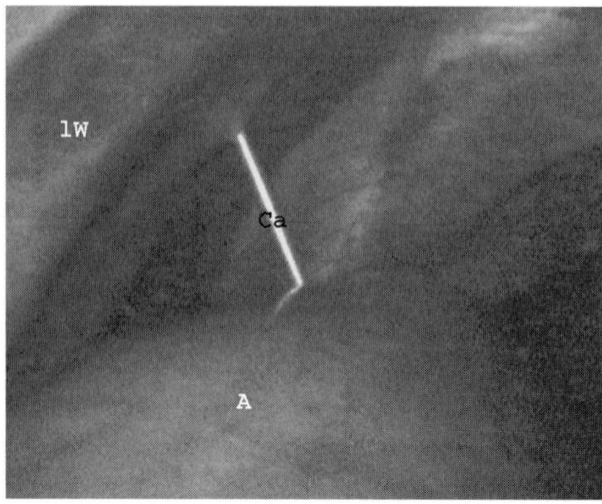

Fig. 26. A long trocar is inserted into the abomasum. Then an adapted toggle pin is slid through the cannula into the abomasum. A, abomasum; Ca, 5-mm cannula with long trocar; W, left abdominal wall.

surgery in a standard fashion along a 20 cm × 20 cm square cranial to the umbilicus. The points of entry for the trocar/cannula units are infiltrated with lidocaine. The first trocar (8 mm) is placed to the right and cranial to the umbilicus. For the second portal, a trocar (5 mm) is placed 10 cm cranial to the first trocar. Both trocars are inserted into the abdomen (Fig. 28). The laparoscope is passed through the first cannula. The two sutures (Fig. 29) are retrieved with grasping forceps and are pulled through the second portal (Maryland dissector). The sutures pierce a roll of gauze bandage and are knotted together with the animal positioned in right lateral recumbency to avoid excessive tension (Fig. 30). The sutures are left in place for 3 to 4 weeks. Janowitz [14] reported that this technique is extremely effective, quick, and relatively safe with a success rate of 98% based on lack of

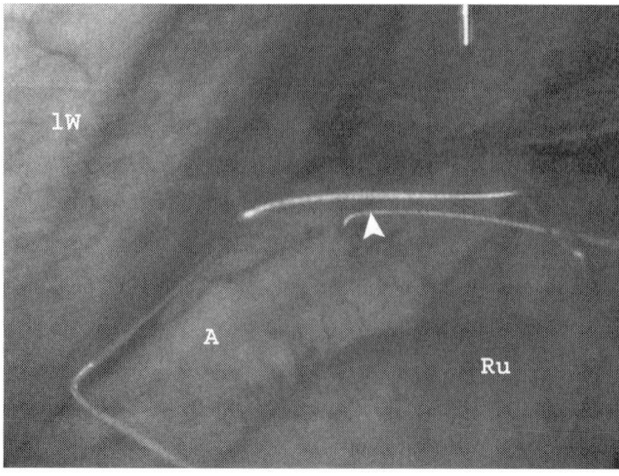

Fig. 27. Abomasum is decompressed, and suture is left free in the abdomen. Arrowhead points to suture. A, abomasum; lW, left abdominal wall; Ru, rumen.

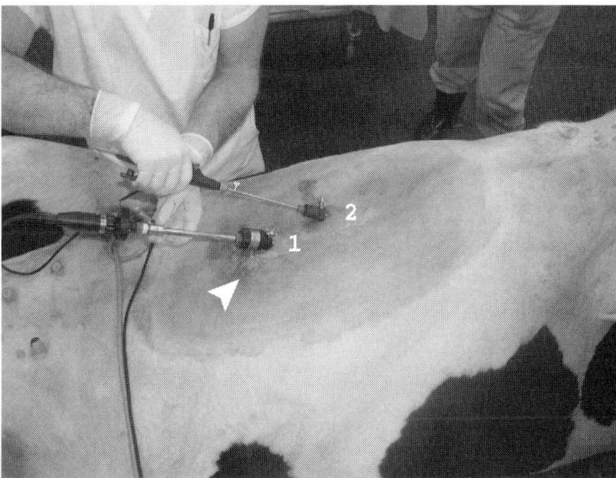

Fig. 28. Second part of Janowitz laparoscopic abomasopexy. The cow is positioned in dorsal recumbency. Arrowhead points to umbilicus. Two trocars are in place: 1, portal site 1 (laparoscope); 2, portal site 2 (5-mm trocar Maryland dissector).

recurrence of left displaced abomasum. No major complications were noted in his study.

Ventral laparoscopic abomasopexy

The ventral laparoscopic abomasopexy technique, described by the authors, is performed on the animal placed in dorsal recumbency and allows the preventive or curative fixation of the abomasum. The cow is sedated with xylazine, 0.1 mg/kg intravenously, and positioned in dorsal recumbency on a hydraulic chute with her four legs tied with cables and the right hind limb slightly extended caudally. The abdomen is surgically

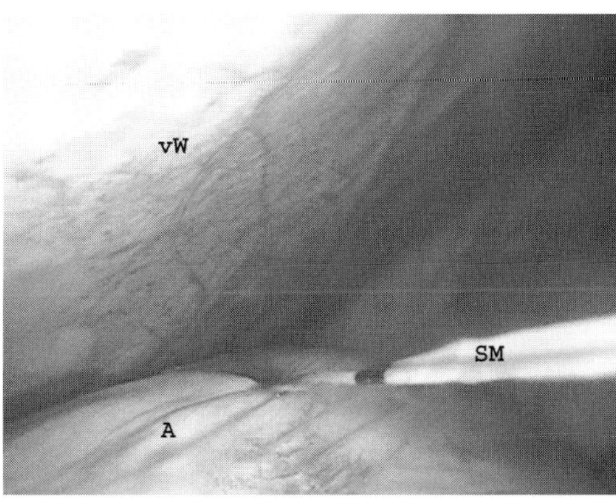

Fig. 29. Ventral view of the abdomen. The suture is grasped with the Maryland forceps to be pulled out of the abdomen. A, abomasum; SM, suture material; vW, ventral abdominal wall.

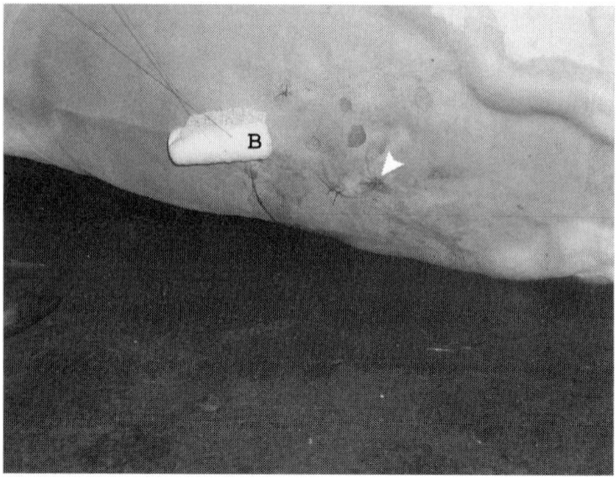

Fig. 30. The cow is placed in lateral recumbency, and two strains of sutures are attached. The sutures are knotted together. Arrowhead points to umbilicus. B, gauze bandage.

prepared from the xyphoid process to 10 cm caudal of the umbilicus and with a width of 20 cm each side of the ventral midline.

Local anesthetic solution of 2% lidocaine is infiltrated subcutaneously at the three portal sites and at the fixation zone (Fig. 31), as follows:

Portal site 1 (laparoscope): 2 cm to the left of the umbilicus
Portal site 2 (grasping forceps): 3 cm caudal and 7 cm to the right of the xyphoid process
Portal site 3 (needle holder): 5 cm to the right of and 3 cm cranial to the umbilicus
Fixation zone: a 12-cm-long line block anesthesia is performed in the body wall 3 to 5 cm to the right of the linea alba centered between the xyphoid process and the umbilicus

A minilaparotomy of approximately 1 cm is performed immediately to the left of the umbilicus to allow the passage of the first laparoscopic

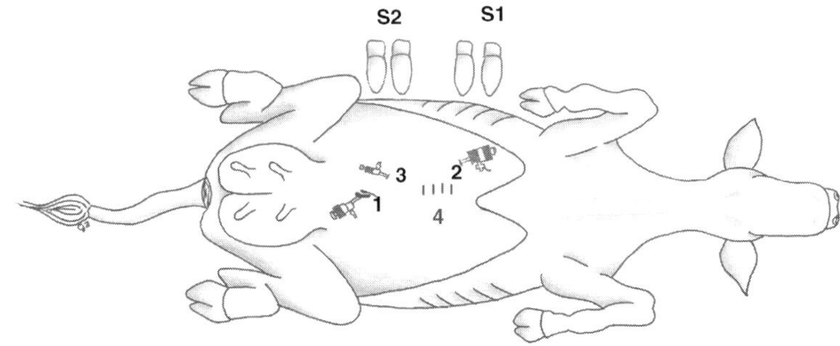

Fig. 31. Position of the surgeons, the portals, and location of the fixation site for a laparoscopic abomasopexy: 1, laparocope portal site; 2, grasping forceps portal site; 3, needle holder portal site; 4, fixation site; S1, surgeon 1; S2, surgeon 2.

cannula. An 8-mm trocar/cannula unit (Dr Fritz GmbH, Tuttlingen, Germany) is introduced in the abdominal cavity aiming cranially with a 45° angle through the abdominal wall without previously creating a pneumoperitoneum. When the first cannula is in place, the abdomen is insufflated with filtered ambient air using an automatic insufflator (Dr Fritz GmbH, Tuttlingen, Germany). This device does not allow for the control of abdominal pressure.

During insufflation, a rigid laparoscope (8 mm in diameter, 0°, and 42 cm long; Dr Fritz GmbH, Tuttlingen, Germany) is introduced into the abdomen through the first cannula (8 mm). The laparoscope is connected to a 150-W halogen light source (Dr Fritz GmbH, Tuttlingen, Germany) and a video camera (Richard Wolf GmbH, Knittlingen, Germany). The abdominal insufflation continues until the viscera of the cranial abdomen are clearly visible, and the abomasum is no longer touching the ventral parietal peritoneum. The abdominal cavity is explored to ensure that the insertion of the trocar has not caused any lesions and to note any abnormalities present.

A 10-mm trocar/cannula unit (Richard Wolf GmbH, Knittlingen, Germany) is inserted through a full-thickness body wall incision performed under laparoscopic guidance at portal site 2. Grasping forceps (forceps 2/3 teeth, 10 mm; Richard Wolf GmbH, Knittlingen, Germany) are inserted through the cannula at portal site 2. The forceps are used first to locate the abomasum and then to grasp it in the middle of its greater curvature, approximately 2 to 3 cm from the attachment of greater omentum (Fig. 32). This site corresponds to the fixation site.

Following a cutaneous incision, a 5.5-mm trocar/cannula unit (Dr Fritz GmbH, Tuttlingen, Germany) is inserted into the abdomen at portal site 3. This site provides the opening for the needle holder (tungsten carbide headed needle holder; Richard Wolf GmbH, Knittlingen, Germany). At

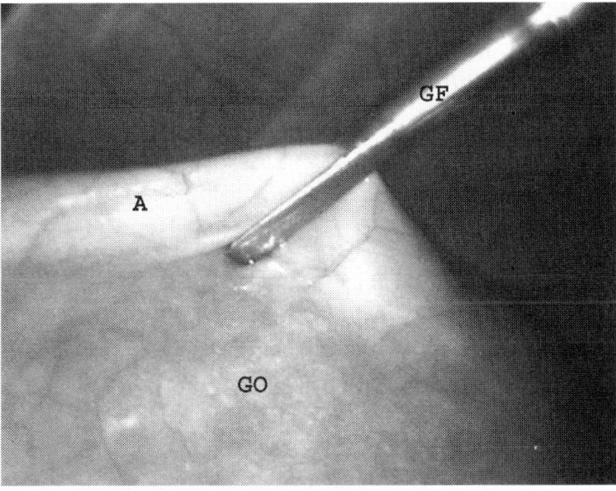

Fig. 32. Ventral view of the abdomen. Grasping forceps are used to hold the abomasum. A, abomasum; GP, grasping forceps; GO, greater omentum.

that time, four 1-cm-long skin incisions are made along the abdominal fixation site. These incisions are spaced 2.5 cm apart and are perpendicular to the ventral midline. The fixation site is 10 cm long and is located between the umbilicus and the xyphoid process, 3 to 5 cm to the right of the ventral midline (Fig. 33).

Both surgeons are placed side by side to the right of the cow. Surgeon 1 handles the grasping forceps and the needle when it was outside the abdominal cavity. Surgeon 2 manipulates the laparoscope and the needle holder.

USP 2 polydioxanone suture material with a swaged-on curved needle (1/2, 40 mm) is used for the abomasopexy. Straightening the needle facilitates intracorporeal and extracorporeal manipulation of the needle. The needle and suture material are introduced into the abdomen through one of the cutaneous incisions and grasped intra-abdominally using the needle holder. The free end of the suture material is held with a pair of hemostatic forceps outside of the abdomen.

The needle and suture material are passed through the serous and muscular layers of the abomasum resulting in a stitch measuring 2 cm and running perpendicularly to the great curvature of the abomasum (Fig. 34). The needle entry site in the abomasum is inspected carefully for the presence of gas or fluid leakage. Each suture is located about 3 cm from the attachment of the greater omentum along the greater curvature of the abomasum. The needle is retrieved using the same needle holder. An 18G needle inserted through the abdominal wall near the entry of the suture is used as a guide to exteriorize the needle and the suture material (Fig. 35). The suture material is pulled out of the abdominal cavity to ensure a good

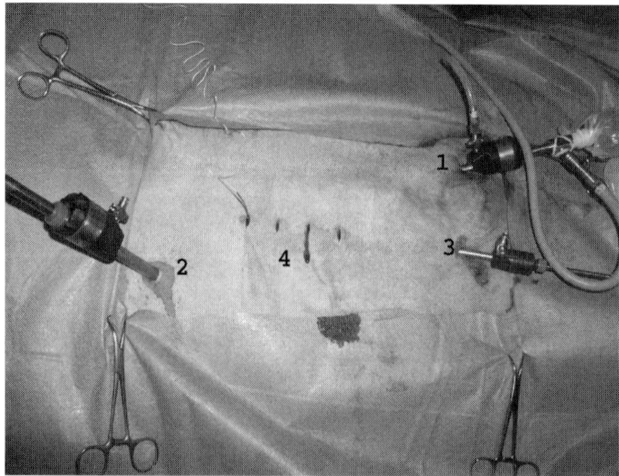

Fig. 33. Positioning of the trocars. Localization of the fixation site (four skin incisions): 1, portal site 1 (laparoscope); 2, portal site 2 (grasping forceps); 3, portal site 3 (needle holder); 4, fixation site (four skin incisions).

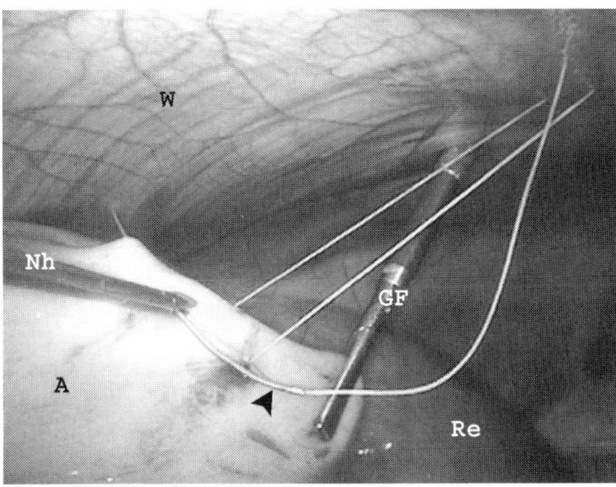

Fig. 34. Suture passage through the seromuscular layers of the abomasum. The first stitch of the fixation is already in place. Arrowhead indicates needle and suture material. A, abomasum; GF, grasping forceps; Nh, needle driver; Re, reticulum; W, abdominal wall.

contact between the abomasum and the abdominal wall (Fig. 36). The two ends of the suture material are held together outside the abdomen using a pair of hemostatic forceps. The three other sutures are placed in a similar fashion. The correct positioning of the abomasum is verified by pulling gently on the sutures without trying to approximate the abomasum to the body wall; this also verifies any inadvertent suture crossing during the procedure (Fig. 37). The air is evacuated from the abdominal cavity by opening the cannula. The sutures are knotted, and the cutaneous incisions are closed using a cruciate suture pattern with polydioxanone material (Fig. 38).

In the authors' study performed on 10 cows, this technique was proved to be safe and quick (30 minutes), and it created durable adherences (Fig. 39).

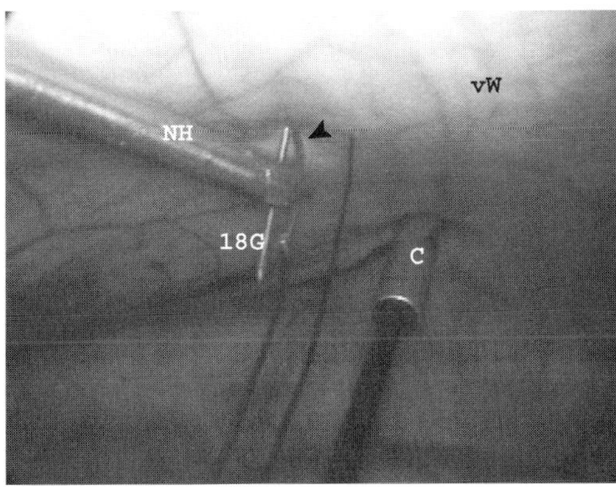

Fig. 35. An 18G needle inserted through the abdominal wall near the entry of the suture is used as a guide to exteriorize the needle and the suture material (*arrowhead*). C, 10-mm cannula; NH, needle holder; vW, ventral abdominal wall.

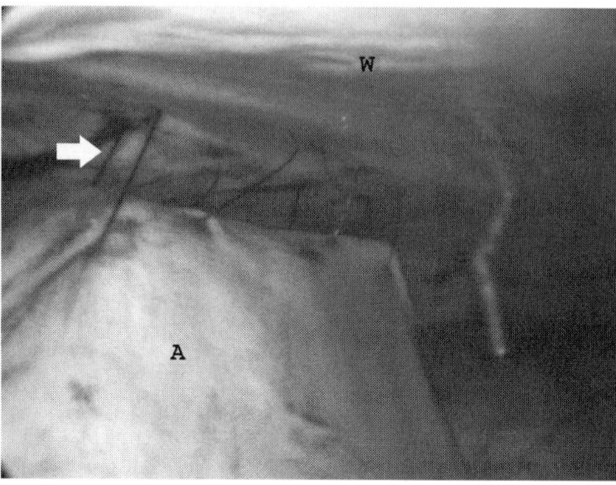

Fig. 36. The four stitches (*arrow*) are in place. After letting out the air of the abdomen, sutures are pulled gently, and the abomasum (A) comes in close contact with the ventral abdominal wall (W).

In a later study performed on 16 cows that had had a previous abomasopexy using this technique to correct a left displaced abomasum, Mulon et al [39] noted that these cows continued to have normal lactations 6 months after the intervention.

Left flank laparoscopic abomasopexy

The left flank laparoscopic abomasopexy technique for left displaced abomasum was developed by Christiansen in Germany and reported by Barisani [40]. This is a modification of the Janowitz technique [14]. A modified toggle pin is inserted as described before (Dr Fritz GmbH, Tuttlingen, Germany) with the exception that the suture is brought ventrally, cranial to the umbilicus, with a specially designed long rod developed in collaboration with Dr Fritz (Dr Fritz GmbH, Tuttlingen,

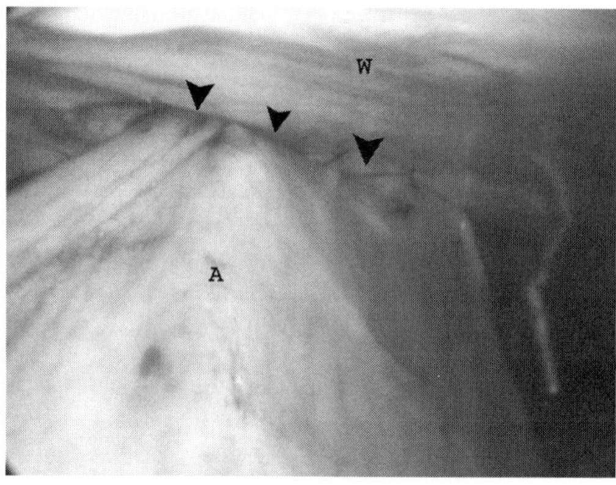

Fig. 37. Approximation of the abomasum (A) to the ventral body wall (W) after the four fixation stitches (*arrowheads*) were performed.

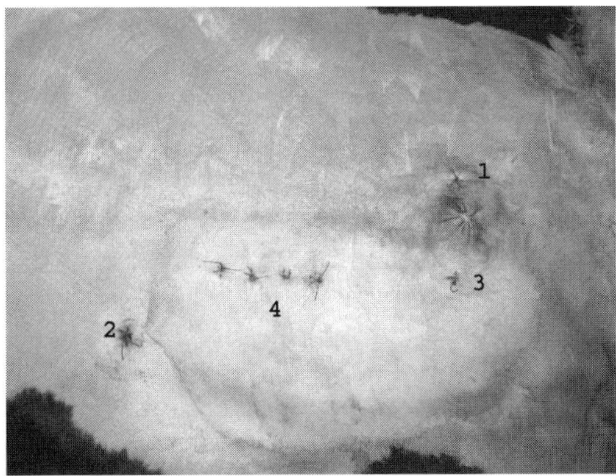

Fig. 38. Skin incision closure. 1, portal site 1; 2, portal site 2; 3, portal site 3; 4, fixation site.

Germany) (Figs. 38 and 39). The end of the rod is equipped with a retractable sharp needle where the sutures are inserted. The entire procedure is performed with the animal standing.

Summary

Laparoscopy in cattle is a promising tool for clinical diagnosis and treatment. The lower cost of the materials available in addition to the possibility of an intervention on an animal that is sedated does not entail more costs than an exploratory laparotomy. The application of this tool during abdominal explorations and biopsies allows the avoidance of invasive and often useless surgical interventions and even with the diagnosis and prognosis of certain conditions. Surgical techniques currently are

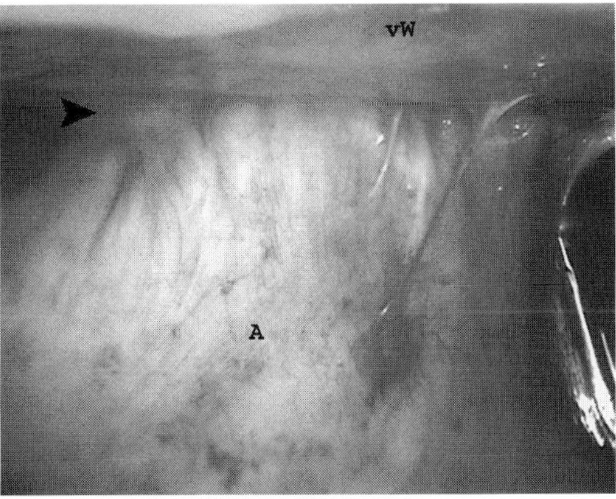

Fig. 39. Adhesions 3 months after the surgery. Arrowhead points to adhesion area. A, abomasum; vW, ventral abdominal wall.

limited to abomasopexies; however, never-ceasing progress and improvements in human surgery are expected to affect the future of bovine surgery.

With the advancements in the multimedia technology used by universities, the use of laparoscopy as a pedagogic tool definitely has a promising future. Endoscopic exploration of the thorax is possible using the same material as for laparoscopy. In addition, diagnostic and biopsy applications are useful. The use of the laparoscope in different body cavities and for different applications would make the purchase of the required materials more cost-effective.

References

[1] Stellato TA. History of laparoscopic surgery. Surg Clin North Am 1992;72:997–1002.

[2] Marlovits H. The history of laparoscopy. Ther Umsch 1997;54:489–91.

[3] Hulka JF, Reich H. Textbook of laparoscopy. 3rd edition. Philadelphia: WB Saunders; 1998.

[4] Gomel V, Taylor PJ. Diagnostic and operative gynaecologic laparoscopy. St Louis: Mosby; 2000.

[5] Luks FI, Logan J, Breuer CK, Kurkchubasche AG, Wesselhoeft CW Jr, Tracy TF Jr. Cost-effectiveness of laparoscopy in children. Arch Pediatr Adolesc Med 1999;153:965–8.

[6] Rosen M, Garcia-Ruiz A, Malm J, Mayes JT, Steiger E, Ponsky J. Laparoscopic hernia repair enhances early return of physical work capacity. Surg Laparosc Endosc 2001;11: 28–33.

[7] Nicholson T, Tiruchelvam V. Comparison of laparoscopic-assisted appendectomy with intracorporal laparoscopic appendectomy and open appendectomy. Journal of the Society of Laparoendoscopic Surgeons 2001;5:47–51.

[8] Maxwell DP, Kraemer D. Laparoscopy in cattle. In: Harrison RM, Wildt DE, editors. Animal laparoscopy. Baltimore: Williams & Wilkins; 1980. p. 133–56.

[9] Anderson DE, Gaughan EM, St Jean G. Normal laparoscopic anatomy of the bovine abdomen. Am J Vet Res 1993;54:1170–6.

[10] Lambert RD. Endoscopy in cattle by the paralumbar route: technique for ovarian examination and follicular aspiration. Theriogenology 1983;20:149–61.

[11] Naoi M, Kokue E, Takahashi Y, Kido Y. Laparoscopic-assisted serial biopsy of the bovine kidney. Am J Vet Res 1985;46:699–702.

[12] Wilson AD, Ferguson JG. Use of a flexible fiberoptic laparoscope as a diagnostic aid in cattle. Can Vet J 1984;25:229–34.

[13] Boure L, Foster RA, Palmer M, Hathway A. Use of an endoscopic suturing device for laparoscopic resection of the apex of the bladder and umbilical structures in normal neonatal calves. Vet Surg 2001;30:319–26.

[14] Janowitz H. [Laparoscopic reposition and fixation of the left displaced abomasum in cattle] [German]. Tierarztl Prax Ausg G Grosstiere Nutztiere 1998;26:308–13.

[15] Anderson DE, Gaughan EM, St Jean G. Normal laparoscopic anatomy of the bovine abdomen. Am J Vet Res 1993;54:1170–6.

[16] Guidoni M, Guintard C, Ravier S, Betti E, Laval A. La laparoscopie de la cavité abdomino-pelvienne chez la vache. Bull GTV 2002;14:87–91.

[17] Naoi M, Kokue E, Takahashi Y, Kido Y. Laparoscopic-assisted serial biopsy of the bovine kidney. Am J Vet Res 1985;46:699–702.

[18] Seeger K. Laparoscopic investigation of the bovine ovary. Vet Med Small Anim Clin 1977; 72:1037–44.

[19] Anderson DE. Laparoscopy. In: Fubini SL, Ducharme NG, editors. Farm animal surgery. Philadelphia: WB Saunders; 2004. p. 82–6.

[20] Carter ML, Dierschke DJ, Hauser ER. Effect of repeated laparoscopic surgery on the bovine estrous cycle. Theriogenology 1981;16:399–405.
[21] Curet MJ, Vogt DA, Schob O, Qualls C, Izquierdo LA, Zuccker KA. Effects of CO2 pneumoperitoneum in pregnant ewes. J Surg Res 1996;63:339–44.
[22] Diaz MO, Atwood RJ, Laufe LE. Laparoscopic sterilization with room air insufflation: preliminary report. Int J Gynaecol Obstet 1980;18:119–22.
[23] Tung PH, Smith CD. Laparoscopic insufflation with room air causes exaggerated interleukine-6 response. Surg Endosc 1999;13:473–5.
[24] Neuhaus SJ, Watson DI. Pneumoperitoneum and peritoneal surface changes: a review. Surg Endosc 2004; in press.
[25] Lambert RD. Endoscopy in cattle by the paralumbar route: technique for ovarian examination and follicular aspiration. Theriogenology 1983;20:149–61.
[26] Bernard C, Lambert RD, Beland R, Belanger A. Laparoscopic investigation of the bovine ovary in the periovulatory phase of the cycle. Theriogenology 1984;22:143–50.
[27] Sirard MA, Lambert RD. In vitro fertilization of bovine follicular oocytes obtained by laparoscopy. Biol Reprod 1985;33:487–94.
[28] Lambert RD, Sirard MA, Bernard C, et al. In vitro fertilization of bovine oocytes matured in vivo and collected at laparoscopy. Theriogenology 1986;25:117–33.
[29] Sirard MA, Lambert RD, Guay P. In vitro development of in vitro fertilized bovine follicular oocytes obtained by laparoscopy. Anim Reprod Sci 1986;12:21–9.
[30] Schellander K, Fayrer-Hosken RA, Keefer CL, et al. In vitro fertilization of bovine follicular oocytes recovered by laparoscopy. Theriogenology 1989;31:927–34.
[31] Fayrer-Hosken RA, Younis AI, Brackett BG, et al. Laparoscopic oviductal transfer of in vitro matured and in vitro fertilized bovine oocytes. Theriogenology 1989;32:413–20.
[32] Reichenbach HD, Wiebke NH, Modl J, Zhu J, Brem G. Laparoscopy through the vaginal fornix of cows for the repeated aspiration of follicular oocytes. Vet Rec 1994;135:353–6.
[33] Nuti L. Techniques for artificial insemination of goats. In: Younquist RS, editor. Current therapy in large animal theriogenology. Philadelphia: WB Saunders; 1997. p. 499–504.
[34] Mylne MJA, Hunton JR, Buckrell BC. Artificial insemination of sheep. In: Younquist RS, editor. Current therapy in large nimal theriogenology. Philadelphia: WB Saunders; 1997. p. 585–94.
[35] Flores-Foxworth G. Reproductive biotechnologies in the goats. In: Younquist RS, editor. Current therapy in large nimal theriogenology. Philadelphia: WB Saunders; 1997. p. 560–7.
[36] Buckrell BC, Pollard J. Embryo transfer for sheep. In: Younquist RS, editor. Current therapy in large animal theriogenology. Philadelphia: WB Saunders; 1997. p. 650–6.
[37] Fischer AT Jr. Laparoscopic biopsy techniques. In: Fischer AT Jr, editor. Equine diagnostic surgical laparoscopy. Philadelphia: WB Saunders; 2002. p. 143–7.
[38] Klein C, Franz S, Leber A, Bago Z, Baumgartner W. [A new technique of laparoscopic biopsy sampling of the small intestine in calves and sheep] [German]. Wien Tierarztl Monatsschr 2002;89:291–301.
[39] Mulon PY, Babkine M, Desrochers A. Abomasopexy by ventral laparoscopic approach in cattle: 15 cases (2002–2004). Vet Surg 2004;33:E16.
[40] Barisani C. Evoluzione della tecnica di Janowitz per la risoluzione della dislocazione abomasale sinistra secondo Barisani. Summa 2004;5:35–9.

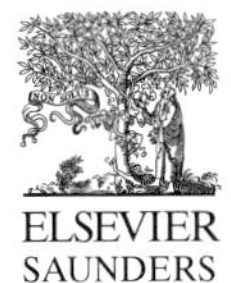

ELSEVIER
SAUNDERS

Vet Clin Food Anim 21 (2005) 281–288

VETERINARY
CLINICS
Food Animal Practice

Index

Note: Page numbers of article titles are in **boldface** type.

doi:10.1016/S0749-0720(05)00013-7

M

N

O

P

R

S

V

W

Changing Your Address?

Make sure your subscription changes too! When you notify us of your new address, you can help make our job easier by including an exact copy of your Clinics label number with your old address (see illustration below.) This number identifies you to our computer system and will speed the processing of your address change. Please be sure this label number accompanies your old address and your corrected address—you can send an old Clinics label with your number on it or just copy it exactly and send it to the address listed below.

We appreciate your help in our attempt to give you continuous coverage. Thank you.

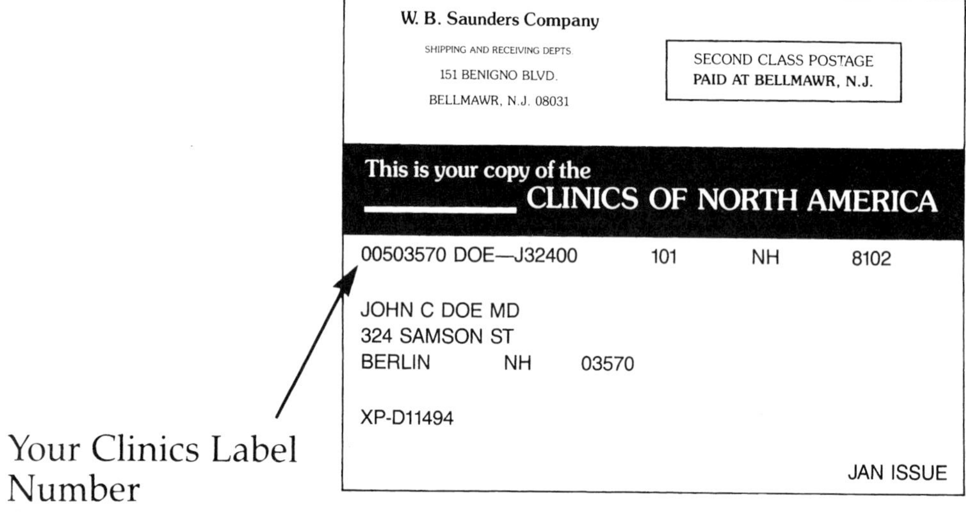

Your Clinics Label Number

Copy it exactly or send your label along with your address to:
W.B. Saunders Company, Customer Service
Orlando, FL 32887-4800
Call Toll Free 1-800-654-2452

Please allow four to six weeks for delivery of new subscriptions and for processing address changes.